CALIFORNIA / MILBANK BOOKS ON HEALTH AND THE PUBLIC

When Walking Fails

Mobility Problems of Adults with Chronic Conditions

LISA I. IEZZONI

University of California Press

BERKELEY   LOS ANGELES   LONDON

The Milbank Memorial Fund

NEW YORK

University of California Press
Berkeley and Los Angeles, California

University of California Press, Ltd.
London, England

© 2003 by the Regents of the University of California

Library of Congress Cataloging-in-Publication Data

Iezzoni, Lisa, I.
   When walking fails : mobility problems of adults with chronic conditions / Lisa I. Iezzoni
      p. ; cm.—(California/Milbank books on health and the public ; 8)
      Includes bibliographical references and index.
      ISBN 0-520-23742-0 (cloth : alk. paper)—ISBN 0-520-23819-2 (paper : alk. paper)
         1. Movement disorders.   2. Chronic diseases—Complications.   [DNLM: 1. Movement disorders—United States. 2. Chronic disease—United States.   3. Gait—United States. 4. Movement disorders—psychology—United States.   5. Public policy—United States. WL 390 I22w 2003]   I. Title: Mobility problems of adults with chronic conditions.   II. Title   III. Series.

RC376.5 .I498 2003
362.4'3'0973—dc21   2002152225

Manufactured in the United States of America

 12   11   10   09   08   07   06   05   04   03
 10   9   8   7   6   5   4   3   2   1

The paper used in this publication is both acid-free and totally chlorine-free (TCF). It meets the minimum requirements of ANSI/NISO Z39.48–1992 (R 1997) (*Permanence of Paper*). ⊗

To Reed

Contents

Illustrations and Tables

Photographs follow p. 104

Foreword

The Milbank Memorial Fund is an endowed national foundation that engages in nonpartisan analysis, study, research, and communication on significant issues in health policy. The Fund makes available the results of its work in meetings with decision makers, reports, articles, and books.

When Walking Fails is the eighth of the California/Milbank Books on Health and the Public. The publishing partnership between the Fund and the Press seeks to encourage the synthesis and communication of findings from research that could contribute to more effective health policy.

This book is about statistics, health services, policy, and the experience of people whose mobility is limited as a result of chronic, progressive diseases or disorders. Lisa Iezzoni conducted more than one hundred interviews in preparation for writing this book. The stories she tells make her analysis of how clinical and financing policy could improve the quality of life for millions of people uncommonly compelling.

Iezzoni brings unusual skill and experience to her exploration of the implications of mobility difficulties for the estimated 10 percent of adult Americans who currently experience them, for the health-care professionals who treat them, and for makers of policy for coverage and payment. She synthesizes evidence and insight that she has acquired as a physician, researcher, and essayist as well as from personal experience in addressing mobility difficulties by, in her words, riding a "battered old scooter held together by bright red airline baggage tape."

Daniel M. Fox
President

Samuel L. Milbank
Chairman

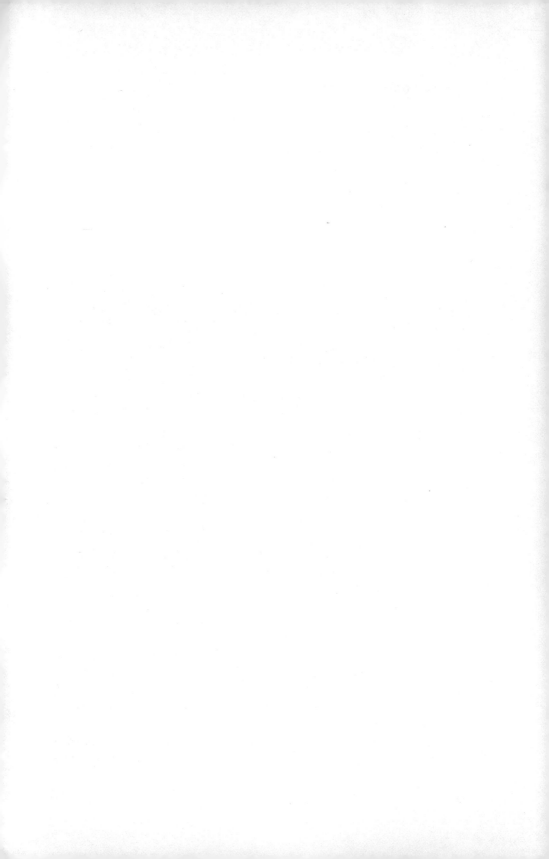

Acknowledgments

The Robert Wood Johnson Foundation Investigator Award in Health Policy Research allowed me to do the project described in this book. Beth Israel Deaconess Medical Center supported me during its writing.

This project involved many people, to whom I am very grateful. In particular, all the 119 persons who were interviewed for this project gave generously of their time, answering virtually every question without demur. Many of them welcomed me into their homes or traveled to my office. This book is about what I learned from them.

Many people recommended potential interviewees and assisted actively in recruiting participants. Lisa LeRoy conducted four focus groups and provided invaluable encouragement and professional guidance on interpreting the results. David A. Stone interviewed ten primary care physicians and offered many suggestions about the findings. Jena Beach, then my administrative assistant, organized several focus groups with reassuring competence. Ron Bouchard, my administrative assistant before Jena, cheerfully drove me many miles north, south, and west, to interviewees' homes and other meetings.

Ellen P. McCarthy, Ph.D., produced the federal survey findings cited throughout the book, with statistical back-up from Roger B. Davis, Sc.D. The Milbank Memorial Fund generously underwrote Dr. McCarthy's efforts. Melissa Wachterman, then my research assistant, now a medical student, found everything I ever asked her for and, with good humor and care, read and proofread my earliest and much, much longer manuscript. Years ago Thomas L. Delbanco suggested the title, *When Walking Fails*, which says it all.

Fred Kent and Mark L. Rosenberg provided photographs, assisted in their array, and helped tell their stories. Mark, a former professor of mine, took the pictures of me that start and end the photo essay. He shot them very early one morning (hence the relatively empty streets and sidewalks) outside a federal office building in Washington, D.C., where several months before we had unexpectedly met again after many years. Fred generously shared some of the photographs he uses to further the mission of Project for Public Spaces (PPS), of which he is president: to create and sustain public places that build communities (more information and photographs documenting PPS's approach and activities are available on their web site at http://www.pps.org).

Special thanks go to Daniel M. Fox for his critical and constructive reviews, and for motivating, engineering, and helping tell the stories of the photographs. Lynne Withey's encouragement and support repeatedly lifted my spirits, as she patiently steered me through the submission and publication process. I also appreciate the thoughtful critiques from thirteen people who reviewed an early version of the book: Susan Edgman-Levitan, Edith Gladstone, Harlan Hahn, Margo B. Holm, Stan Jones, Carol Levine, Don J. Lollar, Patricia MacTaggart, Marcia J. Scherer, Robyn I. Stone, Bruce C. Vladeck, L. Carl Volpe, and Raymond B. Werntz. Again, the Milbank Memorial Fund supported these reviews and other details that made this book possible and provided special creative opportunities.

Finally, I am grateful to my family, friends, and colleagues for their many kindnesses and continuing steadfast support, not just with writing this book, but along the way.

Preface

Before a meeting in Washington, D.C., five springs ago, I hurried to a back room to use the telephone, but a man was already there. We recognized each other immediately. "It's been twenty years," I said. "You taught that wonderful course on living with illness. It helped me decide to go to medical school."

"I remember you well." He paused, eyeing me with momentarily unguarded sadness. "I heard about your troubles."

My mind raced—what troubles? Instantly a student again, I wondered what this professor could mean. Academic troubles? How dreadful! Then abruptly I knew. "Oh, you mean my MS? I don't think of that as a trouble. I'm doing fine."

We spoke telegraphically, catching up on careers, until my meeting began. Later, I rolled onto the mall below Capitol Hill. Although the day was glorious, I could think only about the conversation with my former professor, who seemed saddened to see me in a scooter-wheelchair. Twenty years ago, I ran everywhere. But my reaction puzzled me. Why had I not immediately understood what he meant by "your troubles"? I sensed he wanted to hide his sorrow. This worried me. I didn't want to distress him, nor did I want pity. But his look also conveyed admiration, something that embarrasses me. Given the alternative, the only option is going on. And, yes, it was true. My multiple sclerosis (MS), a chronic neurologic disease, does not feel like "a trouble"—just the landscape I now live in with my motorized chair. How had I arrived at this point?

To say it has taken twenty years seems grandiose. For most of us, the passage between twenty-two and forty-two brings greater equanimity and sense of place in the world. Each of us carries private histories of the hand life has dealt us and how we have survived. As a physician, I know that my hand is much better than that of many people; in important ways, I have been very lucky. But everybody has secret hopes and expectations that, over time, bump up against reality, and I certainly never expected not to walk.

I loved to walk. As a girl and young adult, long walks provided quiet moments for making seemingly monumental life decisions. I also loved to run. It was the only sporting thing I did reasonably well. A tall girl with long legs, I was otherwise gangly and uncoordinated, but I always did OK on the 100-yard dash. While an undergraduate at Duke University, I began jogging daily, rising faithfully at six A.M.—eighteen laps around the old East Campus pool was a mile. I was always acutely aware of the amazing mechanics of walking and running, how strong my legs felt, the powerful sensations of purposeful forward movement. Young people supposedly take their health for granted, but I appreciated my strong, trustworthy legs.

My first definite suggestion of trouble began as I was jogging along the Charles River in Cambridge, Massachusetts—I didn't know where my legs were. Two years previously, I had left Duke for the Harvard School of Public Health, to get a graduate degree in health policy. The mid 1970s were heady times for those wanting to reform what then appeared to be a hopelessly flawed, exorbitantly expensive health-care system. Some political leaders daringly mentioned national health insurance, and the reformers' siren song pulled me. There I met committed physicians like my professor.

I had never considered a medical career. Children of physicians generally sort into two camps: those who choose medicine as their destiny from birth, or those who flee fast in the opposite direction. My father had run a small pediatric practice when I was very young. During office hours, our house echoed with the sobs of children. Who, after all, likes receiving shots, even if they're good for you? Observing this inflicted misery and the all-consuming grip of a medical career hardened my resolve: medicine was not for me. To fulfill undergraduate science requirements, I took "rocks for jocks" geology classes—becoming a paleontologist, combing the world for fossils, had been one career possibility since age eight.

Therefore, the urgings of my professor and several other wonderful physicians that I change directions and consider going to medical school confronted a lifetime of opposition. This shift would require a cataclysmic rearrangement of my entire self-identity. Plus, my spotty science record had significant practical implications: I would have to return to the classroom, learn a lot, and do well. Training would be expensive and lengthy. But these physicians made the compelling argument: if I really wanted to help people, becoming a practicing physician was the absolute best way. I took countless long walks pondering this decision, still jogging at the crack of dawn to exorcise the emotional overload. On the table in my studio apartment, I kept a notepad, vertical line drawn down the middle, listing the pros and cons of doing it on either side. The pros finally outweighed the cons.

Two years after arriving at the School of Public Health, I graduated with my master's degree and matriculated in the "special student premedical curriculum" at Harvard. I would take inorganic chemistry during an intensive summer school program, then calculus, organic chemistry, physics, and biology during the academic year. To reduce living expenses, I moved into the master's residence at one of Harvard's "houses," the dormitory complexes inhabited by undergraduates. In return for a free room on the third floor overlooking the Charles River, I catered periodic social functions that are among the primary duties of presiding masters. That year I made many cookies, discovered wheels of brie, and got to know local liquor stores intimately.

The spooky sensations started that summer, and I attributed them to stress. Without looking down at them, I literally would not know where my legs were in space. My thighs began feeling as if hot branding irons were being pressed into the flesh. The skin was neither reddened nor unusually warm, but the sensation of searing heat felt real.

Such feelings were so odd and hard to describe that I only mentioned them to my father, the physician, after several weeks. Alarmed, he suggested that I go to the emergency clinic at the university health services for evaluation. In retrospect, I can forgive the young physician staffing the quiet clinic that sultry Saturday afternoon for his weary look of incredulity. A summer student, appearing healthy, walks in saying that she doesn't know where her legs are and that her thighs are hot. Without conviction, he suggested that I see a neurologist, but his obvious disbelief seemed reasonable to me. Of course this was stress! What else could it be? It was too weird; it must be all in my head. I did not visit a neurologist, and the sensations disappeared.

Over the next two years, this scenario recurred periodically, with variations in the exact sensations and body parts involved. For four to six weeks strange, unnerving sensations would appear then vanish. I was so busy with school and work that I spent little time even noticing, let alone worrying about, these shadowy visitations, and I always attributed them to stress. I rarely talked about them to friends and barely mentioned them to family. What would I say? None of this made any sense. My last summer before starting medical school, I treated myself to a walking vacation, roaming hills and cliffs through cool mists, from northern Scotland to the outer Hebrides islands. My decision to walk was a deliberate attempt to feel at peace prior to starting untold years of grueling training. I still recall specific, special hours and places from that trip over twenty years ago, when I seek profound quietude. I never walked those long miles again.

I started Harvard Medical School, met Reed (now my husband), and the shadowy symptoms returned—this time with a visible twist. With my internal gyroscope off kilter, I veered randomly into stationary objects, bumping into trees and parked cars. I could no longer attribute these lapses to stress, something "all in my mind." As a second-year medical student, Reed knew twice as much as I did and suggested I visit a neurologist.

The earliest appointment with the university health services neurologist was on Wednesday during final examination week, right before Christmas. I had taken five classes that semester and had one exam each day. When I walked into Dr. John Boyd's office, I was barely conscious of my surroundings or why I was there. I was totally focused on the next day's test, history of medicine (an obligatory humanities class), for which I had barely cracked the book. The dreaded neuroanatomy exam loomed as the finale, on Friday. But John, now a close friend, exuded a calming sense of quiet competence. Gently, without my understanding or realizing the implications, he elicited a classic history of relapsing-remitting multiple sclerosis—neurologic symptoms, affecting multiple parts of the body, coming and going like shadows. The symptoms had actually begun four years earlier: Lhermitte's sign, a tingly sensation, tracking down the arms to the fingertips after you bow your head. The physical examination also showed findings typical of MS, but John was kind and cautious. Like all good physicians, he mentioned several possibilities and said only a careful workup would resolve the diagnosis. I left the appointment with two things, one big, one small. The big message was that a physical cause explained my years of symptoms; they had not been all in my mind. The small message was those initials, MS. What was that?

I didn't spend much time thinking during that Christmas holiday. When I let it, one phrase played repeatedly in my head: "MS, crippler of young adults." Vague recollections accompanied this refrain, advertisements soliciting donations, a young man or woman in a wheelchair. That couldn't possibly be me. In January I returned to Boston for a one-month embryology class about the miraculous transformation from two cells to a whole person. The month was a surreal mix of lectures in cavernous amphitheaters and diagnostic tests. In this time before magnetic resonance imaging, the path to diagnosing MS was circuitous. Early one day I ventured across town for a computed tomography scan of my brain, then hurried back for the lecture, hugging the films in my lap. Another day I traveled to a different hospital for a torturous afternoon of evoked potential tests (little needle electrodes inserted into the muscles, then repeatedly shocked to gauge the muscles' responses). By the end of the month, John asserted unequivocally that I did not have a brain tumor but probably had MS, an incurable disease in which the "white matter," the myelin sheath coating the nerves in the brain and spinal cord, erodes away.

John said something else that became an essential fabric of my existence: the course of MS is unpredictable, so I would have to live with uncertainty. I cannot know now how it will all turn out. Rare tragic cases of MS do progress quickly to profound debility and death, as for Jacqueline Dupré, the renowned British cellist. But the relapsing-remitting form of the disease can stutter along for years, so I might as well go ahead and live my life. This brave statement now belies the bewilderment I felt then. I was more confused, sad, and shocked than angry. Once on the wards, I daily confronted human tragedies wrought by disease, physical and mental, and my own situation seemed comparatively minor. I could still walk, albeit with an unsteady, broad-based gait; I only started using a cane after a fall broke a bone in my foot during my surgery rotation. So I completed the four years of medical school without pause. Although I truly enjoyed interacting with patients, an ineluctable sorrow stayed with me. I remember medical school only in shades of gray.

Confronting the physical limitations and uncertainty of MS was only one step. I also had to deal with people's reactions to me—the "me" they equated with my disease. Harvard Medical School in the early 1980s was a tough place to absorb these lessons. It was poorly equipped to assist students with disabling, chronic illnesses, especially once they dispersed to the affiliated teaching hospitals for clinical rotations. I had only mentioned my diagnosis to a few close friends, primarily because I sought privacy. Now I needed to discuss my situation with officials at the medical school.

At the time of diagnosis, John had warned me that my clinical training would have to be altered. I could not stay up all night in the hospital, "taking call": the risks of exacerbating the MS through long sleepless hours were too great. While I sought neither sympathy nor pity from the academic authorities, I hoped for understanding and some gentleness. I soon learned that those quantities were in short supply. The medical school immediately assigned me to a new academic advisor, a psychiatrist. When I walked into his office for our initial advisory meeting, his words rushed out: "Don't expect me to be your friend. I'm here to give academic advice, not emotional support." The medical school—and some people—have changed, for the better, since then.

I never became a practicing physician. That reality is a sorrow, still raw. Early on, I received frequent hints that my medical career was in jeopardy. On my first day in the operating room during my surgical rotation, the attending surgeon let me hold a finger retractor during a delicate procedure. Once the concentrated silence broke and closing the surgical wound began, the surgeon turned to me, "What's the worst part of your disease?"

Embarrassed by the assembled team of residents and nurses at the operating table, I replied, "It's hard to talk about that."

"Do you want my opinion?" he asked. The scrub nurse rolled her eyes at me sympathetically, and knowing I had no option, I nodded. "You will make a *terrible* doctor," he said. "You lack the most important quality in a good doctor—accessibility. You should limit yourself to pathology, radiology, or maybe anesthesiology." He turned to the anesthesiologist, "Don't you agree?" They planned my career.

Late in my third year I began thinking about applying for an internal medicine residency. At a student dinner, I sat next to a top leader at a Harvard teaching hospital and decided to ask his advice. I would not be able to stay up all night; perhaps I could share a residency with someone else. Few other accommodations seemed necessary. "What would your hospital think of my situation?" I asked.

"Frankly," he replied in a conversational tone, "there are too many doctors in the country right now for us to worry about training handicapped physicians. If that means certain people get left by the wayside, that's too bad." There was silence around the table.

Over the next months, after a wrenching internal debate (joined by Reed, caring and realistic) and with little medical school support, I decided not to battle for an internship but to go straight into research. Four years at medical school left me with one overwhelming lesson: never, ever, talk about *it*, the MS! It can't be cured, so don't mention it. For fifteen years, I almost never did.

I can summarize quickly what has happened since then. First, my walking. When I left medical school, I walked with one cane. At some point, within a few years, I began using two. Two canes offer better stability for the persistent imbalance that sends me veering erratically. Nevertheless, I can still walk short distances. Neither Reed nor I recall exactly how I decided to get the motorized scooter over a dozen years ago. Maybe John first suggested it, but eventually it just seemed the logical thing to do. Initially, I opposed the idea, making all the usual arguments (chapter 12). Only several years later did I find out that when I got the scooter, my work colleagues were frightened, thinking my health was deteriorating. Because I never talked about *it*, they could not know that nothing was further from the truth. My physical functioning was unchanged, just my mind and world had finally opened up. With the scooter, I could get around again. And I loved the freedom!

Work was going well. Here, I was lucky too—the old adage that when one door closes, another opens up. My graduate training in health policy offered an entrée. I spent six years at Boston University, then moved to Beth Israel Hospital (now Beth Israel Deaconess Medical Center) at Harvard Medical School, conducting research oriented toward health policy issues, particularly improving quality of care. I found a small circle of wonderful, supportive colleagues.

I understand the realities underlying my career success. Reed, an academic hematologist and oncologist, does the physical chores around our house—the grocery shopping, the laundry, the lawn, the gardening, the kitty litter—and I work, sitting, writing (I still cook a little, although he appropriately distrusts me with knives). Reed's help allows me to concentrate on my work, at some cost to his own career. Although time restored my spirit lost in the gray hazes of diagnosis and medical school, my subconscious mind remembers my walking past: I still awake occasionally from dreams of running. Uncertainty about the future, John's early warning, is now part of my life's fabric. And that is why, after all these years, MS is not a trouble, just the landscape I live in.

In large measure, my equanimity came with restored mobility—I now go where I want to go in my scooter-wheelchair. This freedom is delicious after years of slowly inching forward, constantly afraid of falling and exhausted with effort. Nowadays, I sometimes grin with the sheer joy of independent movement. On beautiful days, I can track the sun or shadows almost as I used to—a wonderfully freeing feeling, like spring after a housebound winter.

Why am I talking so publicly now? Over time, I came to realize that silence carries consequences. For instance, I could have spared my caring colleagues their fears about my health if I had told them why I had bought the scooter and how it thrilled me. Silence reinforces the stigmatization of disabling conditions, the sense that becoming less able to walk is something to hide—although, of course, *we* can't.

Most important, strangers ask my advice. In my wheelchair I conduct a sort of "rolling focus group," attracting unsolicited questions from strangers, remarks about themselves or their relatives and their difficulties walking. They describe bad knees, bad backs, heart and lung problems, and many other conditions slowing them down. They want advice about restoring mobility or compensating for its loss, getting back out into the world.

I remembered my notepad from twenty years ago, with the vertical line partitioning the pros and cons of going to medical school. The single, overwhelming statement on the pro side of that partitioned page was the opportunity medicine offered to help people. Though my experience wends through this book, I concentrate primarily on the stories of other people whose walking is slowed by progressive chronic conditions. Using their words and those of health-care professionals, I describe both barriers to and opportunities for becoming independently mobile again. Here's my opportunity to help.

1 Mobility Limits

One Christmas my husband and I went to an exclusive shop downtown to buy my father a tie. It is one of those stores where you feel scrutinized by security cameras even if you do not roll in on a battered old scooter held together by bright red airline baggage tape. The saleslady eyed us with barely veiled suspicion as we sorted through the tie rack. When we finally selected a tie and pulled out our credit card, she brightened up and began talking about her mother.

Her mother had had a stroke. She had largely recovered but was terrified of falling, afraid to leave her house. The mother had become isolated and home-bound. On a trip abroad, the saleslady found a four-wheeled folding walker with brakes on the handlebars and a little seat for the user to rest. She brought the walker home, but her mother was still afraid and wouldn't walk outside. What about a scooter like mine, the saleslady wondered. What was it like to use? How could she find one? Would it get her mother out of her house?

Two major themes link this and many similar interactions of my "rolling focus group"—the strangers who talk to me as I roll in my scooter-wheelchair. The first theme is acknowledged loss and sorrow at becoming less able to walk. The second theme quickly follows—hope for returning mobility, even if mechanized. Many confidants are "baby boomers," worried about increasingly limited parents. Others are themselves slowed by chronic conditions, such as arthritis or diabetes. Some, like the saleslady's mother, are isolated, afraid or unwilling to leave their homes for varying reasons, from intractable pain to fear of falling to embarrassment and reluctance to use or be seen with a cane or walker, let alone a wheelchair.

Yet others are simply frustrated. They once traveled the globe and zipped through ever-lengthening spaces—giant office complexes, mega-shopping malls, enormous superstores—but now difficulty walking is slowing them down and circumscribing their reach. They want help getting around, smoothing and speeding their way, if not by walking then by mechanical means. But they don't know where to get advice about restoring mobility.

This book explores the issues that arise when walking fails as progressive chronic health conditions compromise people's everyday lives, partly because of personal physical and emotional consequences and partly because of persisting societal and environmental barriers. This book has two ultimate goals. The first is advocating for over nineteen million Americans who live in their own communities and have some difficulty walking—the plurality of whom have ordinary chronic problems related to aging, like arthritis, back pain, heart and lung disease, diabetes—and the millions who will share these difficulties in the future. Improving people's ability to move freely and independently should enhance overall health and quality of life, not only for these individuals but also for society as a whole. The second goal is informing policymakers about counterproductive health insurance and other public policies that are barriers to improving mobility. I primarily emphasize health-care delivery and payment policy, but the concept of "health" inevitably extends broadly, reaching into homes, workplaces, communities, and the public spaces in which we all live.

For individuals, restored independent mobility offers joy, empowerment, and renewed hope. For society, "designing a flexible world for the many," accessible to all regardless of their mobility ability, will serve everybody well (Zola 1989, 422). But significant personal, societal, health-system, and innumerable other hurdles impede the way. To examine these issues, I addressed three major questions in a project funded by the Robert Wood Johnson Foundation:

> How many adults living in communities have difficulty walking because of chronic progressive diseases and disorders, and what are these health conditions?

> How do mobility difficulties affect people—their physical comfort, feelings about their lives, relationships with family and friends, and daily activities at home and in their communities?

> How do policies, especially for health-care delivery and payment, help and hinder people's ability to maximize independent mobility, through enhancing the ability to walk pain-free and safely, modifying home and community environments, and providing assistive technologies?

These questions assume that getting out in the world is worth striving for, and that strategies exist to help us do so.

Some approaches focus on individuals: reducing pain, obtaining assistive technologies, and redesigning daily activities. Others reach beyond individuals to the broader society. Making our public and private environments and policies—homes, workplaces, educational settings, legal system, communal spaces, transportation networks, health-care providers, and reimbursement policies—easier for and better suited to people with mobility difficulties will improve things for everybody. Future designs should encompass the universe of all people.

I concentrate here on certain people, defined by the extent of mobility difficulties, underlying physical cause, and age. First, mobility limitations cover a broad spectrum, ranging from persons who still walk independently but more slowly and less surely than before to those who require complete assistance with all mobility tasks, such as turning in bed. With the most severe limitations, people need extensive or round-the-clock personal assistance at home or live in nursing homes or institutional settings, raising many complex and important issues. Here, however, I focus on the vast majority of people at the less limited end of the spectrum: persons living in the community without intensive personal assistance at home. Although these people have less severe mobility limitations, their walking difficulties nonetheless affect their daily lives. They rarely identify with others who have mobility difficulties or use services targeting people with impaired mobility. Like the saleslady's mother, they therefore risk feeling alone and unsure of what to do.

Second, I consider persons with chronic progressive diseases or disorders, not people with congenital or acute, generally traumatic conditions, such as spinal cord injury. The experience of growing up with limited mobility or suddenly losing mobility differs from the slow, progressive march of increasing impairment. Responses of the health and social services systems also differ. Persons with congenital conditions such as cerebral palsy, spina bifida, and muscular dystrophy often enter (along with their parents) a bewildering and specialized health and social service labyrinth; these service systems frequently fall apart as children become adults. Persons with spinal cord and serious injuries have obvious needs for assistive technologies and various rehabilitative services. In each instance, unique concerns arise. In contrast, the majority of people with progressive chronic conditions enter the general health-care system, typically through their primary care physicians. Because their limitations increase over time, often slowly, the decision on when to intervene (e.g., with a walker or wheelchair) depends on myriad personal and environmental factors.

Finally, regardless of what caused the mobility limitations, I focus on adults of working age and active older persons. Despite some commonalities, children and adults with mobility difficulties prompt different personal and societal responses. Special issues relating to very old people, especially those with multiple physical and cognitive debilities, fall outside my scope. Many extremely frail persons live in nursing homes or other institutions, raising complex concerns not considered here.

This project used two sources of information: interviews with 119 people, including 56 persons with mobility difficulties and some family members, as well as physicians, physical and occupational therapists, medical directors of health insurance plans, disability rights advocates, and various others; and federal surveys of people living in communities throughout the United States in 1994 and 1995. I tape-recorded all interviews, and this book quotes people's own words (Appendix 1 briefly describes frequently quoted interviewees). Although I cite published autobiographical and scholarly works about mobility limitations and disability more generally, I rely primarily on the interviewees' observations. Appendix 2 lists various sources of information that might assist people with mobility difficulties. (More details about my interviews, the numbers used throughout the book, and how I created the tables are available at http://www.ucpress.edu/books/pages/9456.html.)

Over 10 percent of adults living in communities throughout the United States—an estimated nineteen million people—report at least some difficulty walking, standing, or climbing stairs, according to the federal survey (chapter 2). Whereas these mobility problems increase with age, from 30 to 40 percent of people say their difficulties began when they were younger than fifty years old; they had long lives ahead. The number of people with mobility difficulties will grow in coming decades as the population ages. Thus, walking problems are a major national, social, and public-health concern.

A NOTE ON LANGUAGE AND GUIDING THOUGHTS

Nowadays, some of us who use wheelchairs are bemused by sincere questions from well-meaning people about what "we" want to be called. Perhaps "crippled," "lame," or "gimp" would upset us (unless we use them ourselves), but what about "handicapped," "disabled," "impaired," or "physically challenged"?

My smiling response surprises some questioners. With the exception of phrases "confined to a wheelchair" or "wheelchair-bound"—too laden with imagery of being lashed into place for today's woman to bear—I don't much care. I generally agree with the perspective of the novelist Nancy

Mairs, who uses a power wheelchair because of MS. Mairs does not argue linguistic fine points, refusing "to pretend that the only differences between you and me are the various ordinary ones that distinguish any one person from another. But call me *disabled* or *handicapped* if you like. I have long since grown accustomed to them" (1987, 119). She prefers "cripple," seeing it as "a clean word, straightforward and precise" (118). But that does not mean Mairs views herself as immobile—the very trait prompting others to call her disabled. "Relaxed and focused, I feel emotionally far more 'up' than I generally did when I stood on two sound legs. . . . Certainly I am not mobility impaired; in fact, in my Quickie P100 with two twelve-volt batteries, I can shop till you drop at any mall you designate, I promise" (1996, 38, 39).

But my feelings about language and its implications are not always straightforward. A professional meeting a while back gave me the chance to talk with someone I had not seen in many years. I remembered him with fondness. As a junior faculty member, he had steadfastly supported me during medical school. The last time I saw him, I had walked with one cane. He sat down with a look of concern, saying, "You're really disabled, aren't you?" I produced a socially acceptable, noncommittal response but inside I wilted. We were now professional equals and I'd hoped we would interact on those terms, talking about careers and academic interests. It wasn't the label I objected to, but the implied judgment about my life, the potential pity, and the ineluctable gulf it placed between us.

Near the end of each interview with individuals with difficulty walking, I asked whether they viewed themselves as "disabled." Some laughed as if this were a stupid question: "Of course!" But most paused, observed that others are worse off, and said how much they still do in their lives. They spoke the language that historically has defined our collective national ethos: remaining independent, doing things for themselves, taking responsibility for their lives, not being a burden on others, "standing on their own two feet." Three wheelchair users with MS offered slightly different perspectives but echoed our national themes. Margaret Freemont in her early seventies was an emeritus university professor. "It's ridiculous," she said. "I have some deep denial, I guess, but I don't really feel disabled. I help people, and people help me. I do things for people that are different from things people do for me. There's no one who's universally competent." Louisa Delarte, also in her early seventies, is an artist: "I can't do certain things, so I'm impaired somewhat, disabled, I suppose. I don't think about it. I just cope with it. We can't go around feeling sorry for ourselves." Sally Ann Jones, a retired social worker in her mid fifties, shook her head vigorously when asked about being disabled.

Never. I hate all those words. "Disabled?" What the hell does that mean? The other one is "invalid." An invalid is somebody who's invalid? It's just ridiculous. Other people struggle with straight hair and ugly dispositions, bad teeth, no education, and bad husbands. We've all got our problems. I've got mine. I do the best I can with mine. I do better than lots of other people do with fewer problems. That's because they just don't realize you only live once. This is it.

People of privilege (certainly Nancy Mairs and myself) may too easily dismiss the linguistic debate. Looking especially to the third world, Charlton (1998, 82) compellingly describes persistent poverty, discrimination, and disenfranchisement among many people with disabling conditions, noting that "disability identification takes place as people begin to recognize their oppression." Although outright "oppression" is less apparent in the United States than in the third world, Americans with mobility problems *are* more likely than others to be unemployed, poor, and uneducated (chapter 7).

The catch-22 for those who reject the disability label is that they might need it to live. Sally Ann Jones is a widow and no longer works; she gets Social Security disability insurance (SSDI) and Medicare through SSDI. Many interviewees who deny they are disabled nonetheless seek handicapped placards for their cars and park in handicapped parking spaces, use paratransit systems, or get disability income support. Each person has allowed an external party—physicians and administrative authorities—to label them as "disabled" so they can receive a specific accommodation or benefit.

So a strange dynamic ensues. People must acknowledge "disability" to obtain services that allow them to live the "more normal" lives they want—to not be disabled. One of my earliest interviewees was an older man who used a scooter-wheelchair following extensive surgery for cancer in his leg muscles. When I asked him to describe his trouble walking, he replied that he had no trouble: he didn't walk. He used the RIDE, our local public wheelchair van service, almost daily to go wherever he wished, including adult education, the symphony, and theater. He said he was beginning to feel disabled because he couldn't pull up his pants.

For many decades, people have tried to place the concept of "disability" within broader ideas about how health and physical functioning interact with full participation in societies (Pope and Tarlov 1991; Brandt and Pope 1997; Altman 2001; Williams 2001; World Health Organization 1980, 2001). Even centuries ago, defining disability posed a problem. Disabled people could not hunt, tend fields, or labor to support themselves, and communities decided they merited alms or other assistance. But societies struggled to distinguish deserving from undeserving, fakers from truly disabled people. In the mid 1800s new medical discoveries, insights about disease, and inventions like the stethoscope seemingly provided the solution: "scientific medicine offered the promise of new diagnostic methods that could distinguish between genuine disability (or inability to work) and feigned disability. Clinical medicine . . . gave legitimacy to claims for social aid" (Stone 1984, 91).

This ascendancy of "objective medical science" produced one way of thinking about disability, often called the "medical model." It sees disability as "a problem of the person, directly caused by disease, trauma or other health condition, which requires medical care. . . . Management of the disability is aimed at cure or the individual's adjustment and behaviour change. Medical care is viewed as the main issue" (World Health Organization 2001, 20). Today's health-care delivery and payment systems, such as Medicare, reflect this medical model, largely focusing on treating ailments and making people "better," returning them to "normal." Medical knowledge and treatment advances *have* undoubtedly expanded options for people with disabilities and often enhanced quality of life.

Embedded within this medical model, however, are two assumptions: that disability is something individual people should strive, largely alone, to overcome; and that clinical professionals know what is best for their individual patients.[1] These assumptions defy other realities. Leaders in the disability rights movement observed almost forty years ago that "problems lie not within the persons with disabilities but in the environment that fails to accommodate persons with disabilities and in the negative attitude of people without disabilities" (Olkin 1999, 26). As the wheelchair user Michael Oliver observed, disability is "imposed on top of our impairments by the way we are unnecessarily isolated and excluded from full participation in society" (1996, 22). These arguments coalesced into the "social" or "minority" model of disability. It sees disability not as "an attribute of an individual, but rather a complex collection of conditions, many of which are created by the social environment. . . . The issue is therefore an attitudinal or ideological one requiring social change, which at the political level becomes a question of human rights" (World Health Organization 2001, 20).

These positions girded and motivated critical strides toward disability civil rights in the United States over the last thirty years. Although this model lays responsibility across society, it offers an important message to individuals, articulated by the late American sociologist Irving Zola (1982), a leading thinker of the disability rights movement:

> We with handicaps and chronic disabilities must see to our own interests. We must free ourselves from the "physicality" of our conditions and the dominance of our life by the medical world. In particu-

lar, I refer to the number of times we think of ourselves and are thought of by others in terms of our specific chronic conditions. We are polios, cancers, paras, deaf, blind, lame, amputees, and strokes. Whatever else this does, it blinds us to our common social disenfranchisement. Our forms of loss may be different, but the resulting invalidity is the same. (243)

For many years, proponents of the medical and social models seemed at loggerheads, erecting a "sterile and rather contrived distinction" between the two approaches (Williams 2001, 125). The disability rights activist Jenny Morris (1996a, 181) worried that, in challenging the medical model, "we have sometimes tended to deny the personal experience of disability. Disability *is* associated with illness, and with old age . . . and with conditions which are inevitably painful." In important ways, the experience is intensely individual.

Recent efforts therefore recognize the value of both perspectives, and the interviewees would probably agree. Mattie Harris's arthritis keeps her in constant pain; she cannot play ball in the park with her kids as she wishes. "I don't want to view myself as disabled or as handicapped either," she said. "There's some things I just can't do." Neither the pain nor her inability to play ball have social causes—they are explicitly medical. She wants her physicians to treat her pain. But when Ms. Harris can't board the bus because the step is too high for her painful knees, environmental barriers predominate, furthering her isolation. Thus, life and personal wishes are complex and multidimensional, not tied to one single way of thinking. Both medical and social concerns apply.

In this book, my writing is guided by the framework underlying the *International Classification of Functioning, Disability and Health* (ICF), approved in 2001 by the World Health Organization (WHO). The *ICF* integrates the medical and social models, creating a "biopsychosocial" synthesis of different perspectives on health (WHO 2001, 20). *ICF* identifies three interrelated concepts:

Impairments are problems in body function or structure such as a significant deviation or loss.

Activity is the execution of a task or action by an individual.

Participation is involvement in a life situation. (10)

The *ICF* defines disability as an "umbrella term for impairments, activity limitations or participation restrictions," framing "a person's functioning and disability . . . as a dynamic interaction between health conditions (diseases, disorders, injuries, traumas, etc.) and contextual factors," including environmental and personal attributes (3, 8).

Throughout this book, I use somewhat imprecise language. For brevity, *mobility* refers to independent walking or movement involving the lower extremities, recognizing that some people have mobility troubles isolated to other parts of the body (such as the arms, hands, or head) and that many people (like Mairs) compensate effectively for mobility difficulties using wheelchairs. I use general descriptive words, like *difficulty*, because that language occurs in the federal health survey providing the data. I identify people's diagnoses because, in terse shorthand, they convey volumes about bodily comfort and future expectations about physical functioning. But I quickly follow with people's own words so readers can see people and their experiences as the interviewees see themselves. People's stories fill this book.[2]

Finally, because I hope this book will help people from different backgrounds, I aim for easily understandable language, using common definitions implied in daily speech. When people ask me what phrase other than "wheelchair-bound" describes my mode of moving around, my response is simple: "Just describe the situation. I use a wheelchair; I'm a wheelchair user. No need for metaphors."

2   Who Has Mobility Difficulties

How many people have trouble walking? It's hard to tell from simply looking around. Even just three decades ago, many people with difficulty walking were "somehow made invisible and kept isolated from the rest of the world" (Zola 1982, 95). Nowadays, high-profile celebrities roll in their wheelchairs before the public eye: Christopher Reeve, once a comic book superhero, now an effective albeit controversial advocate of medical research; John Hockenberry, a broadcast journalist, reporting from around the world; Stephen Hawking, an astrophysicist, spinning theories of the universe; and Barbara Jordan, the late congresswoman from Texas, who some said had the voice of God. But highly public people often occupy their positions through special circumstances or intellectual gifts that distinguish them from others with similar physical impairments (Zola 1982, 202). Are "just regular folks" with walking problems more visible in America today?

My eyes tell me that they are. During an early Sunday supper at the local fish restaurant, stacks of collapsible walkers wheeled in by diners covered a long wall. I often encounter other wheelchair users at elevators in accessible subway stations. Visitors to large amusement parks find battalions of scooter users crisscrossing their paths. Wheelchair users now go many places independently and confidently, their way smoothed by new curb cuts and ramps. Power equipment (wheelchairs propelled by battery packs) makes independent travel possible even for people with severe physical impairments. Brianna Vicks, in her mid forties, is almost completely unable to walk because of noncancerous but recurring spinal cord tumors. She lives in a neighborhood of narrow tree-shaded streets and century-old bow-fronted brick townhouses with steep granite steps. Her more modern apartment building, admittedly less charming, is completely accessible to her power wheelchair. Brianna loves rolling independently, going where she pleases.

Some days, if I don't want to catch the bus, I'll ride my wheelchair downtown. I'll just go on my own. I used to work downtown. And if the weather was really nice, not too hot, after work I'd ride my wheelchair home, taking my time: just browse, stop in a store. Don't have no money, but there's a lot of places to go.

Yet some people with walking problems are not on the streets. The saleslady's mother from chapter 1 rarely leaves her home. Mattie Harris, a heavyset woman in her late forties, moves slowly because of severe arthritis. Several years ago, unable to grasp a handrail because of pain in her hands, she slipped down icy steps and hurt her back. She usually stays indoors, caring for her grandchildren and several foster children. "It's terrible that I can't walk and do the things I used to do," Ms. Harris said. "When my kids were younger, I used to take them to the park, bowling, the schoolyard, and play ball with them. I used to be a good ball player. Now I just can't do those things."

"Can you go to church or visit friends?" I asked.

"I don't visit people. I'm so miserable and in pain, and my knee locks like it's going to throw me down. I have to grab onto something or else I'll fall. It's draining. So I don't feel like going out. . . . I stay home." Thus, while many people with walking difficulties do get out, others, like Mattie Harris, remain largely hidden indoors.

HOW MANY PEOPLE HAVE MOBILITY PROBLEMS?

One answer to this question comes from asking people. A nationwide survey in 1994 and 1995 interviewed people in their homes and apartments throughout the community, asking many questions about health and difficulties with daily activities. From this survey, we counted people who use mobility aids or who report difficulties walking three city blocks (about a quarter of a mile), climbing up ten steps without resting, or standing for about twenty minutes.

Roughly nineteen million adults who live outside nursing homes or other institutions—just over 10 percent of persons eighteen years of age and older—report at least some mobility difficulty or use a mobility aid (Iezzoni et al. 2001; Table 1).[1] Many problems probably cause only small irritations or inconveniences, but others suggest substantial impairments. Almost six million adults (3 percent) report either using a wheelchair or scooter or being completely unable to walk three blocks, climb ten stairs, or stand twenty minutes. And 88 percent of them said their problems would last at least a year.

TABLE 1. Adults Reporting Mobility Difficulty

Difficulty[a]	Estimated Number (millions)	Percentage
None	168.32	90
Minor	7.93	4
Moderate	5.23	3
Major	5.82	3
TOTAL REPORTING DIFFICULTY	18.98	10

[a]None = persons who report no difficulty with walking *and* climbing stairs *and* standing *and* use no mobility aid; minor = persons who report some difficulty with walking *or* climbing stairs *or* standing *or* who use a cane or crutches; moderate = persons who report a lot of difficulty with walking *or* climbing stairs *or* standing *or* who use a walker; major = persons who report being unable to perform walking *or* climbing stairs *or* standing *or* who use a manual or power wheelchair or scooter.

Rates of mobility problems rise with increasing age (Figure 1). On average, people reporting difficulties are in their early to mid sixties. But many problems had started years earlier. Almost 30 percent of those reporting major difficulties said their problems began under age fifty and 16 percent under age forty.[2] After we account for age differences, we find that 88 percent of men report mobility problems compared to 91 percent of women.[3] About 10 percent of whites and Hispanic persons report problems compared to 15 percent of blacks, again accounting for differences in age and sex. These gender and racial variations partially reflect differences in rates of conditions causing mobility difficulties. For example, more women than men and more blacks than whites have arthritis (Centers for Disease Control 1994, 347).

Whether the exact percentages and patterns reported in 1994–95 will persist into the next decades is uncertain, especially with the aging "baby boom" generation. Surveys of older persons suggest that rates of serious functional limitations have declined importantly over recent years (Manton, Corder, and Stallard 1997; Manton and Gu 2001).[4] Reduced smoking, better physical fitness, and medical advances have helped improve functioning at older ages (Freedman and Martin 1998; Cutler 2001). Nevertheless, because walking problems are often caused by chronic conditions that increase with age, the sheer numbers of people living in our communities with mobility problems will grow dramatically in the early twenty-first century. Only revolutionary changes in preventing or treating chronic debilitating conditions will slow this trend.

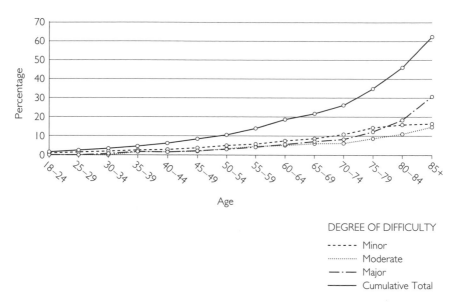

Figure 1. Percentage of adults with mobility difficulty, by age. (From L. I. Iezzoni, E. P. McCarthy, R. B. Davis, H. Siebens, Mobility Difficulties Are Not Only a Problem of Old Age, *Journal of General Internal Medicine* 16, no. 4 [2001]:237. Reprinted by permission of Blackwell Publishing.)

DIAGNOSIS AND CONTROL

Mobility difficulties are generally caused by one or more clinical conditions or injuries, sometimes both. People want to know their diagnosis for two reasons. First and foremost it leads to treatment, even if therapies merely slow progression of impairments. Although few chronic diseases or disorders that cause walking problems can now be cured, some treatments can substantially restore function, diminish pain, and improve quality of life. For example, knee or hip replacements can stop pain and return mobility to many people with arthritis. Diagnoses suggest the future extent of mobility problems and types of symptoms people will have.

Second, the cause often affects how people feel about their walking problems and their sense of control, as well as how society and even medical professionals view them. Knowing the cause allows people to get on with their lives, to plan and make choices, despite a sometimes unpredictable future. Candy Stoops, now in her late thirties, was newly married when her symptoms started nearly ten years ago: "I was dropping things. I had double vision. I'd be sitting watching TV and one eye would shut." Most worrisome, she began falling while climbing the stairs to their third-floor apartment.

The final straw that broke the camel's back was, I was walking up my stairs, and I had something in one arm. My legs just went, and I fell backwards on the stairs. I couldn't even yell or scream. It's almost like your brain is saying, "Do something, do something," and your whole body is not responding. I couldn't talk, I couldn't yell. My dad and my grandfather happened to be over, and they heard this kind of thump. I was very lucky I didn't hurt myself. I kind of fell very gracefully. My husband ran down the stairs and carried me up.

I called my primary care physician. He thought I had MS. He said, "Let's get you to a neurologist," and I said, "OK. We'll deal with this. Just let me see somebody." You're at the point where it's like, just tell me what I've got. I can deal with it. I just want to know what it is. It's that fear of the unknown.

Based on Candy's description of her symptoms, the neurologist immediately diagnosed myasthenia gravis, a disease affecting the junction between nerves and muscles and causing profound weakness. Although the condition is not curable, treatment does reduce the episodes of weakness and risk of falls. Now Candy has "bad days" when she has trouble walking, but only once in a while. She and her husband moved into a one-story house.

Specific causes can also shape perceptions of society and even medical professionals. These public perceptions can, in turn, sometimes affect how people with mobility problems feel about themselves. As discussed later, much of society's concern revolves around whether the person with the mobility problem should qualify for special assistance, such as Social Security disability payments or workers' compensation. The question boils down to who controls the mobility problem.

Questions about control, including assuming responsibility and accepting credit or blame, dominate many discussions in American popular and political culture. These issues also surface when considering basic functions, such as being able to walk. Today's self-help industry ironically casts greater responsibility on individuals to solve problems that even advanced medical technology cannot touch. This perspective affects how people feel about themselves and whether they put up a good fight. Tom Norton, a retired business executive in his early seventies, developed a neurologic problem with his left foot thirty years ago. Mr. Norton's motor neuron disease was beyond his control. Nonetheless, he spent years exercising, "trying to beat it," without success. His wife, Nelda, accused Tom of being "in denial," of deluding himself that he was making a difference. Nelda felt that Tom had wasted time and money on expensive exercise equipment and personal trainers, searching for the perfect exercise cure. But who knows what would have happened if Tom hadn't exercised? Tom notes proudly, "I've never given up."

Three broad stereotypes dominate public perceptions of people with walking problems: people "crippled" from birth or young adulthood by diseases or health conditions; persons debilitated by catastrophic accidents; and elderly people fading away. Each stereotype affixes blame or innocence and suggests whether people have control over their conditions and futures. As usual with stereotypes, fact and fiction intermingle.

People "crippled" from birth or young adulthood by diseases or health conditions are the classic victims, without control over their fates. Tiny Tim, created by Charles Dickens for his 1843 story *A Christmas Carol*, exemplifies this stereotype. Tiny Tim was the son of Bob Cratchit, the hapless clerk working for Ebenezer Scrooge of "bah, humbug" fame. "Alas for Tiny Tim, he bore a little crutch, and had his limbs supported by an iron frame!" (Dickens 1981, 44). Mrs. Cratchit asked her husband how little Tim had behaved at church: " 'As good as gold,' said Bob, 'and better. . . . he hoped the people saw him in the church, because he was a cripple, and it might be pleasant to them to remember upon Christmas Day, who made the lame beggars walk, and blind men see' " (45). As Scrooge metamorphosed, guided by his ghosts, the unhappy fate of Tiny Tim haunted and exhorted him to a better life.

This imagery of unfortunate innocents, struggling to walk, remains potent today, especially among fund-raisers and sloganeers, such as "Jerry's kids" for muscular dystrophy. Stories of persons struck down in youth through no fault of their own evoke powerful, sympathetic responses. Franklin Delano Roosevelt, who contracted polio at age thirty-nine, was virtually never seen publicly in his wheelchair. Yet he became the omniscient, de facto "poster child" of his National Foundation for Infantile Paralysis. Brainstorming about how to raise money from a nation just emerging from economic depression, the radio and vaudeville entertainer Eddie Cantor suggested that people send 10 cent contributions directly to Roosevelt at the White House: "Call it the March of Dimes" (Gallagher 1994, 150). Cantor and the Lone Ranger broadcast Roosevelt's appeal, and within days, envelopes containing dimes overwhelmed the postal service. "The government of the United States darn near stopped functioning," reported the White House mail chief (151).

Such public appeals can undoubtedly support good causes. In 1937 the polio virus was unchecked. The polio vaccine became possible because Roosevelt's foundation raised millions of research dollars (Gallagher 1994). These mass solicitations nevertheless solidify one stereotype of walking problems—blameless people, courageously confronting adversity and struggling to walk, crutches in hand. Despite their exertions, they seemingly have little control over their futures, waiting for the charity-supported research to suddenly sprout a cure. In an America that celebrates independence and self-determination, this stereotype implicitly marginalizes people.

Equally troubling, however, is holding people accountable for their physical impairments in defiance of their disease—a slippery slope between hope and despair. A while back Sam, a colleague, advised his friend Joni to see me. She runs a little shop and had always been very active. For twenty years, she had periodically experienced episodic, unnerving sensory symptoms but never knew why. A physician friend had privately diagnosed MS, but he had not told Joni or her husband. Now all of a sudden, Joni began having serious trouble walking, and the physician revealed his diagnosis. Her husband and his male friends, including Sam, rallied around and mapped out an exercise program "to improve her function." They planned to buy Joni a Stairmaster and start her on daily jogging; one well-meaning enthusiast suggested training for the Boston marathon. Overwhelmed by this onslaught motivated by true affection and concern, Joni felt powerless to make them understand that her legs now felt as if they were encased in concrete, that fatigue drained every scrap of strength. She was failing everybody, she worried. Sam told me later that the husband and his friends had abandoned their physical fitness regime, but I heard doubt in Sam's voice.

The second stereotyped cause, catastrophic accidents, is sometimes shadowed by hinted conjectures about fault—was the person somehow to blame? One "innocent" subgroup is injured either by seemingly random violence, such as being struck by a car, or by mishaps occurring during socially acceptable activities, such as bicycling, skiing, or contact sports. In contrast, a more suspect subgroup involves people injured by their own recklessness, such as driving while drunk.

Persons claiming injuries at work and seeking disability compensation, "workers' comp," are particularly problematic (chapter 9). Soldiers returning from war, however, are a special class of people injured "at work." Almost by definition, injured soldiers are vigorous young people starting their lives. Roosevelt himself, usually unwilling to be seen publicly in his wheelchair, made a special gesture conveying his respect for troops injured in World War II. During a 1944 visit to Hawaii to discuss Pacific strategy, Roosevelt went to an Oahu hospital, and according to an aide,

> The President did something which affected us all very deeply. He asked a secret service man to wheel him slowly through all the wards that were occupied by veterans who had lost one or more

arms and legs. He insisted on going past each individual bed. He wanted to display himself and his useless legs to those boys who would have to face the same bitterness. (Goodwin 1994, 532)

The aide had never seen Roosevelt with tears in his eyes but said the president came close to them as he left the hospital.

Public perceptions of veterans' merit or culpability often depend on views about the war. In 1968 Max Cleland (who became a U.S. senator from Georgia) lost his right hand and both legs to a grenade in Vietnam. As he said, "To the devastating psychological effect of getting maimed . . . is the added psychological weight that it may not have been worth it. . . . The individual is left alone with his injury and his self-doubts" (Cleland 1989, 120–21).

The common element linking all persons with injuries is the suddenness of their change. One minute they can walk; the next minute they cannot. The seeming randomness of the loss generates fear and fascination— this could happen to anyone in a flash. Nobody is exempt or ultimately in control. The overwhelming magnitude of these injuries and their sudden life transformations rivet public attention, especially when they involve celebrities. The 1995 accident of Christopher Reeve while riding his horse Buck in a competition in Culpepper, Virginia, exemplifies that split-second unpredictability and instantaneous impact.

Reeve described that day in *Still Me* (1998), reconstructing details from the accounts of witnesses. He emphasized the care he took before the accident, perhaps to immunize himself from blame for what happened: "I went out and walked the course again. I had already done it twice the day before. But I walked it one more time. . . . I certainly wasn't worried about the third fence on the course" (17–18). According to bystanders, "Buck started to jump the fence, but all of a sudden he just put on the brakes. No warning, no hesitation, no sense of anything wrong" (19). Reeve catapulted over the fence, landing on his head.

Although persons may not control the events surrounding their injuries, controlling their futures is different. Given the frequent circumstances of such trauma (e.g., accidents during vigorous or youthful activities, war wounds), many people with these injuries are otherwise young, strong, and healthy, with the prospect of long lives ahead. Hence their circumstances clash with those of people falling under the first stereotype, primarily around issues of control and self-determination. John Hockenberry became paraplegic in a 1976 accident when the driver of a car in which he was traveling drifted into sleep. In his memoir, *Moving Violations* (1995), Hockenberry recalled his time at a rehabilitation hospital:

> In rehab we were taught never to allow people to push our chairs.
> We were taught to do things ourselves and never ask for help. We
> were proud crips who were going to play basketball and win races
> and triumph over our disabilities. Outside rehab, self-reliance was a
> high-risk proposition. To people raised on telethons, it looked suspi-
> ciously like a chip on the shoulder. . . . No one would think of hav-
> ing a telethon to raise money to build accessible housing for wheel-
> chair consumers or to find jobs for them. (33–34)

Hockenberry recognized that the public, interested in finding cures, was
unlikely to donate the help he really wanted—not a wheelchair pusher but
accessible housing and a job. For those, he was on his own.

Finally, the third stereotype depicts the most common presumptive
cause of mobility problems—elderly people fading away in seemingly inevitable senescence. This stereotype resonates with our own experiences.
Most of us slow down from the ceaseless motion of childhood as we move
into adulthood and old age. Mildred Stanberg typifies this perspective.
Asthma limits her walking somewhat but, more importantly, she fears
falling. She lives alone in an apartment and rarely ventures outside unac-
companied. "I'm eighty-seven," said Mrs. Stanberg. "I figure that it's time.
As my walking slows down, everything else seems to slow down. I hope
my head won't slow down, but everything seems to take longer. I take
longer to dress, I take longer to wash. I shower every morning, so I know.
I'm slow in every department."

The danger of this senescence stereotype is its presumed, inevitable
downward spiral—that nothing can halt or delay the progression and resultant isolation. People may not tell their physicians about these problems,
assuming that nothing can be done, that they deserve no special attention.
Yet, as one physiatrist (a physician who specializes in rehabilitation) said,
"By and large, people with walking problems have some kind of disease process. Trouble with walking is not part of normal aging. Endurance may cut
down with aging—you can't go five miles, you can only go one mile. But
walking should not be a problem. Falls should not be a problem of normal
aging." Generally some medical condition, or sets of conditions, cause walking difficulties.

WHAT CONDITIONS CAUSE MOBILITY PROBLEMS?

The stereotypes do not fit the common causes of mobility problems.
Arthritis is by far the most common cause (Table 2), with back problems in
second place.[5] Together they account for almost 38 percent of mobility dif-

TABLE 2. Common Causes of Mobility Difficulties

Causes[a]	Mobility Difficulty (%)		
	Minor	Moderate	Major
Arthritis and musculoskeletal problems	25	26	24
Intervertebral disk and other back problems and sciatica	14	16	8
Accidental falls	6	7	6
Ischemic heart disease and other heart conditions	5	5	6
Motor vehicle traffic accidents	4	5	4
Chronic bronchitis, emphysema, asthma, and other lung conditions	4	4	4
Cerebrovascular disease, including stroke	1	2	5
Overexertion and strenuous movements	2	3	1
Unspecified accidents	2	2	1
Machinery, firearm, and other specified accidents	1	2	2
Osteoporosis and bone or cartilage disorders	1	1	2
Diabetes	1	1	1
Multiple sclerosis	< 1	< 1	2

[a]This table shows causes reported by at least 1 percent of persons within each level of mobility difficulty.

ficulties, estimated at almost 7.6 million people. The next leading cause, accidental falls, involves many fewer people (just over 6 percent, an estimated 1.2 million persons). The remaining common causes sort into either chronic progressive conditions or injuries.[6] The common chronic diseases are those associated with aging: heart, lung, and cerebrovascular (stroke) disease, osteoporosis, and diabetes. Common causes therefore vary by age, with arthritis relatively more important for older people and back problems relatively more frequent among younger adults (Iezzoni et al. 2001). All types of accidents are more common for younger people. Together, however, chronic conditions far surpass accidents in causing mobility difficulties, regardless of age group.[7]

Oftentimes, disentangling a single reason for mobility problems is impossible. Multiple diagnoses account for walking problems among up to 75 percent of elderly people (Alexander 1996, 438). While most of the interviewees under fifty had a specific disease, such as MS, many older people had more than one condition. Back problems and arthritis frequently occur together, as with Mattie Harris, the woman who rarely leaves her home. Obesity is typically the thread linking these two conditions. Coexisting chronic conditions of aging, such as heart and lung disease, diabetes, and atherosclerosis, complicate the picture. Erna Dodd had more than her fair share of illness. When I first met her, Ms. Dodd said little, concentrating on walking. Her few words carried a Caribbean lilt. She was a heavy woman in her mid fifties, graying hair pulled back tightly from her face, a brace on her left leg. Stopping periodically to catch her breath, she trudged stolidly behind a three-wheeled walker, oxygen canister dangling from the handlebars, its clear plastic tubing snaking up under her nose. She refused our proffered wheelchair, pushing forward herself.

Ms. Dodd had been hospitalized numerous times with many medical problems: emphysema, diabetes requiring insulin, congestive heart failure, seizures, obesity, and arthritis. As she observed, "I end up with everything in life." She held two housekeeping jobs many years ago when her major problems started.

> I was working in the hotel. That was my second job. I fall down and busted my knee, the ligament. They had to operate on my leg and take out my ligament. The doctor told me that arthritis had set into my leg. I couldn't work in the hospital, and I couldn't work at my other job. I couldn't walk. I already had emphysema, then I had seizure. I fell down with seizure. After that, my boss told me he was going to put me on disability because I was going to lose my job.
>
> So I been wearing braces on my knees for years and years. The brace just keep the knee tight so I don't feel too much pain. But it doesn't help you all together. It cut up my leg, so I only wear one. The left leg is worse than the right leg. If I ever make a mistake and walk without the brace, I fall down. Like the bone shifts or something, and I fall down. And I don't want to get hurt real bad.
>
> I don't feel because a person is sick, you should sit down and just give up. You still have to try, and that's what I do. If I can't walk and my breathing is bad, I stay home and go on my breathalyzer machine till I get calmed down.

Arthritis and emphysema clearly slowed Ms. Dodd's walking, the first causing pain and mechanical difficulties, the second reducing her endurance. I cannot say which condition contributed more to her walking difficulties. The reality is that arthritis rarely kills people; emphysema does. Nearly six months after we spoke, Erna Dodd died from lung failure.

As the stories of Erna Dodd and Mattie Harris suggest, one condition deserves special mention—obesity. About 55 percent of adults living in the

United States are overweight and 22 percent of them are obese (Atkinson 2000, 3237). Obesity is the second leading cause of preventable deaths in our country and it severely limits daily lives. Being overweight is associated with several common causes of walking problems, most notably arthritis, back pain, and diabetes.[8] Carrying excessive weight frequently initiates and exacerbates degenerative arthritis of the knees through wear and tear on the joints. People with mobility problems are more likely than others to be grossly overweight—around 30 percent of people with mobility problems are obese compared to 15 percent of others.[9]

Obesity is problematic for several reasons. First, it is hard to control. Despite spending $33 billion annually on diet programs, exercise regimens, and low-calorie meals and dietary supplements, Americans remain overweight, and rates of obesity are increasing (Freudenheim 1999, A11). Second, especially once it results in painful joints and fatigue during exertion, obesity initiates a vicious cycle, slowing or halting the very exercise that would help weight loss. Finally, obesity carries stigma in our youth-oriented society, owing, at least in part, to the issue of control. Many believe that having a slender body merely requires self-control, cutting caloric consumption, but recent findings relating to fat metabolism in other mammals, and thus presumably humans, suggest that the issue is much more complicated. Nevertheless, overweight people who have trouble walking feel keenly the stigma attached to obesity.

Marianne Bickford, in her early fifties, has had trouble with her weight for a long time. In high school, she had dreamed of being a nurse: "I passed the test, but the nurse who interviewed me said I had to lose 50 pounds, and she was heavier than me!" Ms. Bickford became a secretary. Now, years later, she is overweight, but she also has a painful back and knees. She always uses a manual wheelchair, even in her apartment. Her primary care physician, Dr. Greenberg, told me that he does not understand why she uses the wheelchair. Dr. Greenberg speculates that her obesity is a major factor and said she gets upset every time he brings it up.

Ms. Bickford, in contrast, is frustrated that Dr. Greenberg concentrates exclusively on her losing weight. She feels as if she is working on it: "Every time he talks about walking, me being confined to a wheelchair, it's always about my weight. That annoys the daylights out of me. Maybe it would make a difference, but I don't feel it's going to make a big difference. If you have knees that are degenerate, what is losing weight going to do? They're not going to get any better unless they're operated on, and the bone's taken off the bone, and the knees are built up again. The medical profession, they push you to walk, and they make all the suggestions." Tears welled in her eyes.

"A lot of times I don't say anything, because if things get too out of control with my doctor, then emotionally I'm drained for the rest of the day. They just think that you don't *want* to walk. You just want to be in the wheelchair—it's comfortable. Well, you try it!" Ms. Bickford and Dr. Greenberg seem at loggerheads. In this stalemate, both sides are right. It would help for her to lose weight, but weight loss is difficult and won't necessarily fix her painful back and knees.

3   Sensations of Walking

Most people walk without giving it a thought. Their legs automatically and painlessly obey the myriad impulses zipping to and from their brains, moving them effortlessly at will. These complex commands and compliant responses do not penetrate consciousness until something goes wrong. Reynolds Price, the novelist and radio commentator, described warning signals sent by his still-hidden spinal tumor as he rushed one afternoon, late for an appointment: "I should hurry along. I know I thought *Run,* a conscious signal, but I couldn't run. The command had got no further than my brain. Some bridge was out. I stalled . . . inexplicably paralyzed." Momentarily, he walked again "at normal speed, though I had to concentrate not to veer or stumble" (1995, 6). Within a month, Price took his last "free walk." He now travels widely with his wheelchair.

The physical sensations and biomechanical forces that accompany or impair mobility vary by the underlying cause. For people with progressive chronic conditions, four types of problems arise:

- biomechanical problems involving knees, hips, and other joints, ligaments, and tendons, and typically producing pain
- abnormal neurologic function or deficient communication between nerves and muscles, generally causing weakness, imbalance, distorted sensations, and loss of control over movements
- limited endurance and lower physical conditioning involving the heart, lungs, and/or blood vessels supplying the legs, causing shortness of breath, chest pain, leg or calf pain, or generalized weakness
- missing lower limbs or toes, amputated because of progressive chronic diseases (e.g., diabetes mellitus)

This chapter describes the sensations and biomechanical forces that accompany and compromise walking. Stories about four men with different
conditions exemplify these problems. All men were white and in their
early to mid sixties, but their personalities, sensory experiences, and responses to their physical situations varied widely. The chapter concludes by
discussing falls and incontinence, which frequently complicate living with
mobility problems.[1]

THE GAIT CYCLE

Walking upright is a complicated feat of bioengineering. Gait is the physical action of walking—a repeating cycle of movements going sequentially
from side to side. A complete cycle lasts from heelstrike to heelstrike of the
same foot. An average man without any impairment has a gait cycle of 1.03
seconds and walks 117 steps per minute, roughly 2.8 miles per hour
(Malanga and DeLisa 1998, 4). The average woman takes five steps more
per minute; steps are shorter and quicker with high-heeled shoes (Inman,
Ralston, and Todd 1981, 28). Stride length generally shortens as people age.
    The gait cycle involves two phases: the stance phase, about 60 percent of
the gait cycle; and the swing phase, the other 40 percent (Figure 2). The
stance phase splits further into the double-leg stance (both feet contacting
the ground) and the single-leg stance (one foot only contacting the
ground). At average walking speeds, the double-leg stance takes up about
10 percent of the gait cycle. This percentage falls as speeds increase and dis-
appears altogether when running. During the stance phase, various muscles work to prevent the supporting leg from buckling.
    Legs not bearing weight are in their swing phase. This phase starts when
the foot of the swing leg lifts from the ground and moves forward by flex-
ing the hip and knee, along with uptilting the foot by the ankle. The swing
leg then aligns with the stance leg and moves forward so the foot strikes
the ground, with specific muscles operating as shock absorbers at heelstrike. Then, normally, the opposite leg enters its swing phase, and the
cycle repeats, propelling people forward. Swinging arms, usually moving
opposite to the pelvis and leg, aid balance and smooth forward movement.
    Human anatomy requires us to shift our weight continually during the
gait cycle. The center of mass (COM) occurs midway between our hip
joints. During the gait cycle, the COM moves rhythmically up-and-down
and side-to-side, while transferring weight from one leg to the other. People naturally adjust their limb and trunk muscles and walking speeds to
minimize COM movements. Abnormalities that increase these distances

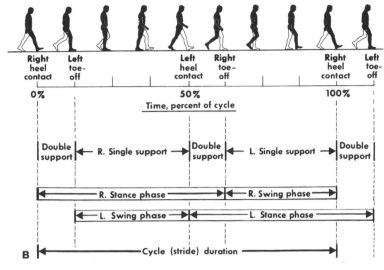

Time Dimensions of Walking Cycle

Figure 2. Gait cycle. (From V. T. Inman, H. J. Ralston, and F. Todd, *Human Walking* [Baltimore: Williams and Wilkins, 1981], 26.)

or distort smooth wavelike COM movement increase the energy required to walk.

Quiet standing requires about 25 percent more energy than lying down (Rose, Ralston, and Gamble 1994, 52). At the average, comfortable walking speed of people without impairments (about 80 meters per minute), the body consumes roughly four times the energy used at complete rest (Kerrigan, Schaufele, and Wen 1998, 168). Walking faster and running demand more energy, but so does walking slowly—for muscles and other structures to provide additional balance. At their respective, comfortable walking speeds, people with and without walking difficulties expend about the same energy during the same amount of time. But people with impairments walk more slowly. Therefore, people with mobility problems consume more energy while walking the same distance than do others.

Efforts to avoid pain typically distort smooth COM movement, increasing the energy required to walk a given distance. Keeping joints stiff because of pain requires more energy to swing the limbs forward. Typically, people with hip arthritis avoid bearing weight on their painful joint, reducing the stance phase on that side. Lurching their trunk toward the affected hip, often by dipping their shoulder on that side, they move the COM over the joint, decreasing stresses on it. During the swing phase, people flex their hip slightly, and they avoid jarring and painful heelstrikes.

These maneuvers consume considerable energy and are tiring, however slowly people walk.

Abnormalities of nerves or their communication with muscles can impair gait, sometimes also by distorting patterns of COM movement. Problems with coordination can cause staggering, lunging gait, with legs placed wider apart than normal. People with strokes involving one side of their brains frequently have a "hemiplegic gait." They reduce the time spent and amount of weight shifted to the affected side during the gait cycle; the arm on that same side is flexed and rotated inward, not swinging freely. Gait is slow, with prolonged stance phases and shortened steps. To walk the same distance, people with hemiplegic gaits consume 37 to 62 percent more energy than those without gait problems (Kerrigan, Schaufele, and Wen 1998, 170).

People with lower-extremity amputations need external support (e.g., from a walker or crutches) during the portion of the gait cycle involving the missing limb. Eventually, many people learn to walk well with prostheses, artificial or mechanical legs (Leonard and Meier 1998). People with amputations on one side typically walk faster with prostheses than those with bilateral amputations, whose slower speed demands more energy. Persons with below-the-knee amputations generally ambulate more easily with prostheses than those with amputations above the knee.[2] Shifting weight onto the prostheses and maintaining balance while ambulating require considerable training. Maintaining the health of the stump (skin integrity, in particular) is crucial.

Walking depends on many important factors beyond lower-extremity functioning, including people's cognitive status and judgment, vision, other problems affecting balance (such as vestibular or inner ear function), upper-body strength and mobility, global physical endurance and fitness, and overall health. People with mobility difficulties are more likely than others to report vision problems, dizziness, imbalance, and poorer overall health (Table 3).[3] Any of these factors worsen gait.

PAIN FROM BIOMECHANICAL CAUSES

"My knee was so painful. You could feel bone rubbing against bone," Mattie Harris recalled. Biomechanical problems, such as worn or inflamed knee or hip joints, compressed nerve roots exiting the spine, and collapsed or shifted vertebrae, typically cause pain. Pain can develop slowly and insidiously or appear suddenly and relentlessly. It can be all-consuming, keeping people awake at night, preventing even the most trivial-appearing activi-

TABLE 3. Other Physical Problems

	Physical Problem (%)[a]			
Mobility Difficulty	Poor Vision	Dizziness	Balance Problem	Poor Health
None	2	1	1	1
Minor	8	7	10	13
Moderate	12	13	16	28
Major	15	13	26	38

[a]Poor vision = serious difficulty seeing, even when using glasses or contact lenses; dizziness = dizziness that has lasted for at least 3 months; balance problem = problem with balance that has lasted for at least 3 months; poor health = poor overall health.

ties. Stella Richards retired early from her secretarial job when a back problem, spondylolisthesis, laid her out flat for almost six months.

> I was in misery! If I went into the bathroom, I just had time to wash my hands and hobble back to the bed. It was so excruciating. You should have seen me trying to take a bath. I knew that I only had so many minutes to get in that tub and out. If I was in there to go to the bathroom, I could never stay long enough to brush my teeth. I had to go back and make a special trip for that.

People with arthritis often describe immobilizing and painful stiffness, especially on awaking in the morning or after prolonged sitting. Like the tin woodsman from *The Wizard of Oz* after a rainfall, they feel rusted in place, painfully unable to flex, bend, or move. Some "work out" this stiffness and pain by exercise. Jimmy Howard, in his late forties, feels "like somebody's in there with a hammer and a chisel, just chiseling away. Every way I move is pain." At first he didn't know why. "I'd be walking, and I'd feel a pain in my hip. So you walk it off, and it goes away. Months went by. It wouldn't bother me, then all of a sudden, it would act up again. I wouldn't pay it no mind. Then one day I was walking, and, whoa, it really started—excruciating pain. You'll feel like your hip is going to give out." Exercise helps. "After I get up every morning, I read my Bible for a couple of hours, and then I ride my bike to loosen up before I start my day."

Other people report similar experiences of hips or knees almost collapsing beneath them, joints "locking" into place, almost toppling them over. Mattie Harris is embarrassed by this. "The knee locks on me like it wants

to throw me down. It doesn't want to move when I want it to move. Sometimes I almost fall. I'd be in the supermarket, and I'd have to grab onto people I don't know. They're looking at me like I'm crazy. I have to apologize.
I can remember one time I was walking to catch the bus. I got halfway, and
my knees locked, and I couldn't move. People I knew walked by and said,
'Mattie, you all right? You want us to help you?' 'No, thank you, I'll be all
right.' "

"Why didn't you want them to help you?"

"Because my knee has to unlock on its own. If I tell them to help me,
and my knee's still locked, I can't go no place. I still might fall."

Some describe misimpressions that outsiders have about their ability to
get around. Cynthia Walker, in her mid thirties, has two children under five
years old. Her rheumatoid arthritis primarily affects her ankles, knees, and
wrists. Friends suggest that she crawl when all else fails.

> With rheumatoid arthritis, when you're immobile, when you lie on
> the couch, on a bed, your joints are very relaxed. But when you go
> to stand up again, you can't. You really have to put pressure on the
> floor for quite a while for your joints to hold your weight, to put
> one foot in front of the other, and sometimes you just can't stand up
> anymore. You have to sit down.
>
> If a child yells for you or you need to be somewhere fast, it's a
> problem. . . . I'll stand up off the couch and, pardon me God, I can't
> stand up! And the child is screaming, and the crutches are upstairs
> because you left them upstairs that morning. You want to get just
> two rooms over, but that two rooms might as well be two miles. But
> you do it. Now some people say, get down on the floor and crawl. I
> can't. My knees don't work, and if I get down on the floor, how the
> hell am I going to get back up?

People try many things to control their pain, including medications
(e.g., nonsteroidal anti-inflammatory drugs), physical therapy, exercise,
mobility aids (canes or walkers to lessen pressures on painful joints), and
ultimately surgery. They also attempt steroid injections, acupuncture,
heating pads or cold compresses, pool therapy, massage, and prayer. Sometimes physicians explicitly say they can do nothing more for the pain, leaving people angry, frustrated, and disheartened (chapter 8).

Nevertheless, most people say they are stoic, refusing to "give in" to
pain. Despite her older children's protests, Mattie Harris sweeps her
kitchen floor when it's dirty; she can't "sit there and see something that
needs to be done." People say they learn to live with pain, acknowledging
that if they didn't, their lives would become unacceptably limited. Even
those with self-described high pain thresholds may eventually try surgery

in an attempt—sometimes successful, sometimes not—to eliminate pain and restore function. Deciding exactly when to operate is often hard. Mike Campbell was a case in point.

Mike Campbell

Mike Campbell, a retired maintenance man in his mid sixties, had osteoarthritis of both knees. He and his wife, Betty, occupied an in-law apartment upstairs in their daughter's home outside a New England picture postcard town. We met on a perfect autumn day, crimson and golden leaves swirling in the wind, pumpkins on every stoop. The air smelled wonderful and woodsy when I and Ron, my administrative assistant and driver, emerged from the car onto a bed of needles from towering pine trees. From the driveway, we saw only the side of the house, with steep, wooden stairs leading to a second floor door. How had Mr. Campbell climbed those stairs with his incapacitated knees? Ron reported that we were meeting in the daughter's living room downstairs.

Mr. Campbell, a big man, ruddy in a hale and hearty way, sat in a wing-back chair at one end of an immaculate living room dotted with china figurines. Having had his second knee replaced several weeks previously, he had crutches propped against the wall, and his left knee appeared thickly padded. Betty joined us, a calico cat cuddled beside her. Mr. Campbell had not planned on retiring from building maintenance two years previously. "I was going to work another two or three years. But my legs got so bad that I figured I'd take early retirement and get done with it. The pain got so bad at the end that I could only walk 35, 40 yards, and then I'd stop and rest.

"I know I had the arthritis coming on for years. Sitting in a straight-backed chair, I had to get halfway across the room before I could get straightened up and my legs working. I think it's hereditary. My mother had it. Her father had it before her, and my brother just had his second knee replaced. My mother was always crippled. For the last thirty years of her life, maybe forty, she rarely ever went out."

"Mike didn't want to be housebound like his mother," said Mrs. Campbell.

"She let it happen to her. One day, she weighed over 300 pounds, and she never really tried to do anything. That's one thing that I worry about. I have no intention of getting caught that way."

"When the problem started for him, he took off about 40 pounds," said Mrs. Campbell. "The arthritis didn't go away, but it alleviated the pain back then. He has a very, very high tolerance for pain."

"High tolerance?" Mr. Campbell repeated. "I can ignore it!"

"So you were determined to go on?" I asked.

"It wasn't a question about being determined or going on," Mr. Campbell laughed. "You gotta make a living. And I had a hard job doing that." Mr. Campbell had a high school education and had worked from childhood.

"When I got to the point where I couldn't do my work and do it right anymore, I figured it was time to get out." I asked how Mr. Campbell had decided to have his knees replaced.

"He was to the point where he was losing cartilage in between the knees," Mrs. Campbell replied. "Last year, the X rays showed there was no cartilage at all in one knee. Bone on bone. The other one had just one side of cartilage left. He could only go up and down the stairs in this house one time a day. He was pretty housebound to the apartment."

"About eight years ago, I was going to have these operations done. But then the doctor said they couldn't guarantee me more than fifteen years, and fifty-five is kind of young to get something like that done." Orthopedists typically put the lifetime of knee prostheses, the hardware that replaces the knee, at about fifteen years. "All of a sudden, it cleared up a lot! Not completely, but enough." Mr. Campbell delayed surgery for six or seven years. "I thought I'd wait as long as I could. Then when I couldn't get around anymore, it just seemed like the practical thing to do."

Now he hoped newer prostheses would last longer, but I also felt that he was joking, darkly, about whether he would last for fifteen years. Mr. Campbell patted his right knee; that replacement had worked like a charm. He and Betty planned to return to long walks at the local shopping mall. "I don't have any pain at all in my right leg. I got a little bit in the left one, but that's going to be here until the swelling goes down. The only thing I would advise other people is, when they start having troubles and their leg starts acting up, get it checked out. Don't fool around like I did."

Two years afterward, I called Dr. Josh Landau, Mr. Campbell's rheumatologist, to see how he was doing. Dr. Landau responded swiftly and sadly. The left knee replacement had alleviated his pain and restored his ability to walk, but Mike had died a few weeks before my call from an unusually aggressive pneumonia. Dr. Landau sounded shaken that he could not save this man he had known for fifteen years.

NEUROLOGIC PROBLEMS

Given the diversity of neurologic conditions, people's physical experiences vary widely, ranging from being unable to move a leg paralyzed by a stroke to the eerie sensory disturbances of MS. People describe weakness, overwhelming fatigue, imbalance, tripping or careening into objects, stubbing toes on tiny bumps and cracks, and having trouble initiating, maintaining, or controlling movement. They have difficulty describing their sensations to loved ones, friends, and physicians. "It was hard on my husband because there's no way to describe what I'm going through," said Candy Stoops, who had fallen on the stairs when her legs collapsed. "There's no way my husband could have a concept of doing something and then suddenly not being able to do it, but thinking you're doing it all the time."

Nonspecific sensations like weakness and profound fatigue can be explained so easily by other aspects of daily lives—hectic schedules, demanding responsibilities, unwelcome consequences of aging—that they are often dismissed until they can no longer be ignored. Walter Masterson, in his late fifties, was a business executive flying frequently abroad for exhausting negotiations. He disregarded the initial symptoms of amyotrophic lateral sclerosis (ALS), Lou Gehrig's disease.

> I started being bothered by the limp in the summer but didn't go to the doctor until that fall. I didn't think twice about it because it had happened before. I would go overseas for two, three, sometimes even four weeks at a time, which meant I was carrying damned near everything I own and running through airports with this massive bag banging against my knee. I would very often come home with a limp. After a week or so, it would go away. So I never really thought much about it except that this one didn't go away. After a bit of pushing by my wife, I finally went to the doctor.
>
> I came in for a variety of torture tests, which were essentially measuring the nerves' response to being stabbed and jolted. The net result of all that was that an expert diagnosed me with ALS. At that time, the limp was bad enough that I had to have a cane. Progressively, I had to have braces on one leg and then both legs to help me stand up. I briefly tried crutches—that just didn't work at all. Shortly thereafter I got a wheelchair for outside and a tricycle walker for home. Just recently, I got an electric wheelchair for outside. So, that's the state of things. Increasing weakness in my legs that has taken me from limping to not being able to walk at all.

Feeling unbalanced is another common sensation. Lester Goodall, in his mid fifties, had long-standing diabetes requiring insulin. A manager in a Fortune 500 company, Lester's recreational passion was throwing darts in leagues organized at local pubs.

> This is how I discovered I had MS. I used to throw darts, and I was pretty good if I say so myself. I would pick up my darts and try to get into the right position holding the darts, but I couldn't. That was strange. Then I'd stand on the line like you normally do, and the

next step lose my balance. I'd sort of fall. I attributed this to my diabetes acting up, my blood sugar being high because I wasn't controlling it like I'm supposed to. Then I noticed my vision. It was like
someone had taken the contrast on a TV and turned it up as bright
as they could, and I couldn't see the contrasts. So they put me
through all of these tests, a vestibular test for the balance, this test,
that test. MS was diagnosed through a process of elimination. At
that point I changed some things. I really got control of my diabetes.

Mr. Goodall's MS started with two characteristic symptoms of the disease—imbalance and difficulties with vision. This combination is especially
troubling since vision problems compound the risk of falls. Mr. Goodall's imbalance often leads people to think he is drunk: "It always appeared that I was
inebriated and losing my balance. I didn't know myself what was wrong back
in those days, so I just figured, hey! I know there's times when I'm walking
and people look at me and think this man had too much to drink."

Even without overtly losing balance, people say their gait has changed.
Instead of planting their feet firmly where they used to, striding purposefully forward, their legs splay outward and their steps veer erratically.
Often these changes reflect the nervous system's attempt to restore or
maintain balance in the face of neurologic deficits. The characteristic gait of
a person with MS is described as "broad based"—feet planted far apart,
trying to keep the walker erect.

Neurologic problems can also generate pain. "People don't understand
that it's painful to walk," said one woman. "My legs always burn, like
they're burning from the inside out. How do you describe it? It's ironic. I
can't feel pain and temperature. Yet my legs are always burning." The
nerves that communicate actual pain and temperature sensations to the
brain often malfunction in neurologic disease, sending erroneous messages. Neurologic pain and distorted sensations are difficult to treat.

In contrast, diabetes mellitus can lead to "peripheral neuropathy," a nerve
problem that diminishes sensations in the lower extremities (toes, feet, and
legs). That is one reason why periodic foot examinations are recommended
for persons with diabetes, who may not feel injuries or sore spots, leaving
wounds inadequately treated. Arnis Balodis had peripheral neuropathy from
decades with diabetes and had had both legs amputated because of encroach-
ing gangrene. Using mirrors, he carefully checked the stumps of his legs
where they fit into his prostheses. "I don't feel pain," Arnis reported. "If I get
blisters, then they take at least two weeks to heal up."

By their nature, neurologic diseases often affect many aspects of bodily
and mental functioning beyond mobility. Especially with illnesses that compromise cognitive function or the ability to communicate, walking prob-

lems may appear relatively manageable, particularly if they can be compensated for with mobility aids. An example is Parkinson's disease, first described by James Parkinson over 180 years ago. Affecting more than one million people in North America, its cause is unknown, although genetics and aging play a role (Lang and Lozano 1998a, 1998b). Parkinson's disease not only produces progressive debility, often including dementia, but it also shortens longevity. No current treatment reliably slows the progression of Parkinson's disease. As did his father, Barney Fink has Parkinson's disease.

Barney Fink

Barney Fink is a retired optometrist in his early sixties. He offered to talk at my office, observing, "I feel like I'm at the hospital every other day. I have so many doctor appointments." Dr. Fink has a shock of white hair, ruddy face, and Puckish grin, although his features frequently freeze in a sad, suspended expression. His voice is soft, breathy, and blurred, sometimes trailing away entirely. He walked independently, without using a cane or holding onto his wife, Rachel, although he shuffled and lurched slightly to one side. When we reached my office, Rachel left us to explore the neighborhood.

Starting about five years ago, a two-year period began during which Barney experienced vague problems—difficulty writing, trouble walking, a feeling that "something is not going right." He did not have specific tremors and movement disorders that often accompany Parkinson's disease, and his primary care physician dismissed the diagnosis. Barney finally consulted a neurologist, who noticed that his face had a "fixed, glazed look," a common appearance with Parkinson's disease. After an extensive evaluation, the neurologist confirmed the diagnosis and started levodopa treatment.

As is typical in Parkinson's disease, Barney's biggest walking problem is "Getting started, getting over the inertia. Once I get started outdoor walking, I'm fine. Like getting up from this chair. I find it difficult." He admits he is slow, but he still goes mall walking with Rachel. "They open up the mall around 8:00. Even before the merchants get there, the employees get there, we usually get there one day a week. But once, I tripped and fell. I was going down. As I fell, I put this arm out to break my fall, and that's when I ripped this." Barney pointed to his shoulder joint, the so-called rotator cuff, for which he contemplated surgery. "When I start walking with Rachel, I start shuffling. And if there's something on the floor, I'll catch it. Just trips me up. I have seen it progress and progress in the last year and a half." I asked how his problems had changed.

"It's so vague. The last time I went to the neurologist, he says, 'You're doing great, you're doing great.' I might have been doing great for that short time that I was in his office, but in the long run, it's been going down." Dr. Fink remembered his father's experience with Parkinson's disease. "My dad was falling all over the place. In fact, we got him hockey pads. Elbow and knee pads. It hasn't come time for that for me, yet. I presume in time it will. My father carried a cane, too, but he never let it touch the ground. Later Dad used a wheelchair. I took him out in it. For a ride. He'd get around that way in the summer. Spent a lot of time together. It was wonderful. But it took its toll on him."

I asked Dr. Fink what was hardest for him about his Parkinson's disease. Walking is certainly problematic, but other things go to the core of his identity. "The talking, communicating. That's where it went really downhill. There are things I want to say, and I just can't get them out. . . . I really clamp up. I get very tense, and it really bothers me." Barney worried that he might be giving substandard care, so he retired from optometry. Although the fixed income from disability insurance is tight, he feels relieved to no longer practice. Nevertheless, "I do get depressed. Not suicidal or anything like that. I just go into myself.

"So I try to do something with my time. To make it worthwhile. There's more to life than playing golf. I decided three years ago that I'd become a hospice volunteer. So I do that. I've had patients for four or five months, and I become very attached to them. It's something that helps, it's been marvelous. I'm able to separate my life. I don't bring work home. People say, 'How the hell can you do it all the time?' I talk about quality of life and dying with dignity." I sensed Barney was talking about himself.

Two years later, I asked his primary care physician how Barney was doing. "About the same," the physician said.

LIMITED ENDURANCE

Walking consumes considerable energy as each gait cycle shifts weight from side to side and moves people forward. Medical conditions that compromise global physical endurance therefore affect walking. Heart and lung conditions are the fourth and sixth most common causes of mobility problems among adults (see Table 2). These conditions and circulatory difficulties of almost any type limit the capacity for physical exertion and activities demanding energy and oxygen, such as walking. During exertion, heart and lung problems often produce difficulty breathing or shortness of breath. As Nan Darnelle, a former nurse in her early forties, observed, arthritis hurts but being short of breath really stops her.

I had an operation on my knees for arthritis. I have arthritis in my spine and in my shoulders. It hurts. It's hard to do anything. I do one thing, and I'm totally out of breath. I have to just stop and sit down. I have to go shopping for myself, and I have to walk to the store because I don't drive. And there's no bus from my house to a store. It used to take me twenty minutes. But now it takes me an hour just to walk to the store, and I only carry maybe two things at a time. So I have to go to the store, come back with that. Sit down and wait, catch my breath, then go back to the store, just to get dinner. A piece of meat or a can and whatever. It's hard.

Smoking contributes to both heart and lung disease. For people without mobility problems 27 percent report tobacco use, with slightly higher numbers for persons with impaired mobility (28 to 30 percent).[4] Fred Daigle's occupational exposures to asbestos compounded his lung damage from smoking.

Fred Daigle

Fred Daigle, in his early sixties, retired in his late forties from being a painter and all-around handyman. His lungs and heart had failed.

Ron drove me to the Daigles' house on a February day, the sun pale in a clear cold sky. In the old Massachusetts mill town, abandoned storefronts and empty brick factories told a grim economic tale. The houses on Pleasant Street were shabby and run-down, their landscaping ragged and unkempt. From a distance, the Daigles' house appeared a jauntily incongruous lemon yellow. Up close, the house was dingy and shuttered, all shades drawn, with broken storm windows patched by packing tape. Mr. Daigle motioned us to come in the back way. We opened the door in a stockade fence encircling an aboveground swimming pool, a puddle of ice on its cover. Faded plastic toys lay scattered about the small concrete patio.

The back door entered directly into a tiny kitchen, an early American, cherry-wood table where we sat filling the space. Mr. Daigle was of medium height and slight build, with the frailty that often accompanies chronic illness. Oxygen tubing wound from some recess in the house to the nasal prongs under his nose. His clothes were worn, but the loose cardigan and leather slippers retained the newness of Christmas presents. His wife, Martha, fussed around the sink, disappearing periodically into another room. She had a cast on her left wrist, a watchband stretched over it. Preoccupied, she said she had acquired a cold from a grandchild so didn't want to come near.

"What kind of work did you do?" I asked Mr. Daigle. As he described his first job, almost fifty years ago, Martha got antsy. She sat down at the table and cut to the chase. "He was a spray painter. He got asbestos in the lungs. He smoked. They did a biopsy of his lung. The doctor said there's nothing they can do. Start putting him on oxygen. He couldn't breathe. We've faced that fact. You never give up the hope that maybe something will come. One doctor said, 'You've got to put in an asbestos law suit.' I said that's not going to give me back my husband. I would do it if the money could give my husband new lungs. But it won't.

"He stopped smoking for Lent because he was getting heartburn and having a hard time breathing. I told him to go to the doctor. That's when the doctor told him he needed a heart bypass and valve replacement. That's what retired him. The heart and his breathing. He's been fine up until three months ago. He'd retired, but he had his little jobs. He'd go and paint a room, just to keep busy. But then about three months ago, he was having a hard time breathing. After three days, we went to the hospital, and we discovered the lungs had started to get worse. And now he can go only from here to there." Mrs. Daigle indicated a distance of about 20 feet.

"I get up in the morning from that room," said Mr. Daigle, pointing toward the front of the house. The Daigles had made the living room into Fred's bedroom because he couldn't climb stairs. The bathroom was behind the tiny kitchen. "If I make it to the bathroom and back here, then I have to sit down." He paused, catching his breath. "I had to learn to be slow, to pace myself. I've always been in a hurry. Got to get there quick! I didn't know why when I'd get there."

"The last doctor was just truthful," Mrs. Daigle stated. "He said there's nothing they can do. I'd rather he was up front with us. I have to go back to work. This is what's bothering me. I know Fred. He'll just sit, and that's the worst thing in the world. He'd get in a rut." Mrs. Daigle was a housekeeper at the local hospital but had taken time off following her wrist fracture. "I'm hoping when the weather gets better, we'll drive the kids and walk around Castle Island." Mrs. Daigle described outings with their grandchildren to the ocean-side park south of Boston. "I'm going to ask Fred's primary doctor if we can get him a wheelchair.

"In the summer time, God willing we're still here, we can go to Castle Island. I can push Fred in the wheelchair or he can learn to use his hands. That will get him out. Even if he says, 'I've got to walk,' we'll push the wheelchair along. When he gets tired, he can sit down. Then he can get up again after about five minutes. I think with the wheelchair, it's better than him just sitting at home. He's got to get out."

"We'll take me for a ride," said Fred.

"We like to go down to Nantasket Beach. Once a month, they have a band for us old fogies, and they play all the old music."

"Have to schedule a day out. We work all our lives looking for me and her to retire, and what happens?"

Mrs. Daigle looked at her husband with tears in her eyes. "Don't worry about it. As long as I have you, that's all that counts."

I tried later to find out how Mr. Daigle was doing, but the physician who had recommended that I talk to him had left our hospital. I logged onto our computer system and found appointments and emergency room visits, packed close, until about two months after our interview—no visits since.

MISSING LIMBS

Amputations generally occur in one of four scenarios: extensive trauma, beyond surgical repair; cancerous tumors; invasive infections unresponsive to antibiotics; and various conditions that compromise blood flow. Unlike the slow chronic progression of other conditions, the functional impact of an amputation is instantaneous. Typically, however, the conditions leading to the amputation have lasted years. Today, roughly 95 percent of amputations are caused by peripheral vascular disease (blockage or narrowing of arteries, often associated with atherosclerosis, smoking, severe hypertension, or elevated cholesterol) or complications of diabetes (Feinglass et al. 1999, 1225). In peripheral vascular disease, amputations become necessary when blood flow is so limited that tissues actually die, when pain is severe and intractable, or when infections (such as gangrene) defy standard treatments.

How much to amputate depends on the situation. Obviously, when dealing with cancer or infections, surgeons aim to remove all diseased areas, ensuring that only healthy tissue remains. People walk better with prostheses when less is amputated. Therefore, someone with diabetes may have gangrened toes amputated first, followed by higher amputations as the disease progresses up the leg. Fitting a prosthesis requires care, ensuring a comfortable connection around the stump and proper alignment of the equipment during the stance and swing phases of the gait cycle (Radcliffe 1994; Leonard and Meier 1998). With prosthetic limbs, many people, especially younger persons with trauma or cancer, resume virtually normal lives after amputations, skiing, running, and performing other vigorous activities almost as before. Often, older people must also contend with other effects of their progressive conditions, such as limited endurance from diabetes-related cardiovascular diseases.

Despite new prosthetic technologies, many view losing a lower limb with dread. Several years ago, I caught a taxi in Washington, D.C., heading to National Airport. The woman driver, noting my scooter, started talking about her brother who had had diabetes. In his late fifties, he had developed gangrene and needed an amputation. Her brother said he would rather die than not be able to walk. He was unmarried and believed he would become a burden. The taxi driver had pleaded with him, discussing artificial limbs and motorized wheelchairs. But her brother refused the amputation and died of gangrene. The driver did not visit him during his final days, too upset that he "would not listen to reason" and insisted on dying.

Now in his mid forties, Boris Petrov was a young surgeon in the former Soviet Union when he developed thromboangiitis obliterans, in which blockages or thromboses arise in numerous arteries. He has had many amputations moving progressively upward, finally losing both legs up to his hips as well as most fingers. During his first episode, Dr. Petrov developed life-threatening sepsis, an infection in the bloodstream caused by dead tissue, before agreeing to surgery.

> I was performing a routine appendicitis operation one night, and I started feeling pain in my right leg. I didn't understand at first what had happened. I felt so successful. I was married and everything was in front of me. And I am a Jew! Finally we got the diagnosis and learned I might lose this leg. I waited three and a half months with the thrombosis. I didn't want to lose my leg. I decided that my life was finished. Many people, I thought, poets and composers, had died before my age.
>
> I was in the hospital with sepsis, and I could see through a window. The snow was dirty, but there was green grass coming up through it, and children were playing. I remember this moment very well. I thought, "What am I? A piece of leg?" They couldn't operate without my permission unless I became unconscious and three surgeons signed the order, saying my life was in danger. That night, I started thinking differently, that I was more than just a leg. The next morning, I gave the surgeon permission, and he removed my leg in half an hour.

The most dramatic physical sensation caused by amputation is the "phantom limb"—the feeling that the missing limb is still there and behaving as before. Beyond the phantom limb, perhaps the most important physical feeling is actually the absence of normal sensation. Without the real limb in place, the brain no longer receives the subconscious neural messages positioning the body in space and assisting upright balance. People with amputations learn quickly not to walk in the dark. Most need their vision to assist in maintaining balance. Through hard work and physical therapy, many learn to walk upright with artificial limbs but may still need canes or crutches for balance. Arnis Balodis knew all about this.

Arnis Balodis

Arnis Balodis, in his early sixties, had had diabetes since childhood, resulting in amputation of both legs below the knees. Arnis and I met one afternoon at my office. When making the appointment over the telephone, Arnis spoke in a bounding, staccato voice: "Afternoons are better. In the mornings, I have to get mother settled. She's ninety-five. You'll recognize me. I'm 6 feet tall. Weigh 200 pounds. Call me Arnis."

Arnis matched his description, although from my scooter I am not an exact judge of heights. He had a round face, deep-set dark eyes, and a small wiry mustache. His stiff-legged, slightly lumbering gait caught me off guard. He had legs! He was standing sturdily above me, albeit carrying an elaborately carved cane. Given his self-assured movements, it took me a few seconds to remember that his lower legs were artificial.

My eyes went to his ankles, thick, smooth, and pinky-flesh-colored. Why hadn't Arnis worn socks to cover the prostheses? Subsequently I understood that he viewed prostheses as tools, functional inanimate objects to be scrutinized dispassionately for their mechanical performance. The outer aspect of his cotton pants had eight-inch zippers for easy access to the prostheses. During our interview, Arnis unceremoniously unzipped the right pant leg to demonstrate how his stump in its white knit sleeve fit into the upper "clam shell" of the prosthesis. Later, he unzipped the left pant leg to show how the newer prosthesis was slightly off kilter. At several points, he tapped the artificial limbs with the wooden cane he had carved himself. No, it couldn't hurt. Those legs weren't "real."

Arnis seemed willing to talk, although with a wait-and-see skepticism. From eastern Europe, Arnis, his parents, and twin brother were put by the Nazis into a camp for "foreign detainees. At the end of the war the Americans came. The American army, with its tanks, was sitting and eating oranges. That was the first time I ever saw an orange. By that time, I was skin and bones. I couldn't figure out that oranges had skin that you didn't eat. The soldiers showed me how to peel it apart. When the Russians advanced, the American army said anybody who wants to come with us can come. So we were piled onto military trucks like sardines, and that began the journey to West Germany."

When he was ten years old, Arnis was diagnosed with diabetes at a German clinic. "They gave me a bottle of insulin and a hypodermic and they said, 'This is your life. How long or how short, we don't know.'" Several years later, the Balodis family came to the United States. His parents could afford to send only one son to college. "So we flipped a coin. I went to work. My twin went to school. And then he decided to become an officer and a gentleman." He was very proud of his brother, who rose to a high military rank, but Arnis repeatedly referred to himself as uneducated, smart in the "raw materials" sense only. He always thought he would die young and did many reckless things—boxed, drove fast cars, worked dangerous security jobs. He seemed fiercely proud of his lifetime working and was realistic about his choices.

"There was a lot of discrimination. The diabetes limited you to certain kinds of work. If you put diabetes on an application for a better job, they assumed you couldn't do nothing. That's why I didn't get a couple of nice jobs. But why lie about it? I'm diabetic. I wasn't a weak diabetic. I could press close to 300 pounds. I boxed, and I wasn't a very gentle person," Arnis laughed. "I have never blacked out from diabetes, just when I get punched in the ring boxing."

Arnis controlled his diabetes on the edge. For seven years he didn't see physicians; he thought they knew less about his disease than he did. He finally connected with a diabetologist, Dr. Steve Greenfield, with whom he achieved a relationship of mutual respect. About ten years ago, "I knew the circulation in my legs wasn't that good because they would not heal. I used to always wear cowboy boots to protect my feet. All of a sudden, my toes turned black, and the heel split. I called Steve and said we got a big problem." After tests found blocked blood flow, a vascular surgeon performed a bypass of an artery in his leg, "which helped for six months. Then it collapsed.

"I was on a strong dose of antibiotics. 'You can hold onto it,' the surgeon says. 'I'll give you a year. Then you're creating problems with getting all kinds of bad things in your system. The impurities.' So I said you can take it off." Arnis showed not even a slight frisson of emotion while talking of his leg. About a year later, the surgeon amputated gangrened toes from the other foot, then subsequently amputated the second leg, again below the knee.

Arnis viewed his legs and prostheses with the critical eye of an engineer. The surgeons had left his second leg with a short stump, giving him "trouble because the leg floats around. I've got to be very careful when I step. If it's a stair, I got to make sure I aim close to the edge. The stump is so short that it's not stable. It's like a pendulum on a clock. It swings, and you don't know if you're going down."

"Can't the biomechanics people make a better leg?"

"There are better legs. On television I've seen people who can run. When I cross streets, I've got to judge traffic and wait for some good samaritan that will stop, because I've wound up twice on the hoods of cars."

"What prevents you from getting a better prosthesis?"

"Medicare. Money."

"Are you afraid of falling?"

"This year I took two tumbles. I went to a Christmas party with friends who have a living room with a plush carpet plus the foam padding. When you put down the artificial foot, you can't feel it. So you're not sure of yourself. You're floating, you're trying to balance on one leg, and of course you pop out of the clam shell."

"Did you hurt yourself?

"I just let myself go. I'm not ashamed of it. The only thing is usually, if it happens at home, I get on a chair. I push myself up." His ninety-five-year-old mother couldn't help given her arthritis and heart problems.

"Did you ever marry?"

"No, I figured out my life expectancy. If I had known I'd live this long, I would have. I did some silly things in my younger days. I always had fast cars, and I didn't mind having a lead foot on the accelerator. And I mean a lead foot. Diabetes is a very misunderstood illness because you don't look sick. I could step in the boxing ring with an equal and hold my own."

"Had you known all along that there was a chance you would lose your legs?"

"Yup. I took a gamble. No, it wasn't a gamble. It was a calculated risk."

"And was it hard when the surgeon said we need to take off the leg?"

"No, I'm very realistic. The surgeon said, 'You've got two choices: getting gangrene or losing the leg.' And so I said, 'I think I want to live a little bit more.' "

I asked Steve recently how Arnis was doing. He had just died from an irregular heartbeat that perplexed my colleague, but it could also have been "a broken heart." He had never recovered from his mother's death a few months earlier and his days had become empty.

FALLS

All types of mobility problems predispose people to falls, which have huge health, emotional, and financial costs. In 1997 falls were the most common cause of injuries nationwide, and the only cause with higher rates among females than males.[5] Almost 37 percent of falls occurred on level ground, with 12 percent and 10 percent happening on stairs or steps and sidewalks or curbs, respectively (Warner, Barnes, and Fingerhut 2000, 18–19). The chance of falling each year rises to 50 percent by age eighty (Tinetti and Williams 1997, 1279). Falls increase with worsening mobility: whereas about 25 percent of people with mild walking difficul-

TABLE 4. Falls during the Last Year

Mobility Difficulty	Fell	If Fell in Last Year (%)		
		Fell More Than Once	Had No Help Getting Around	Was Injured
Minor	25	48	6	56
Moderate	33	58	12	52
Major	41	62	22	57

ties report falling in the prior year, 41 percent of those with major difficulties fell (Table 4).

Falls can be fatal, if not because of the acute injury then through the longer-term progressive debility and deterioration, and they dramatically increase the likelihood of being admitted to a nursing home (Tinetti and Williams 1997). Falls heighten fear, anxiety, and social isolation, as people become less willing to leave their homes. Most assume that falls occur only while people are walking or actively moving around. The truth can be much less dramatic. Men described falling while dressing at their bedsides. "I fell as I was trying to pull up my pants myself," said one man. "I was trying to hold onto something, but you can't pull up pants one-handed. . . . I always want to make sure I'm close to the wall."

Even sitting in an unsteady chair, especially one with wheels, can result in falls. Since many people with mobility difficulties cannot do sustained weight-bearing exercise, they are especially prone to osteoporosis or thinning bones, increasing their chances of fractures. One woman in her forties fractured her hip when her rolling chair tipped over on a polished hardwood floor. Jeanette Spencer, a former schoolteacher in her late seventies, recounted many years of "unreliable knees. I would just collapse. All of a sudden I was down on the sidewalk." She later had a mild stroke and Parkinson's disease, producing a "drunken walk" requiring her to "stay close to the wall, so I can grab onto something." Gradually, as her debility progressed, she rarely left her house. One day several months after our interview, she fell and fractured her hip while moving from her bedside chair onto her bed. Mrs. Spencer died a few months afterward without ever returning home.

Houses are obstacle courses for people with mobility problems. During interviews in people's homes, I observed innumerable accidents waiting to happen, such as slipping area rugs, stairs without railings, and general stuff piled on the floor, blocking travel routes. Although people admit tripping, they do not like to change their homes (chapter 10). Trade-offs between safety and quality of life may arise. As one woman remarked ruefully, "I have a cat that likes to nap on the back doorstep. I've stepped on her a couple of times, but I've managed not to fall. What do you do with a cat? She's a beloved pet."

Among people with major mobility problems who fell in the prior year, over 22 percent said they fell because they didn't have help getting around (see Table 4). About half of people who fall require assistance getting up and about 10 percent of people lie longer than one hour undiscovered (Tinetti, Liu, and Claus 1993, 65). Rather than turn from a supine to prone position (i.e., from their back to their front), crawl to a strong support, and pull themselves up, some people, panicked after a fall, often try unsuccessfully to rise from the weaker supine position. Failure inflames fears, sapping strength, exacerbating the situation.

Numerous people voiced concerns about being unable to get up after a fall, even when they live with other people. One man's wife calls 911, summoning the police, when she cannot lift her husband. He constantly carries a portable phone whenever his wife leaves home so he can call for help. Brianna Vicks lives alone, but the day she fell, her daughter was visiting.

> I was using my walker, and . . . my shoe got caught on the rug. I fell flat on my butt, but this leg was turned in. My daughter got upset, but I said to myself, I'm gonna stay calm. Just pull my leg up, and I'll be fine. I told my daughter to go knock on my neighbor's door. My neighbor's grandson picked me up and put me up on the couch. I called my doctor, and she called the ambulance. I was starting to shiver and get chills. They said, "You broke your leg." And that's when I lost it. I think now my subconscious is a little bit afraid. Maybe that's why I don't walk that much and I use my wheelchair in my house. I'm afraid of falling. But I keep my Lifeline around my neck all the time.

Brianna pointed to a small, plastic device that summons help at the push of a button.

Falling in public is a double-edged sword for some. People might be around to assist, but their actions—while well intended—may not be helpful. When my legs collapse, it's like a hard disk crash on a computer. Everything completely shuts down. I need time literally to "reboot": after a few minutes on the ground or floor, my strength returns. During those minutes of shutdown, however, I am totally dead weight, without strength to assist in rising. It is better for bystanders to let me sit for those minutes, but their natural inclination is to pull me up. Conveying this reality without appearing ungrateful or irrational is challenging.

Falls often mark a downward transition in the gradual progression of debilitating disease. Walter Masterson, the man with ALS, described how he first knew he needed a cane.

> I came to the cane because I started falling down. In fact, at most of these transitions where some new piece of equipment has been necessary, I've always pushed things too far before I accepted the change. And the result of pushing things too far is, very often, falling down or some equally unpleasant experience. . . . One day I was trying to make it from the building to my car in the parking lot with a large bag of papers, and I didn't make it. I learned that once fallen, it's very difficult to get up! So I started taking falling a lot more seriously. Not just the jolt of landing, but then how do you get back up?

A number of people said they were used to falling and no longer worried about it: "If it's gonna happen, it's gonna happen. . . . I've learned to relax when I fall. You're not going to get as hurt as when you're tense." Various interventions can reduce the risk of falls: doing exercises for strength and balance, using canes or other mobility aids, minimizing medications that cause drowsiness or dizziness, adding home modifications such as handrails, grab bars, and raised toilet seats, and eliminating low-lying furniture (Tinetti et al. 1994, 822). These strategies must recognize people's other health problems. Mattie Harris says that railings offer little support because her hands, with their painful arthritis, cannot grip the rails. Even if people do not fall, the fear of falling is a powerful impediment to leaving home, resulting in increasing social isolation. These fears may be well founded: most of my interviewees live in New England, and many are afraid of slipping on ice and snow and do not leave home in winter. Arnis Balodis tumbled on black ice one morning and skidded the full length of his steep driveway; passing cars could not see him lying behind the snowbank. He did the "doggie crawl" up to his house.

Other fears can have more subtle roots but are equally isolating. Mildred Stanberg, in her late eighties, lost her husband several years previously. Her caring children suggested she sell the home she had inhabited for over fifty years and move two hundred miles away to an apartment designed for elderly people. Although Mrs. Stanberg now lives near her children, they have full professional lives and can spend little time with her during weekdays. Numerous shops, synagogues, a library, and movie theater are within a block or two, but she rarely leaves her apartment, virtually never alone.

"I think I developed some kind of a fright of walking or falling," Mrs. Stanberg said. "Being on my own now and being without the people I knew all these years, it's made me afraid. I had lived in a big house, my own home, and I got around pretty well. . . . Then, when I came here, I suddenly felt even walking to the corner was difficult unless I had somebody with me. My daughter was worried and took me to the doctor." The physician found mild asthma, and Mrs. Stanberg had a cataract removed from one eye. Otherwise, she was in good health.

"Unfortunately, I don't have enough friends to keep me busy and going out."

"Would it help if you lived with somebody?"

"I really like my privacy. I don't mind being on my own."

"What would make things better?"

"Somebody to adopt me and take me for a walk every once in a while."

INCONTINENCE

People with mobility problems, especially elderly persons, often become incontinent. Aging changes the bladder and lower urinary tract, increasing the likelihood of incontinence even in people without specific health problems. About one third of older people residing at home and half of those living in institutions experience urinary incontinence (Resnick 1996, 1833). Women are incontinent more often than men, although gender discrepancies narrow with age. Incontinence contributes to pressure ulcers, falls, infections, and death.

Immobility and neurologic problems increase the chances of incontinence. Many neurologic diseases that cause walking problems, such as stroke, Parkinson's disease, and MS, exacerbate incontinence through faulty neurologic signals to the bladder or bowel. Such conditions as diabetes and back problems can compromise one's ability to compensate for age-related changes to the urinary tract. Being unable to move quickly for whatever reason heightens anxiety about having an accident; this emotional stress can exacerbate the situation. As one woman said matter-of-factly, "You can't rush to the bathroom. Accidents do happen."

In our society the stigma, embarrassment, and humiliation attending incontinence are obvious and overwhelming. People with walking problems feel especially degraded, unable to control yet another basic function presumably mastered in earliest childhood. Several interviewees with neurologic conditions find bladder and bowel control more troubling than walking difficulties. "The thing that frustrates me more than anything with MS is trouble with my urinating and my bowels," Lester Goodall said. "I could live with anything else. Especially my bowel tract. Because of the nerves, I have a problem evacuating myself."

"Have you ever had an accident in public?"

"Once. At my office. I told my boss this hasn't happened to me since I was in diapers. I was sitting in the office working. It was almost like you could feel things coming on and you try to tighten up and hold on. This one I just had no control over. I was running to the bathroom. I was trying to get my pants down and before I got them down—I just had no control whatsoever. So now I don't wait. If the urge comes any time, I just go right away."

The good news about urinary incontinence is that with "a persistent, creative, and optimistic approach, most patients experience substantial improvement if not complete restoration of continence" (Resnick 1996, 1838). Treatments are often multifaceted, including bladder training and other exercises (to prevent incontinence associated with actions that increase intra-abdominal pressure, such as coughing), surgery, various medications, and use of absorbent pads and undergarments.[6] Improved urinary continence helps bowel control, along with other strategies to encourage regular bowel movements. Some interventions require a physician's input, but most interviewees confronted these problems on their own.

Near the end of the focus group involving ten women and one man, the participants brought up incontinence after a women mentioned interminable lines at ladies' rooms. (The sole man objected, "Men, too. You can't discriminate!") In a lively exchange, participants eagerly shared strategies and basically agreed that urinary incontinence can be handled.

"It's better to use some pad," said a nurse in her mid forties, "than be on the street and see urine going down your leg or saying, 'I've got to go home now because I've got to change my clothes.' You know what I'm saying? That limits the time that you have to enjoy being out."

"I bought me a package," said a woman in her late sixties, naming a leading incontinence pad, "and I put mine on today. I thought, I'm going out, and I might not get to the bathroom in time. And you know what? It's not a Pamper. It's nothing to be ashamed of." Having found other people who understood and shared their experiences, everybody nodded and agreed.

4 Society's Views of Walking

"Lena Walks!" my sister announced excitedly on the subject line of her e-mail message. Her little daughter had astonished parents and daycare workers alike by taking her first independent steps at eight months. After initial forays, she retrenched and resumed crawling, but that was too slow. Lena soon walked again, then started running lickety split. Two months later we observed this phenomenon firsthand. Lena ran everywhere, joyously climbing stairs, jumping delightedly, and laughingly being swept from the precipice of disaster by vigilant parents. After two days, merely watching made me weary. "Don't you wish Lena had walked a little later?" I asked my exhausted sister. Her response initially surprised me.

"No, we were really glad when she started walking. Lena was so frustrated before. She'd get really upset when she couldn't get things or go where she wanted. She's much happier now, getting around all on her own." On quick reconsideration, that logic makes perfect sense. Humans were not designed as sessile organisms, fixed in place, passively watching the world float by. More than any other species, we actively navigate and shape our environments. Walking is our private means of transportation, completely under our control. In our personal microenvironments, walking moves us efficiently wherever we want to go. Lena's walking allows her to act and act quickly, independently fulfilling her inscrutable infantine desires. No wonder she was frustrated before.

But as the sociologist Michael Oliver (1996, 97) observed, "Walking is not merely a physical activity which enables individuals to get from place A to place B. . . . It is also culturally symbolic." Bipedal locomotion, not intellect, defined the first human ancestors 3.6 million years ago. Our national ethos assumes citizens free to move at will, acting independently, being self-reliant, taking control and responsibility, not burdening others. Upright movement permeates American aphorisms, connoting independence, autonomy, perseverance, strength, achievement—"standing on your own two feet," "walking tall," "standing up for yourself," "taking things in stride," "climbing the ladder of success," "one small step for a man, one giant leap for mankind." After seriously injuring his left leg, the neurologist Oliver Sacks observed, "erectness is moral, existential, no less than physical" (1993, 107). Finally regaining the ability to walk without conscious struggle, Sacks found

> the joy of sheer doing—its beauty, its simplicity—was a revelation: it was the easiest, most natural thing in the world—and yet beyond the most complex of calculations and programs. Here, in doing, one achieved certainty with one swoop, by a grace which bypassed the most complex mathematics, or perhaps embedded and then transcended them. Now, simply, everything felt right, everything *was* right, with no effort, but with an integral sense of ease—and delight. (121)

Therefore, perhaps it is not surprising that societal views of walking problems remain a complex tangle of fears, discomforts, sorrows, rages, and uncertainties. Much of society still holds people with mobility difficulties individually responsible for problems they have in daily life (for example, with employment, transportation, housing), rather than crafting physical environments and public policies to accommodate mobility differences (Oliver 1996). Among some, the sense persists that, "if we fail, it is our problem, our personality defect, our weakness" (Zola 1982, 205). People with walking problems face the fallout of these perceptions daily.

The nineteen million adults who report at least some mobility difficulty do not necessarily face harsher public attitudes or barriers to full participation in society than do persons with other disabling conditions. At least fifty-four million Americans have some disability, including mobility problems (U.S. Department of Health and Human Services 2000, 6–4). Having studied disability worldwide, Charlton (1998) argues that blind and mobility-impaired people are better off than those with other disabling conditions. He asserts that, regardless of country or continent, "a hierarchy of disability" puts persons disabled by mental illness at the greatest disadvantage, followed by deaf and hard of hearing people (97). He finds that persons with physical and visual impairments have the strongest support systems and greatest political, social, and economic opportunities.

Nevertheless, walking difficulties are the quintessential "visible disability"—they are hard to hide. Often problems are obvious to onlookers, even from far away. Many of us are slow or need personal assistance, offering ample opportunity for conversational openings and breaching our precious zone of privacy. This visibility and availability attracts strangers to tell us their opinions and to ask whether they can help. Therefore, people with mobility problems (and probably blind people, too) have more interactions with strangers around their disability than do others, allowing us to get a good sense of societal attitudes.

Deciding when and how to respond to strangers requires split-second judgments. One morning several years ago I was waiting at Logan Airport for an early flight, and an older man in uniform walked up to me. Short and dapper, proud of his black hair minimally touched by gray, he had recently been promoted from wheelchair pusher to guard at the security station. "Can you tell me," he asked, "what is wrong with you?" Having seen me many times before, he seemed genuinely concerned, although decidedly curious. I saw an educational opportunity.

"I have MS. Multiple sclerosis." He still looked perplexed. "A disease of the nerves."

He reached to a cord around his neck and fished out a cross. "Jesus, Mary, and Joseph," he said, kissing the cross. "Can it be cured?"

"No," I said.

"I'm Italian," he said, "I'll pray for you." He walked away, shaking his head. This conversation did yield unanticipated benefits. Still at his post, the man eagerly smoothes my way through airport security, a particularly slow and intrusive process for wheelchair users.[1] Having shown me his hands, joints swollen by painful arthritis, he happily accepts my sympathetic return. But it told me again how some strangers view me.

Nevertheless, much has improved in the last thirty years, making physical spaces and public venues more accessible and even welcoming to people with mobility difficulties. A vigorous disability rights movement catalyzed these changes and engineered the 1990 Americans with Disabilities Act (ADA, P.L. 101–336). Other authors have chronicled the fascinating history of this movement (West 1991b; Shapiro 1994; Pelka 1997; Young 1997; Francis and Silvers 2000; Longmore and Umansky 2001). Here, I touch only briefly on history relating specifically to mobility difficulties, then recount interviewees' stories about their interactions with strangers. Many persons report positive encounters, but others—especially African Americans and poor people—note less happy experiences.

Society's views of walking difficulties are deep-rooted, often dark, and complicated. Tracing their historical origins is hard (Longmore and Umansky 2001). People with impaired walking have always been shadowy figures, hidden or living on the fringes. Their implied moral culpability compounded this isolation. Leviticus (16:18–20), in the Old Testament, cataloged "blemishes" that precluded persons from joining religious cere- monies: "a man blind or lame, or one who has a mutilated face or a limb too long, or a man who has an injured foot or an injured hand, or a hunchback, or a dwarf."

As societies developed, they depended on people to work, both to sup- port themselves and give something back to their communities. But people were assumed to dislike work and shirk labor by exaggerating their physi- cal problems. "Hence, the concept of disability has always been based on a perceived need to detect deception" (Stone 1984, 23). The legacy of these views persists today in insinuations about whether people can control their walking difficulties (chapter 2). Fourteenth-century English laws held that "honest beggars"—those who deserved alms—came involuntarily to their plights, forced by circumstances beyond their control (Stone 1984). Once proven, walking problems were granted immediate legitimacy. A 1536 En- glish statute allowed citizens to give alms directly to "lame" or blind per- sons, but not to other beggars in the street. In late-nineteenth-century En- gland, "lameness" qualified people as "defective" but deserving, meriting special vocational training.

In seventeenth-century America, the physical demands of exploring and settling rough and rugged country "meant that early colonists put a premium on physical stamina" (Shapiro 1994, 58). Initial settlers opposed immigration of persons who might need community support; people with physical or mental impairments could be deported (Baynton 2001). By the time of the Revolutionary War, these attitudes had eased somewhat, al- though most disabled people remained hidden, cloistered indoors. In 1781 Thomas Jefferson reported that Virginians without "strength to labour" were "boarded in the houses of good farmers," supported by tithes from local parishes (Jefferson 1984, 259). Only in "larger towns" might such people be seen, begging on the streets.

Wounded soldiers from America's wars merited special consideration (Scotch 2001). The Civil War inflicted roughly 60,000 amputations, about 40 percent involving lower extremities (Figg and Farrell-Beck 1993, 454, 460). In 1862 Congress passed the first of several laws to assist injured vet- erans, including granting $75 to purchase a prosthetic leg for each "loyal" Union soldier in need. Southern states bore prosthetic expenses for Con- federate veterans, with Mississippi spending 20 percent of its state rev- enues in 1886 on artificial arms and legs (Shapiro 1994, 61). By World War I, improved medical care allowed veterans to return home with even more severe impairments, prompting federal legislation in 1918 and 1920 to provide vocational training and job counseling. These programs also benefited growing numbers of persons injured by industrial accidents.

Nonetheless, people disabled by disease—not war injury or accident—remained largely hidden from public view. Into this environment came Franklin Delano Roosevelt. In August 1921 at his Campobello resort, Roosevelt "first had a chill . . . which lasted practically all night" (Gallagher 1994, 10). Roosevelt never took another true step. He also never complained or talked about his impairment to friends or family, including his wife, Eleanor. How much Roosevelt deceived himself remains unclear, but he knew he must deceive the public to get votes. So he crafted a fiction. After arduous practice, Roosevelt appeared to walk, when he actually threw his legs sequentially forward from the hips while basically being carried by his arms. His goal was to "walk without crutches," to "stand easily enough in front of people so that they'll forget I'm a cripple" (63).

At the time, Roosevelt's denial of his disability served his nation well. Before polio, Roosevelt had appeared cocky and arrogant; after polio, he connected with people. The public accepted the story that Roosevelt had overcome polio and was now just a little lame. Even the White House photography corps willingly hid Roosevelt's wheelchair use. From the unseen wheelchair and almost without respite, Roosevelt led the nation through the darkest days of the twentieth century before he died, as Winston Churchill observed, "in battle harness, like his soldiers, sailors, and airmen" (Gilbert 1991, 836).

Roosevelt's legacy relating to disability is complicated. The March of Dimes, using Roosevelt as its behind-the-scenes poster child (chapter 2), raised more money than any other health campaign, eventually leading to discovery of the Salk polio vaccine. Roosevelt understood that rehabilitation of polio patients "was a social problem with medical aspects. It was not a medical problem with social aspects" (Gallagher 1994, 53–54). In 1929, as governor of New York he exhorted the legislature to recognize the state's obligation "to restore to useful activity those children and adults who have the misfortune to be crippled" (78). As soon as the original Social Security Act passed in 1935, Roosevelt contemplated expanding the program, possibly adding medical and disability benefits (Stone 1984, 69). The demands of World War II allowed disabled persons—as well as women—to work in record numbers, although they lost these jobs when peace arrived (Linton 1998, 51). Yet Eleanor Roosevelt conceded that her husband "has never admitted he cannot walk" (Gallagher 1998, 208).

Especially among older people, Roosevelt's attitudes still resonate—or perhaps, more simply, Roosevelt's attitudes exemplify certain national values that transcend his individual example: "stiff upper lip, good soldier to the last" (Gallagher 1998, 209). Nelda Norton accused her husband, a retired business executive, of denying the motor neuron disease that seriously

weakened Tom's left leg. "For five years no one, not anyone in the family except myself, could know that he had been diagnosed with a disease," Nelda
Norton said. "It's one of the worst five years of my life. I couldn't tell friends.
The children would say, 'Why does dad walk so funny?' and I couldn't tell
them." Mr. Norton finally started falling. "When he was having a hard
time," Mrs. Norton recalled, "one of his sons said to him, 'You know, Dad, we
had a president in a wheelchair.' "

"I started using the cane about eight years ago," Mr. Norton interrupted.

"What happened then?" I asked.

"I retired from my company. Since I'd retired, the cane wouldn't inter-
fere with my image. Company presidents don't use canes." His son's reference to Roosevelt failed to move him.

CHANGING ATTITUDES

With Roosevelt's silence, a "teachable moment" was lost. Societal attitudes
changed little. In 1963 the sociologist Erving Goffman published his classic
book on stigma—attributes that leave people "discredited . . . facing an un-
accepting world" (19). Being "lame," "crippled," or "multiple sclerotic"
qualified as stigmatized attributes (along with minority race and religion),
which taint, discount, or discredit people in their own and society's eyes.

But something *has* finally changed. Reading Goffman's book a few
years ago, I entered a time warp. Here are some examples:

> When the stigmatized person finds that normals have difficulty in
> ignoring his failing, he should try to help them and the social situa-
> tion by conscious efforts to reduce tension . . . to "break the ice," ex-
> plicitly referring to his failing in a way that shows he is detached,
> able to take his condition in stride. (116)
>   Unsolicited offers of interest, sympathy, and help, although often
> perceived by the stigmatized as an encroachment on privacy and a
> presumption, are to be tactfully accepted. (118)
>   The nature of a "good adjustment" is now apparent. It requires
> that the stigmatized individual cheerfully and unselfconsciously ac-
> cept himself as essentially the same as normals, while at the same
> time he voluntarily withholds himself from those situations in
> which normals would find it difficult to give lip service to their simi-
> lar acceptance of him. (121)

I do not argue specifics of some of Goffman's assertions. Many interviewees use humor to diffuse discomfort, and courtesy is certainly preferable to

rudeness. Stigmatization may dissuade people from taking inappropriate advantage of economic support programs, such as disability insurance (Minow 1990, 91). Nevertheless, "the stigmatized" today would shrug aside Goffman's depiction of what they should do (especially to help out "normals").

Nowadays people with disabilities often find themselves not only included but celebrated. Centers for independent living, run by people with disabilities, address daily concerns within communities and teach self-empowerment; state and local governments sponsor offices on disability to ensure accessibility to services and spaces; disability rights centers offer legal counsel and advocacy; hundreds of internet sites provide disability-related services, advice, information, and support; numerous companies market products, from customized wheelchairs to accessible vacations; wheelchair users roll through television shows, commercials, and movies; dance troupes and other cultural organizations feature artists using wheelchairs; wheelchair athletes compete at elite levels; and a vibrant community of disability scholars carefully observes and chronicles societal attitudes.

The disability rights movement, which began several decades ago, deserves credit for this change (West 1991b; Shapiro 1994; Pelka 1997; Young 1997; Francis and Silvers 2000; Longmore and Umansky 2001). Early victories were often personal. In 1964 Gallagher (1998, 111–13), a wheelchair user, served as legislative assistant to Bob Bartlett, U.S. senator from Alaska. Gallagher occasionally needed to conduct research at the Library of Congress, which was not wheelchair accessible. Senator Bartlett contacted Quincy Mumford, librarian of Congress, requesting that a ramp be built at the back entrance that only had two steps. Mumford responded that adding to the library's physical plant might need a specific act of Congress. Frustrated by Mumford's stonewalling, Senator Bartlett inserted $5,000 explicitly for the ramp into Congress's budget, and the ramp was built. Gallagher's efforts culminated in the Architectural Barriers Act of 1968, which required all buildings constructed with federal funds to be physically accessible.

The disability rights movement, however, reached beyond individual battles to seek broad societal recognition of basic human and civil rights for people with disabilities (Bickenbach 2001). The hard-won achievements of racial minorities and women in the mid 1960s offered little to persons with disabilities. Unlike during these civil rights movements, disability rights advocates had not filled the streets. The critical precursor to the ADA, Section 504 of the Rehabilitation Act of 1973, was "a stealth measure in the midst of a backlash against civil rights" (Young 1997, 12).

> Section 504 of the Rehabilitation Act of 1973 was no more than a
> legislative afterthought. . . . At the very end of the bill were tacked

on four unnoticed provisions—the most important of which was
Section 504—that made it illegal for any federal agency, public university, defense or other federal contractor, or any other institution
or activity that received federal funding to discriminate against anyone "solely by reason of . . . handicap."

. . . Congressional aides could not even remember who had suggested adding the civil rights protection. But the wording clearly
was copied straight out of the Civil Rights Act of 1964, which ruled
out discrimination in federal programs on the basis of race, color, or
national origin. There had been no hearings and no debate about
Section 504. Members of Congress were either unaware of it or considered it "little more than a platitude" for a sympathetic group.
(Shapiro 1994, 65)

For four years, successive administrations (under Presidents Ford and
Carter) resisted implementing Section 504, fearing its potential costs. In
April 1977 frustrated disability activists, lead by wheelchair users, took
over federal offices in San Francisco, holding them for twenty-five days.
When one administration official suggested setting up "separate but
equal" facilities for disabled people, the proposal, with its unfortunate
phraseology, backfired. The civil disobedience tactics surprised the nation,
but this victory marked "the political coming of age of the disability rights
movement" in the United States (Shapiro 1994, 68).

The ADA was not enacted until many other battles were won. The diversity of disability advocates and difficulties identifying with each other
occasionally threatened their success. Political fears about costs, litigation,
and burden on business posed perhaps the biggest hurdle.

The ADA is unique in the context of civil rights legislation because
it requires that businesses and government do more than just cease
discriminatory actions. They must also take proactive steps to offer
equal opportunity to persons with disabilities, commensurate with
their economic resources. The ADA is distinctive in the context of
disability legislation . . . in its comprehensive nature and application
to much of the private sector. (Young 1997, xx)

Ultimately, the power of the disability rights movement came from
sheer numbers, the "hidden army" (Shapiro 1994, 117). Most people either
have a disability or know someone who does: the cause seems universal.
The ADA passed with strong bipartisan support.

The full legacy of the ADA is still unfolding (Francis and Silvers 2000),
with the U.S. Supreme Court increasingly circumscribing its reach.[2] Anti-
ADA sentiments arose almost immediately. Unlike prior civil rights legislation, the ADA requires businesses to take positive steps, to make "reasonable

accommodations," which they assume will cost money. Some accommodations cost nothing, as when the Supreme Court required the Professional Golfers Association to allow Casey Martin, who has painful swelling of his right leg, to ride a cart while competing in tournaments.[3] Over 70 percent of workplace accommodations cost less than $500 (Olkin 1999, 147).

The courts are also being asked to define disability.[4] In its spring 1999 session, the U.S. Supreme Court heard two cases from people claiming disabilities, neither related to mobility.[5] In their 28 April 1999 arguments, the justices publicly struggled with defining disability under the ADA, and they ultimately ruled against the persons claiming disability, giving employers the right to determine when potential employees qualify for jobs (Young 2000). The National Council on Disability, a federal agency, warned that the Supreme Court had left millions of Americans "with significant mental or physical impairments unprotected against egregious discrimination" (Silvers 2000, 128). With other ADA cases pending, these definitional debates are far from over.

Today, when the public equates claims of disability with expectations of entitlement—even for something as minor as a parking spot—hackles rise. Drivers in crowded malls can almost come to fisticuffs over perceived usurpation of handicapped parking spots. Disability's appearance in *New Yorker* cartoons marks a cultural shift. In three recent sketches (Figures 3 to 5), a peg-legged sailor leaves his skiff at a mooring marked with a wheelchair symbol; an elderly man rolls his scooter down a grocery store aisle, followed by the grim reaper, scythe held aloft, also riding a scooter; and a stout woman crosses a street with her cane, arm grasped by a Boy Scout who says, "I also do suicides." These cartoons do not evoke easy smiles.

No single viewpoint encapsulates today's attitudes toward disability in general, walking problems in particular, or the ADA. Attitudes are evolving, probably soon to be shaped by aging "baby boomers." But few could deny that the situation has improved. Over three decades after Erving Goffman's 1963 injunctions on how "cripples" should behave, the 1996 comments of the novelist Nancy Mairs, who uses a wheelchair because of MS, offer an eerily parallel counterpoint but with an entirely different sensibility.

> If I want people to grow accustomed to my presence, and to view mine as an ordinary life, less agreeable in some of its particulars than theirs but satisfying overall, then I must routinely roll out among them. Inevitably, my emergence produces some strain. I must be "on" all the time, since people seldom glance down to my height and so tend to walk into me as though I were immaterial. Most who notice me are willing to help, and I never spurn an offer. . . . I can use all the help I can get. (104)

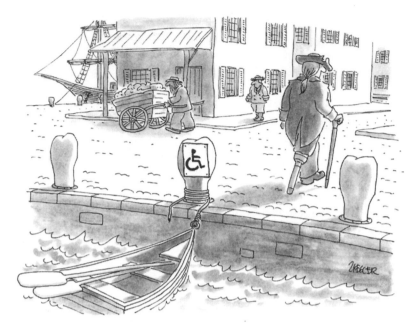

Figure 3. Peg-legged parking. (© The New Yorker Collection 1997 Jack Ziegler from cartoonbank.com. All rights reserved.)

Of course, would-be helpers must be taught how . . . They must also be dissuaded tactfully when their efforts are worthless. . . . The pedagogical role required can wear thin. (104–5)

Regardless of structural and attitudinal modifications, I am never going to be entirely at ease in the world. Unless paradise is paved into a parking lot, most of the earth's surface is going to be too rough for my wheelchair. . . . To some, for reasons outside my control, I will always be a figure of pity, scorn, despair. (105)

These are my realities, and some of them nearly break my heart. Some of them don't. I will never wield a mop again, after all, or scrub another toilet bowl. My grief is selective. But it is not the world's task to assuage whatever genuine sorrows darken my spirit. . . . In asking that the entrance to a building be ramped . . . no one expects all impediments to be miraculously whisked away. In insisting that others view our lives as ample and precious, we are not demanding that they be made perfect. (105–6)

INTERACTIONS WITH STRANGERS

The interviewees recounted many interactions with strangers, reflecting the complexities of today's societal attitudes. Discomforts entangled with

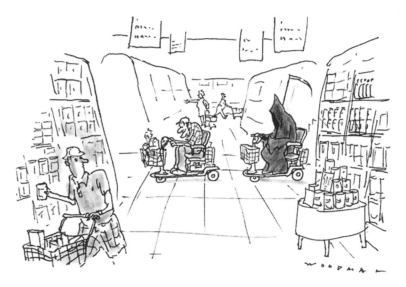

Figure 4. The phantom shopper. (© The New Yorker Collection 1997 Bill Woodman from cartoonbank.com. All rights reserved.)

race or ethnicity can further complicate views about disability; therefore in this chapter I indicate interviewees' race or ethnicity. Researchers typically try to find overarching themes tying such comments together, but here I could not—numerous threads emerged. They do fall broadly into two camps, good and not-so-good. The same interviewee could suddenly turn 180 degrees, one minute lauding the consideration of strangers, the next decrying their insensitivity. "Good" experiences can have troubling subtexts and vice versa. These contradictions probably reflect reality.

"Can I Help You?"

Many people, especially older white women, described strangers as "nice," "kind," "willing to open doors." One elderly white woman recounted attending a concert in Harvard Square. "Someone came up behind my husband at the car and asked if he could help with the scooter. He was Governor [William] Weld. That was nice of him, really sweet." Strangers react kindly even when interviewees overstep usual bounds. Mattie Harris, a black woman who suddenly has "to grab onto people I don't know," finds that strangers, initially taken aback, relent when she explains about her locking knees.

Strangers sometimes seem anxious to offer assistance but hesitate, afraid of offending. No interviewees viewed such offers as patronizing or pitying. One white man observed, "A lot of people think, 'That person's in a wheelchair. I want to help him but I'd better not ask, because they're

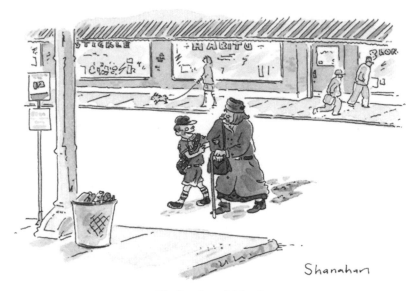

"I also do suicides."

Figure 5. The ultimate Boy Scout. (© The New Yorker Collection 1998 Danny Shanahan from cartoonbank.com. All rights reserved.)

going to feel that I'm talking down to them.' " Strangers need instruction. As one wheelchair user said, "People are very decent, really want to help. But very few of them know what to do, and so they have to be guided. It's very rare that I get a door deliberately slammed in my face. People do not see me—it's not ill will."

Some people will never ask for help. When help comes unsolicited, especially when people fall, negotiating the impulses of strangers can prove challenging (chapter 3). One white woman admits that she hasn't "been that nice" to strangers who reach down to lift her when she falls.

> I'll say, "Leave me alone," kind of in an angry way. When I didn't have strength in my legs, it was actually not helpful for somebody to pull me up. They'd always take me by the arm, but I needed my arms to get up. So, I'd say, "No. Just let me do it myself." It wasn't the whole independence thing that I wanted. It's just how it had to be for me to get up. Afterward I'd think, "Boy, that poor person. They're trying to be helpful." And I wish I could go back and apologize.

Curiosity—generally a negative attribute—can have positive sides. Children frequently sidle up to scooter users, anxious to learn more about their interesting conveyance. Parents often whisk them immediately away, signaling avoidance and shame (Murphy 1990, 130). Or parents exhort the child, "do not stare." Some children persist, as finds this white woman and scooter user,

> Children come up to me. . . . They usually ask questions: "How do you steer it? How do you turn it?" They almost always want to get on, take a ride. Of course I wouldn't dare do that because of the liability—the child might push the wrong buttons. But I explain it to them. I say, "I can walk, but I need this for help. It gets me around a lot faster. I can do all my errands without taking a long, long time. This is great for me." And they understand it. Children are very accepting.

Adult stares sometimes presage requests for information. The woman the governor helped sometimes uses a rolling walker, attracting questions from strangers: "People ask me about the walker. They're very interested because they've got a relative who doesn't have such a nice walker." Gerald Bernadine, a white man, has a bright red scooter. Saying they wish they had one, strangers ask him where he got it, how much it cost. He gives them his telephone number, telling them to call for more information. Mr. Bernadine relishes this role: "It gives me the opportunity to help other people, which is a plus I hadn't anticipated."

"People Walked by Me"

Numerous experiences are less positive. At the outset looms a contradiction: even though people do not and will not ask for help, they are nevertheless upset when strangers ignore their distress and fail to offer assistance. "I don't count on people," said an elderly white man and scooter user. "People go out a door and slam it right in your face. One time I was trying to go over a curbstone in my wheelchair, and I got stuck. I really thought somebody would stop and give me help up. Maybe ten to fifteen people walked by me. I can't go around begging for help. I don't ask people for anything."

Small things assume enormous importance, reflecting general societal incivility and disregard for others. A woman with severe back pain resents people who take more items than allowed into express check-out lanes at grocery stores. Able to stand only briefly, she must speed through check-out and is delayed by persons flouting the rules. Lester Goodall, a black man and cane user, summarized these views:

> I think the average John Q. Public is oblivious to common courtesies that we took for granted when we were younger. On the train, for instance, the seats by the door have a placard, These Are Reserved

for People Who Have a Problem. I got on the train yesterday morning and was halfway sitting down, when someone ran and jumped in the chair. There are some people who will get up and offer you their seat on the train. That's the exception, not the rule, and I don't expect it. The public just don't care. . . . It's a total lack of values and morality. People don't respect anything. They don't respect each other.

Mr. Goodall recognized that having mobility problems compounds the general disregard: "You don't want anyone to dote on you. You just want people to give you the same chances and opportunities that they would expect. Because I walk funny, doesn't mean I'm not capable, and I think people think you're not capable."

The theme of not being noticed recurs in multiple guises. Strangers seem unaware; strangers don't see; strangers don't listen; people with walking problems become invisible and unheard. People interpret this in many ways, primarily as disrespect or invalidation. A striking example of this phenomenon involved a physician colleague of mine, Megan Martin. After Megan fractured a bone, her orthopedist insisted that she stay off her foot for six weeks. I encountered Megan on her return to work, and she was exhausted. How could she get around our huge hospital on crutches? "Rent a scooter," I suggested.

As expected, Megan initially responded unenthusiastically: "People will think I'm a wimp." But within two days, she rented a scooter and later acknowledged she couldn't have managed without it. Nevertheless, Megan remained uncomfortable, rarely riding the scooter outside the hospital.

The few times I did take it out, it was almost impossible to get through a crosswalk before the light changed. I'd be sitting right at the curb, waiting to go, and somebody would walk right in front of me and then just stand there and chat for a while. Well, *they* can run when the light changes. People don't want to see you.

One day after the six weeks ended, Megan stood outside my office, balanced on crutches. Nick, another physician, approached her. "Megan, did you do something to your foot?" he asked kindly. Nick had been around when Megan used the scooter. Why hadn't he noticed? Megan found that many people reacted this way: they did not inquire about her injury while she used the scooter, but when she resumed crutches, they asked whether she'd hurt herself. "The whole time it was *really* uncomfortable for people."

We also are not heard. Returning to Boston after a business trip, a colleague pushed my airport-issue wheelchair to the gate. The agent processed our tickets, then addressed my colleague, "Here's a sticker to put on her coat," gesturing toward me with a round, red-and-white striped sticker.

"Why?" I asked.

"It will alert the flight attendants that she needs help," the agent replied to my colleague.

"Thanks. If I need help, I'll ask for it."

"But the sticker indicates she needs assistance."

"When I need help, I'll ask for it."

"So she won't wear the sticker?"

"No, I won't."

"Why won't she?"

"Because I can ask for help."

"She won't wear it?" This was going nowhere. I looked at my colleague, imploring her to stop this silliness. "Because it's demeaning," she said and rolled the chair up the ramp.

Eleanor Peters, a black woman who uses a power wheelchair, told a story repeated by others. In restaurants, "the waiter or waitress will ask the person that I'm with, 'What will she have?' It can only happen once, because I just won't allow it." Similarly, Walter Masterson, a white man and wheelchair user, found,

> I'll go into a store with my wife and say, "I want to see thus and such." The clerk will speak to my wife and say, "What size is he?" And I'll say, "I'm 15 1/2." And he says to my wife, "Long sleeve or short sleeve?" It's actually funny now, but I was absolutely struck dumb the first time it happened. Not simply being ignored, but not being acknowledged to exist. My nose is at tabletop level, I guess. I have to wave to get noticed.

Some people reported outright hostility or explicit invalidation. "They figure that people with disability should just stay home and be like a bunch of dunces, just looking out the window," said Lonnie Carter, a black woman and wheelchair user in her late forties. "A lady said to me, 'I wish most of you would stay in the house and don't come out.' They think you have something they can catch. But we who are disadvantaged have to go out— we cannot just stay in the house. We have to let people know that we are capable of being somebody."

Yet, ironically, when people with mobility problems are not seen, people assume they don't exist. Sally Ann Jones, a white woman who uses a scooter, has fought her town for years to improve physical accessibility. Town officials tell her "there are no handicapped people in our town." Mrs. Jones responds, "Maybe nobody comes downtown because you can't get into any shops or restaurants." She suggests another explanation for why others don't notice people with mobility difficulties:

> Handicapped people remind people of what they don't want to be. It's like being very old. You have to make yourself more cheerful than you are, more independent than you want to be. . . . People think, "You cost a lot of money to keep going; you're a problem; you clog things up." It gets worse as you get older because then you get that double whammy of being old and handicapped. People lose their compassion and, of course, lots of people don't come with much compassion to begin with.

Poverty exacerbates societal attitudes about disability, in addition to its obvious impact on daily life and access to services described in later chapters. Erna Dodd was the black woman in her mid fifties with many medical conditions. She had worked two housekeeping jobs until she was laid off after a bad fall.

> They put me on disability because they say I couldn't walk right anymore, dragging my leg. At the time, I didn't know what disability was. I just wanted to work because I never had nobody to handle anything for me. . . . Sometime people out on the street look at me like I don't exist, like I'm not human. Sometime people think, "Oh, you are living off of us. You are living off welfare, off disability, off my money." And it get to me sometime. I don't want to be like a nobody. From the time I was 14 years, I was working and helping my parents. I like to work and if I could work, I would work, even if it was just with my hands. . . . When you're sick, it seem like a beholden thing.

Relying on others is sometimes unavoidable but compounds feelings of losing control. Service workers, such as wheelchair pushers at airports, can seem insensitive—after all, it's just a job. "One trip recently, I was traveling alone," recalled Tina DiNatale, a white woman in her mid forties with MS, "and the [wheelchair pusher] just parked me at the connecting gate. The gate agent wasn't there, and I needed to go to the bathroom. But I couldn't wheel myself. I couldn't control it. When they went to board me, I looked down at the wheelchair, and there was a little puddle. It was humiliating."

Yet people reject outright expressions of pity. Joe Warren, a white wheelchair user in his early forties, finds, "You can tell the people that are real from the people that overcompensate, trying to be friendly to you because you're in a chair."

"How do you tell the genuine people?"

"They talk to you normally. A lot of people say they don't even see the chair when they're talking to me, and I can tell. Other people try to pretend like the chair doesn't bother them, but it really does, and they're over-friendly. And there's some people that can't deal with it at all. I'm going down the street, and they just look the other way. The fake ones are the worst. They're overzealous, buddy-buddy, and hanging onto you."

Strangers, however, are not the only ones to express pity or sympathy—so did interviewees for persons more impaired than they. "When I see somebody in a wheelchair, I feel for them," said Jimmy Howard, a black man who uses a cane. "A lot of their lives has been taken away, especially if they were a person that's used to going all the time—getting up and doing what they want. Then all of a sudden they're confined. They got to depend on people." While interviewing Arnis Balodis, a white man, I fielded such views. Arnis had made choices, not tightly controlling his blood sugar level and knowing that amputations might result. But—big but—he would not tolerate a wheelchair. Arnis gazed at me sideways, obviously calculating, before saying, "I know you're in a wheelchair, and I don't mean to make you feel bad, but people view you as dependent—that's just the way it is. I couldn't take that."

One final irony in the post-ADA world is that some people want what they perceive as the "perks" of disability. Restrooms are a particular battle-ground. As one scooter user said, "All the time you go in and the stalls are empty except for the wheelchair one. Somebody's in there. So I wait and wait and wait, and then this husky eighteen-year-old comes out." My strangest among countless such experiences happened at a museum in western Massachusetts. Standard restrooms are down a flight of stairs, and the only wheelchair accessible bathroom is a unisex facility on the first floor. I waited outside until a young man emerged, glancing at me before moving off with a grossly distorted gait. Later I saw him in the museum walking just fine.

EXTRA BURDENS FOR MINORITIES

The public response to black interviewees with mobility difficulties seemed qualitatively different from that to whites. During a focus group of eleven African Americans, ten women, they explained why black people have much higher rates of mobility difficulties than do other races (chapter 2). "Lifestyle," asserted Paula Wright, a nurse in her early sixties. "I mean housing. I mean jobs. I mean other opportunities. There's a high level of stress with black people. Hypertension is there. When you think about the things that people have gone through, the hard work. Many black women have been on their hands and knees scrubbing floors and working hard. They've got arthritis in their fingers and their knees. So lifestyle. Just living. It's only been since the civil rights movement that a change of life for black people came about. A real significant change." Everybody nodded.

In another focus group, Lester Goodall linked civil and disability rights: "I equate this struggle with the struggle of minorities. You have to persevere, to sometimes have civil disobedience. You're viewed as a few that want to be accepted. 'Why should we accept you? Just stay home; don't go to work. Why should we change what we do, just to accommodate you?' You're going to get that sort of kickback. We're up against some of the same subtleties as the civil rights struggle."

"It's not just black either," responded a white man and scooter user. "Try being gay and going into the gay community when you're handicapped. Sorry! I'm not welcome in the bars anymore and many of the restaurants my brothers and sisters own and work in. There's prejudices against blacks, gays, women, still. And it's obvious. Nothing is hidden."

Several black interviewees recounted falling or being assaulted in some way without people rushing to their assistance. Their stories contrasted starkly with those of white interviewees, who sometimes complained about crowds gathering, anxious to help. Even without conclusive evidence of racism, dismissing these discrepancies is hard. "I take my cane with me when I go out," said Jackie Ford, a human services counselor in her early fifties with MS. "When you're walking, you feel like you're a burden to other people, because they're rush, rush, rush. One time I was on the train and when I was ready to get off, for some reason I just fell. Do you know that people just walked right over me? Literally just walked right over me! If it wasn't for one old white man who helped me up, I would have still been on that ground."

"I take a lot of buses because I don't drive," said Nan Darnelle, a former nurse in her early forties. "One day I walked down the hill with my cane to catch the bus. I just had an operation on my knee, and I'm hurting. I'm standing there waiting for this bus, and a little boy and his mother went by, and the little boy snatched my cane. I almost fell on the ground. The little boy just snatched the cane out of my hand."

"What about his mother?"

"His mother didn't say nothing. And I'm not prejudiced about people, but they were white. The lady said, 'Come back, child, with that cane.' And that's all she said. The boy ran a block. I'm standing there. Praise God for the wall. I would have been on the ground. I just had got a shot in my knee—you know how that hurts! So I'm in pain. My back's hurting, my knee's hurting, and I'm standing there about to pass out. And the mother didn't say anything. She went and got it, and just went like this." Ms. Darnelle pantomimed tossing the cane.

Late in the focus group, Jackie Ford had a message:

> A neurologist told me that because of my gait being off, I should walk with my head down. I said, "Never." He said, "What?" I said, "Never. I will not walk with my head down." He said, "But your MS puts you in a situation where you have to watch where your feet go." I said, "No. I do it my way." Walking with my head down makes me feel less of a person. Doctors have to listen to us.

For Ms. Ford, holding her head erect conveys her self-respect.

Roughly one-third of the people I interviewed had never heard of the ADA. Another third merely knew of the law's existence, without any substantive understanding, and the final third knew both the law and its purpose. Those who understood the ADA generally had professional or personal reasons for awareness. Only one interviewee had actually read the ADA—Boris Petrov, the surgeon in his mid forties who had emigrated from the former Soviet Union. "What do you think about the ADA?" I asked.

"I can tell you by the words of President Bush," Dr. Petrov responded. "Someone asked him what he was most proud of that he had done through all his public service. He said, 'That I signed the Disability Act.' And I believe that this *is* most significant. You know, when we're all gone, this country will be changed by that act. For the first time in history, this act was not dictated by—I don't know the right word—pity. Not by pity, but to give people the chance to live who do it in a different way."

5 How People Feel about Their Difficulty Walking

Many years ago, when I still walked with one cane, a close friend took Reed and me to her new boyfriend's house for dinner. We'd heard good reports about this fellow and wanted to like him. Such meetings are often awkward, and after several forays, conversation finally focused on travel. The new boyfriend recounted well-researched ventures to distant, exotic destinations. In concluding, he asserted that he wanted to travel while he still could, before he got too old and slow. "Frankly," he said, turning to me, "I wouldn't want to live like you."

In deference to our friend, we let his statement hang in midair. Such confident pronouncements tapped into my uncertainty as a relative newcomer to disability. Was he not merely rude but also right? Weakness, imbalance, and fatigue made getting around with the cane tough; I could only go so far. The minute-by-minute realities of my bodily sensations seemed leagues away from the empowering assertions of disability rights advocates—that "disability is something imposed on top of our impairments by the way we are unnecessarily isolated and excluded from full participation in society" (Oliver 1996, 22; cited in chapter 1). Yes, our friend eventually jettisoned the guy.

This chapter examines how people with progressive chronic conditions feel about their difficulty walking. These feelings cluster on the darker end of the emotional continuum. No interviewees expressed happiness, joy, pleasure, or glee as their walking failed. More often they felt sad, wistful, frustrated, angry, stoic, resigned. Hope remained—sometimes as only a thread. But hope is complicated, as people with chronic illness "are impelled at once to defy limitations in order to realize greater life possibilities, and to accept limitations in order to avoid enervating struggles with immutable constraints" (Barnard 1995, 39). Disability rights activists might urge them to frame their experiences within the broader social context

(Oliver 1996; Charlton 1998; Linton 1998; Barnes, Mercer, and Shakespeare 1999; Albrecht, Seelman, and Bury 2001)—"it is not the inability to walk which disables someone but the steps into the building" (Morris 1996a, 10). But the interviewees spoke in intensely personal terms. And as Jenny Morris, who had a spinal cord injury, wrote,

> Insisting that our physical differences and restrictions are *entirely* socially created . . . [denies] the personal experiences of physical or intellectual restrictions, of illness, of the fear of dying (Morris 1996a, 10).
>
> Even if the physical environment in which I live posed no physical barriers, I would still rather walk than not be able to walk. . . . To be able to walk would give me more choices and experiences than not being able to walk. This is, however, quite definitely, *not* to say that my life is not worth living, nor is it to deny that very positive things have happened in my life *because* I became disabled. . . .
>
> We need courage to say that there *are* awful things about being disabled, as well as the positive things. (71)

CHANGES

Every interviewee described fundamental transformations, although along diverse dimensions. Once quick, they are now slow. Once independent, they now depend on others. Once in control, now constrained; once fearless, now fearful; once mobile, now "stuck"; once working, now "on welfare"; once busily occupied, now at loose ends; once engaged, now isolated; once athletic, now on the sidelines; once stylish, "loving high heels," now wearing "flat, sensible shoes." Two comments personify these transformations. Cynthia Walker, in her mid thirties, never expected her diagnosis.

> It was June four years ago, and I was literally doing cartwheels in the yard teaching my daughter. That's when the sensations all began. I was diagnosed in October with rheumatoid arthritis, and by December I had difficulty walking. I'd been extremely active. I walked everywhere; I ran everywhere; I rode a bike; I did everything. And all of a sudden, I couldn't do it. I was foolish enough to believe that arthritis only happens in older people. . . . So now I am physically impaired. It can be tough. But it can be a challenge to help me grow rather than sit by and say, "Pity poor me."

Salvador Marquis, in his mid fifties, can't understand why it happened to him.

> I'm from Alabama. My father always told me, "Just go to work, and everything will be all right in your life." They tell you, "Keep a job;

don't steal, don't cuss; respect everybody—and your life will be all right." I did all that, I worked, and now I'm like this. Nobody ever said nothing about no stroke. I can't catch the bus because I'm scared I'm going to fall, and if I trip, I know I can't get back up. I don't much go nowhere by myself.

People's feelings about their walking difficulties do vary by medical condition. Recently diagnosed with progressive ALS, which carries a grim, short-term prognosis, a woman in her mid forties said that she most feared becoming unable to swallow and breathe. Walking problems are troubling but ultimately manageable. Nevertheless, the daily frustrations of her current walking difficulties are stressful and have fundamentally changed her life. She recently quit after working with the same company for over twenty years.

Before detailing the perceptions of interviewees, I must acknowledge an important limitation of my project. I spoke to most people only once. Yet, by definition, this book is about change—progressive chronic conditions. Attitudes change over time. About three to five years after disability begins, people typically stop talking about how it happened—"it's a moot point" (Olkin 1999, 60). People's perceptions evolve, although research suggests that attitudes are unrelated to the extent of physical impairments. The value that people place on their physical abilities shifts over time, as they become used to progressive impairments (Eklund and MacDonald 1991; Kutner et al. 1992; Dolan 1996). While others may perceive persons as having "poor" health, they themselves may prize their health "since they have adjusted their life styles and expectations to take account of their condition" (Dolan 1996, 559). These shifts in self-perceptions and expectations become especially apparent when someone finally decides to use a wheelchair (chapter 12). Ostensibly the quintessential symbol of defeat and despair, wheelchairs often restore independence to people who have long felt "stuck" in place (Scherer 1996, 2000).

Experts have studied how people "adjust" to impairments, the "stages" they pass through to reconcile themselves to physical limitations. But people do not proceed, lock step, through neat stages, instead varying widely in their responses (Olkin 1999, 47). In chronic illness especially, physical abilities and sensations continuously shift, unlike for injured people (where deficits are fixed, although functioning can alter with secondary conditions). One large challenge is learning "to live with ongoing and permanent uncertainty" (Toombs 1995, 20). Rhonda Olkin, a psychotherapist who uses a scooter because of polio, became increasingly uncomfortable as she read articles on rehabilitation.

I do not believe there is such a thing as "adjustment to disability."
That is, the response curve, while steeper at first, does not ever level

off at some mythical stage of adjustment and acceptance. Rather, it continues to wend its way, often up, sometimes downward, throughout the life-span in a continuous process. (Olkin 1993, 15)

Other experts have studied "coping styles" and people's perceptions of control over their lives. Two coping styles emerge: "problem-focused," confronting the difficulty, seeking relevant information, and devising management strategies; and "emotion-focused," denial, escape, avoidance, or reconfiguring the problem to appear more positive. While most people use both strategies, one style usually predominates. Sometimes clinicians pressure people "not only to cope but to cope correctly," thus implicitly criticizing those "who are doing the best they know how under trying circumstances" (Olkin 1999, 124). Oftentimes people with mobility problems are poor, unemployed, and uneducated (chapters 6 and 7). "Coping" against such disadvantages takes on an entirely different connotation.

I, for one, do not know how to respond when people ask me, "So, how are you coping?" If I say, "Just fine," will they believe me? My friend's former boyfriend, seeing me now using a wheelchair, certainly wouldn't. Some people's negative views of mobility problems remain firmly entrenched. If I say I'm fine but frustrated by not finding wheelchair-accessible taxis or confronting heavy doors without automatic openers, how will people react? I can try changing minds, but I can't do so unless I appear "well adjusted" and content —perhaps harking back to Goffman's exhortations from forty years ago (1963; see chapter 4). Although the notion of adjustment may prove chimerical, today's reality holds that

> A positive attitude of the person with a disability toward disability in general—as evidenced by self-acceptance, open acknowledgment of the disability, and disclosure about self—has a positive effect on others' attitudes. . . . This places a burden on the person with a disability to take the lead in putting others at ease. . . . Holding a positive self-view does not fully protect one from incurring prejudice, stigma, or discrimination, although it may lessen their frequency and, importantly, their psychological impact. (Olkin 1999, 67–68)

COMMON FEELINGS ABOUT WALKING PROBLEMS

Studies confirm that people with disabilities are just like other people—no overall personality differences exist. No surprise! They share the same vast array of aptitudes, attitudes, foibles, and fears as other people. The interviewees expressed many varied feelings about their walking difficulties, as described below.

"I Don't Know My Body Anymore"

Walking difficulties break a trust forged in infancy: the unquestioned confidence that our legs will reliably, without conscious effort, carry us wherever we want to go. Getting around now requires conscious effort, often accompanied by pain, exhaustion, fear, and other unwelcome and sometimes spooky sensations (chapter 3). Walking problems transform people's images of their corporeal selves. As one woman said, "I don't know my body anymore."

Intractable pain arrives as an unwelcome intruder, a stranger inside one's body. "It's like somebody's in there with a hammer and chisel, chiseling away," explained one man with arthritis. "There's no description of pain," said another. "It's like a thunderstorm inside your body. Sometimes it just rumbles." Some people refer to their bodies in the third person, as does Sally Ann Jones: "I say to my feet, 'Move, damn it!' And they say, 'No. We're on strike.'" Candy Stoops experiences an eerie dual reality: "It's almost like your brain is saying, 'Do something! Do something!' And your body is not responding. In my mind, I'm doing something, but in reality, my limbs are not moving."

People are constantly reminded of their impairments. "Every time you exercise," said one woman in her mid forties with rheumatoid arthritis, "you come face-to-face with the limitations of your body. You face everything that has been lost." After being diagnosed with MS, S. Kay Toombs found, "My body could no longer be trusted. Nor could it be ignored. I needed to be on guard, to watch and listen to my body's rhythms, its sensations, its movements" (1995, 12). Women, in particular, recognize that they cannot meet cultural norms of attractiveness, desirability, and sexuality (Fine and Asch 1988; Morris 1996a; Toombs 1995). Aging compounds these perceptions, as for Sally Ann Jones:

> I went with my sister to the mall, and we went to the Liz Claiborne shop. They have thousands of lovely things, really pretty. It was Christmas. I just wanted to sit and cry. I thought, even if I could afford all these yummy things, where would I go? It's a combination of being a widow and having a disability. Some of those things overlap. But I'm not angry at anybody about that. I always say to everybody: you only get to do this once, so you better do it the best way you can. I mean life. I would have preferred to be a prima ballerina in the Bolshoi, but it didn't work out that way.

Men also confront fundamental questions about their bodily images, with societal views of masculinity "inextricably bound up with a celebration of strength, of perfect bodies" (Morris 1996a, 93). Several women volunteered that men with walking difficulties are worse off than women because of these cultural expectations. Boris Petrov, the former Soviet surgeon, finds, "It's much more easy for me to think about my soul separate from my body."

"How does that help you?"

"If you don't separate your soul from your body, you will always be ill. . . . Unfortunately sometimes I look in the mirror! I do not shave every day. When they ask me why, I say because I do not like to shave, but actually I do not like to look at myself in the mirror."

"How do you feel when you see yourself?"

"Sorry for Sonya," Dr. Petrov quipped about his girlfriend.

People can become frustrated when others do not appreciate their physical limitations. "The usual comment when people look at me is, 'You look great!' " noted an elderly woman with Parkinson's disease and a small stroke. "The implication is there's nothing wrong with you. I've gotten so I don't say anything back to people. I once would say, 'Well, I don't feel so good.' But people certainly didn't want to hear that." Others grow weary of hearing "complaints," so silence ensues. Those in pain must convince people their pain is real, so intense they cannot walk. People sense subtle suspicion, disbelief, accusations of malingering, hints that nothing is seriously wrong, they're simply not trying hard enough.

Although their bodies have changed, people often fight to retain their former appearance to themselves and the outside world. They acknowledge "vanity." Because their vanity targets a socially laudable goal—walking independently and upright—they accept it. But vanity sometimes gets in the way. "If I fall, I'm going to be a hell of a lot worse off than losing a little vanity," recounted Gerald Bernadine. "Vanity had prevented me from using the cane. You surely don't feel very good about yourself as you struggle up a hallway and people look at you with sympathetic eyes and hold the door open for five minutes till you get through it. If you're worried about vanity, try having MS. It vanquishes vanity and gives you humility. But humility is a good thing, isn't it?" Gerald laughed ruefully.

Others use vanity as motivation. "I have inner battles with physical impairment versus vanity," said Cynthia Walker. "This is a very real relationship to me. In the long run, I'll stop being so foolish. However, vanity is giving me the drive to move forward and say I'm going to be damned if this is going to get the better of me. Yes, when I need it, when I don't have any other choice, and to help others around me, I will use a cane. But right now I choose to push forward."

Arthritis has changed Cynthia's body. "When you're used to having feet that are straight and legs with a certain amount of shape and a hand that goes out straight without having this horrendous bump," she held up her wrist, "it's a vanity issue. My body doesn't look the way it used to. I don't feel as good about myself as I once did. This disease is changing my physical appearance, and I resent that incredibly. But I'll be darned if I'm going to let this disease get the worst of me. So I learn to accept this after a lot of inner conflict. You have to go through the stages of denial and anger before you can move forward. My husband looks at me lovingly and says, 'But honey, I'll love you no matter what you look like.' 'Well, I love you, too, darling, and in a perfect world, I'd really feel good about myself, but turn out the light! I'm not comfortable.' "

So people's bodies become strangers, with wills of their own. A middle-aged woman with heart problems recapped the prevailing wisdom of one focus group:

> There's things that I want to do so much, but I can't. I try to do them, and I can't. So I get called lazy and everything else. But we have to take one day at a time. My favorite saying is, "the spirit is willing, but the flesh is weak." That sums it all up.

"I'm Very Independent"

When that trust forged in infancy breaks and people's bodies no longer carry them, independence is the first casualty. Once independent, moving at will, people now face limits and need help, human or mechanical. Almost everyone raised this issue in some way: regardless of their impairments, they want to remain as independent and self-sufficient as possible. Their sense of personal worth is linked, inextricably, to doing for themselves. Almost blind from diabetes and with two bad hips, Lonnie Carter was "very independent—always have been. I was brought up that way by my parents. They taught the four of us children not to depend on anybody else to do it for us."

A subtle shift occurs in views of independence. Especially when walking problems progress, reality intervenes. People are caught between needing help (mechanical or human) and their desire for independence. Many interviewees recalibrate their perceptions of what constitutes independence: they aim toward trying as hard as they can rather than actually doing everything themselves. Independence becomes attitude rather than action. Lonnie Carter, for instance, was a disability advocate for minorities. She sought all services to which she was entitled and filed grievances, usually successfully, when denied. Despite her various supports and services, she still viewed herself as independent—she certainly worked hard leading her life. (Ms. Carter died about sixteen months after the interview from complications of diabetes.)

Requesting personal assistance is difficult. "I could always do stuff for myself," said one wheelchair user. "It's hard to ask, but you have to put down your pride and just go for it." Some people worry that seeking help starts a downward slide toward dependence, giving up. Jimmy Howard warned,

> If you start depending on people, then you get in that mood: "I don't feel like doing it; I know someone who can do it for me." But if you can do it for yourself, why depend on somebody else to do it for you? I'm not being judgmental, but a lot of people don't do every-thing they can for themselves. If you depend on others, what are you going to do when nobody's around? Now don't get me wrong. Everybody needs help sometime. I'm not too proud to ask for help, not if I need it. But if I can do it myself, I do it myself. I'll put in my last breath to try. That's just the way I am.

Discussions about independence offered the perfect opportunity for people to mention environmental and societal barriers—to say their inde-pendence would be enhanced by ADA-type accommodations or other de-vices or services. A few people did, like Lonnie Carter and Sally Ann Jones, a disability advocate and social worker, respectively. Others interviewees, however, spoke of their chronic conditions and walking problems as per-sonal battles, fights for themselves alone, extending possibly to their inti-mate family. Nevertheless, they do not appear to accept the "individual model of disability," of being marked by tragedy, a victim, "in need of 'care and attention', and dependent on others" (Barnes, Mercer, and Shakespeare 1999, 21). Quite the contrary. In fighting their individual battles, they pre-serve their sense of independence. They adapt. As one man with MS told me, "If this is the worst I get, I can live with it."

"It's a Lonely Case"

Isolation is both physical and emotional. Some people find themselves con-fined within their homes; some have no one to talk to—who will listen? Erna Dodd was short of breath, in pain, and exhausted: "I don't go out nowhere. I just stay home." She didn't even attend her cherished church. "I don't like to be bothering someone because I'll always be telling about my sickness. I have some rough time, especially in the night. Sometimes I re-ally don't know what to do, who to call. When I'm home alone and I be by myself, it's a lonely case."

Most interviewees who felt isolated also confessed they were afraid, pri-marily of falling. According to the federal survey, people with mobility dif-ficulties *are* more likely than others to report "unreasonably strong fear where most people would not be afraid" (Table 5). While 3 percent of peo-

TABLE 5. Fear and Depression

Mobility Difficulty	Emotion (%)[a]	
	Fear	Depression
None	3	4
Minor	12	20
Moderate	16	30
Major	18	31

[a]Fear = unreasonably strong fear where most people would not be afraid; depression = frequently depressed or anxious.

ple without mobility problems admit such fears, 18 percent of persons with major mobility difficulties are afraid.[1]

Even couples can become profoundly isolated. Esther Halpern has spinal stenosis (a back problem), and her husband, Harry, has cancer. Mr. Halpern's oncologist had forbidden Harry from driving because of his extreme frailty and falling. The Halperns live in a modest, one-story home north of Boston—no railing on the front step, piles of yellowing papers and other "stuff" cramming every corner of space. They seemed thrilled to have a visitor, saying this was their social event for the week. The elderly couple careened dangerously to and fro in their obstacle-filled home. They offered cookies, a hot drink, a cold drink, or Mrs. Halpern's newly made fudge; they showed me photographs of grandchildren. The Halperns had been married forty-nine years and neither finished a sentence during the entire interview—the other intervened. The most heart-wrenching moments came when they talked about their isolation.

"The kids had already decreed it—" said Harry.

"That he shouldn't drive a car," said Esther.

"So we asked the doctor—"

"And he agreed."

"But I need a haircut," Harry fingered his wispy white hair.

"He's not in a position to drive," argued Esther.

"But I will again," said Harry. Later he mentioned isolation once more. "The biggest thing, almost the biggest thing, is that we don't see people."

"We don't see people," nodded Esther. "Not very often."

"And this is a major—"

"Social visit."

"Barring everything. We're seeing somebody. Normally, we don't see anybody."

"Don't see anybody."

"Because you're home alone all the time," I observed.

"All the time," they concurred. It was very hard to leave them.

The Halperns' daughter does live nearby but she rarely visits. "She is so busy," explained Mrs. Halpern. "If we absolutely need something, if it's an emergency, she can get away." The Halperns would never ask for more.

People make self-sacrifices, big and small, rather than "burden" others, especially their children. Mildred Stanberg, in her late eighties, lives near her children, but they rarely see her on weekdays. "One weekend my grandson was here," Mrs. Stanberg recounted, "and we all went to the Arnold Arboretum," a 200-acre park within metropolitan Boston. "The place is huge. They all went walking, looking at the trees. I sat on the bench because that way I didn't spoil it for them. I walk very slowly, but I really enjoy being outdoors." Three years later her daughter took her to Spain with a rented wheelchair, and Mrs. Stanberg (then ninety years old) saw almost everything.

"I Had Some Dismal Thoughts"

According to the survey, people with mobility difficulties are much more likely than others to be "frequently depressed or anxious" (see Table 5). While 4 percent of people without mobility problems report these feelings, 31 percent of those with major mobility difficulties do. Perhaps this is not surprising in light of pain and physical discomforts, societal attitudes, and isolation. Some people spoke openly about depression, as did Barney Fink, who has Parkinson's disease (chapter 3). Others said they were more "sad" than depressed. "When I first got it," said Candy Stoops of her myasthenia gravis, "it changed my vision of myself. I wasn't as mobile as I would have liked to have been. You have to understand. We had a third-floor apartment; we couldn't afford to move—we had gone from two paychecks down to one. The only way that I could get out of the building with my son was if somebody helped me out. So yeah, I had some dismal thoughts." Gerald Bernadine described being almost in suspended animation.

> When I was diagnosed with MS, I was scared, I was so frightened. Not so much in the beginning, but then I got fired. They waited until after Christmas, because you don't fire anybody at Christmas time. Then I really was totaled, emotionally a basket case. And my father had just died a couple months before. So I was diagnosed with MS, then my father died, then I got fired. Between those three

things, my self-esteem was at an all-time low. I remember going to an ATM machine at the bank to make a withdrawal. I spent fifteen, twenty minutes doing it. My self-confidence was just zero.

The comments of Candy Stoops and Gerald Bernadine highlight a critical issue. Often people with mobility problems have many other things going on in their lives. In addition, according to the survey, people with mobility difficulties are much more likely than others to say that their overall health is "poor" (see Table 3). People with mobility problems are much more likely to be poor, unemployed, uneducated, divorced, and to live alone (chapters 6–7). Once we account for these various factors, people with mobility problems are roughly twice as likely as others to report being depressed or anxious.[2] Depression is often treatable, regardless of its cause. Unfortunately, clinicians frequently fail to recognize depression, especially in persons with chronic illnesses (Olkin 1999).

However, roughly 70 percent of people with major mobility problems are *not* frequently depressed or anxious. Yet because of widespread expectations that depression is inevitable, fanciful explanations often purport to explain why people are not depressed.

> The logic goes as follows: "You have a disability. Having a disability is awful. Therefore you must be suffering. I see you as suffering. Ah, but you are not suffering, in a situation in which suffering should occur. Why not? It must be because you are brave, courageous, plucky, extraordinary, superhuman." . . . Virtually all persons with disabilities I know have been told how brave they were, sometimes for *simply getting up in the morning*. (Olkin 1999, 79)

Recently, an elderly man spoke admiringly of my bravery for "getting up and dressed every morning." Still taken aback, I haven't yet perfected my reply but generally use the old George Burns line about birthdays: "consider the alternative."

"Sometimes I Get So Irate"

Some interviewees admitted being angry and frustrated. More often, however, people seem less angry at their physical limitations than at the attitudes of people around them, especially when people feel invalidated, that others don't believe or respect them. Anger is particularly acute among people in pain or with stigmatized conditions, such as obesity.

"Sometimes I get so irate," said Marianne Bickford. "I get in an ugly mood." Getting around her neighborhood and finding wheelchair-accessible transportation frustrates her. She chafes when her personal assistant shows up late and doesn't seem motivated to help. She feels that her physicians don't understand her situation or why she uses a wheelchair, that they believe she just isn't trying. "I'm not here for the fun of it!" she admonished. "When it comes to the wheelchair, I get very annoyed. People think it's a party, that it's an easy way of getting out. It's not; it's a struggle."

Interviewees recognize that expressing anger openly can alienate others. They risk appearing ungrateful and antagonizing the very persons they need for assistance. Ms. Bickford recounted falling in public and needing help: "Sometimes you have to use humor. So I'd say, 'I like falling on the floor. It's nice to see what the floor looks like up close.' " Outsiders can see anger as the failure to adjust properly (Olkin 1999, 78). "The unsound of limb are permitted only to laugh. The rest of emotions, including anger and expression of hostility, must be bottled up, repressed, and allowed to simmer or be released in the backstage area of the home" (Murphy 1990, 107). People keep anger to themselves.

"You Find Strength You Don't Know You Have"

With many complexities in their lives, people still must get through the day, and they find things that help. Humor is important. Religion and faith sustain many. Through her faith, said one woman, "you find strength you don't know you have." Brianna Vicks admitted many emotions:

> I'll be honest. Sometimes I get down. I'm not always chipper. Things do bother me, but I don't let it come out. My friends know something's really wrong, and they'll ask me about it. But I don't like to tell my troubles. That's just me. You can't let things bother you. If you do, you're gonna be feeling sorry for yourself. I have a lot of faith, and I believe in God. God brought me through all the things I've been through. They said I was gonna die. He pulled me through that and a lot of other things. So I just go day-by-day, and I go to church. I have a lot of faith that He'll bring me through.

Encounters with organized religion are not uniformly uplifting. Jody Farr is a physician in her late thirties with an unusual form of progressive muscular dystrophy. She only recently began using a wheelchair and thinking about spirituality. "I can't sit in the synagogue and say, 'God is great, God is good,' " Dr. Farr said. It just didn't feel right to her. So she went to a rabbi who seemed uncomfortable with her from the outset. "He started by telling me that he knew I was angry. It was this weird conversation in which he told me what I must be feeling. He projected all his own feelings onto me. It was useless, and afterward I felt very down. So I called my mother's closest friend who is very wise. And she said to me, 'So, you're angry? What the hell! What are you going to do next? Let's get moving.' " Jody laughed. "It was the best thing she could possibly have said."

THE INNER SELF

With few exceptions, walking difficulties do not change how interviewees feel about themselves as people. Yes, their legs no longer carry them, but their core inner beliefs about themselves remain basically unchanged. Despite probing questions, most interviewees denied that their walking difficulties had permanently altered their basic sense of self, although they may have had rough times. Eleanor Peters, in her late forties, finally started using a power wheelchair because of worsening limitations related to childhood polio.

> Some of us still have attitudes. Some of us are still going through denial; some of us are still dealing with the disability. Some of us are still angry. So I think once we get over that initial anger or sorrow or madness, then we can learn to live with the disability. Because either we're going to learn to live with it or we're going to have a hell of a hard time.

Reynolds Price anticipated Eleanor's comments by a statement and two questions that have guided his own "new life" since becoming paraplegic: compared to who you were before, "you're not that person now. Who'll you be tomorrow? And who do you propose to be from here to the grave, which may be hours or decades down the road?" (1995, 182).

While bodies and external identities (e.g., career, relationships) clearly can change, fundamental inner beliefs about self remain intact: independent, self-reliant, stoic, autonomous—"central values in American culture" (Murphy 1990, 199). But with mobility difficulties, the strategies required to be independent, self-reliant, stoic, and autonomous inevitably change. As Barnard notes, "for persons with chronic illnesses and disabilities (or without) the illusion of total self-sufficiency may be among the most destructive. It not only cuts us off from very practical gains to be made in solidarity with others, it radically distorts our view of the human situation" (1995, 55). New tactics for getting through each day can alter how people interact with others and how they see their role in life.

The interviewees did acknowledge changes in their personalities and feelings about themselves, albeit not their core convictions. One woman admits being "disappointed" in herself that she's afraid. Another woman wishes she could "deal with things better," be less angry. One man who formerly kept his feelings to himself now realizes, after divorce, that he must talk openly about his emotions. Another man wants to feel more reconciled to "not being able to do the things I used to do." Unnoticed or disrespected by store clerks, taxi drivers, and passersby in general, people now must sometimes speak up. Once reticent, they become feisty, albeit recognizing that self-advocacy sometimes appears shrill, strident, narcissistic, or rude. They take that risk, often surprising even themselves, beginning perhaps to identify with other disabled people. They set limits. "I'm in *non-denial*, OK?" said Lonnie Carter. "I used to be in denial. If I don't feel like doing something, I ain't doing nothing I don't have to do."

Life's existential inquiry now has a clear target: why me? "I'll be fifty next year," said Sylvia Thomson, a former secretary who uses a scooter. "I've had diabetes my whole life, insulin dependent. In my mind, I want to do what I used to do. It stinks, and I don't like it. I know deep in my heart that there was a reason for this happening, but I always still think, why me?" Others assert they have moved on. "What I refuse to say," stated Lester Goodall, "is, why me? I think that's self-defeating. I'm from the school that these are the cards that I've been dealt, and I have to do the best I can with these cards. It's not that I accepted it or embraced it with open arms, but I say this is it, and I just have to go on. So the old cliché, a positive outlook." Several interviewees cautioned against feeling sorry for oneself. "You have to be realistic," said one woman. "Don't go around wanting things you can't have."

People often comfort themselves by observing that others are worse off than they. "As bad as you might feel someday," said one woman with arthritis, "somebody comes to you with a bigger problem. It helps you, it really does." It gives people perspective. Sometimes those who are "worse off" embody people's fears for their own future, but they also can offer hope. Even if the "worst" happens, life goes on. Although Lester Goodall still walks with a cane, needing a wheelchair is never far from his mind:

> I think about it especially when I see people on the street in a wheelchair. When I see them, it seems like it's not the worst thing in the world that can happen. They're still able to function and do things. It lessens the overall impact of the "what ifs?" What if it happens to me? It doesn't mean that my life is over. I can still get around. I see they're active, they're on the train, they're doing jobs, and they're in a lot worse shape than I am. . . . I feel for those people, but in a way it makes my plight a lot easier.

An unspoken subtext to many comments was the question about when to adopt a "disability identity"—incorporating disability into their core self-image. Near the end of our interview, I asked people if they were "disabled," and I got three types of responses: about two-fifths of people said "yes"; a comparable fraction said "no"; and the remaining fifth answered both "yes" and "no." Some people who said "no" are wheelchair users, while some who said "yes" still walk, albeit with difficulty. The federal survey asked people two questions about perceived disability:

Do you consider yourself to have a disability?

Would other people consider you to have a disability?

While the percentage reporting disability increases with worsening mobility difficulties, substantial numbers reject this label even among those with major mobility problems (Table 6).[3] Of people reporting major mobility problems 25 percent say they do not see themselves as disabled; 18 percent of manual and 10 percent of power wheelchair users do not consider themselves disabled.[4]

The interviewees offered varied explanations for whether they see themselves as disabled. Those who do typically say that they cannot do physically what they wish to do. Those who deny being disabled generally see disability as associated with complete physical incapacity. As Jimmy Howard observed,

> Maybe I need a little more time to do things, but I've never really used neither of those words, "disabled" or "handicapped." I just call it an "inconvenience." That's how I looked at myself. Things are a hindrance to me, but it's not like I'm bedridden, that I can't get up and do nothing. That's what I consider being disabled—that if you want to go to the bathroom, you got to call somebody to help you or wipe your butt. That's what I call bad. But I never looked at myself like that, never.

About one-fifth of interviewees said they both are and aren't disabled—recognizing the contradiction but explaining it by distinguishing the mind from the body. "Let's put it this way," said Lonnie Carter. "I am disabled in a physical way but not in a mental way. I'm able to do things other people wouldn't even try to do, like going to school even though I'm almost forty-nine years old. And I just got a new job."

As did Lonnie Carter, most interviewees continue looking ahead to their futures, acknowledging that their chronic conditions and walking difficulties affect their plans. Two feelings predominate: first, the need to live with uncertainty; and second, the intention to deal with whatever happens. Only two or three interviewees (admittedly a selected group) seemed to have given up, retreated from the world. Instead, some felt their health problem had jolted them out of complacency, stimulated them to be better people. Helping others, doing whatever one can, gives meaning to lives. "I can help

TABLE 6. Perceptions of Disability

	Self-Perception (%)	Others' Perception (%)
Respondent's mobility difficulty		
None	4	3
Minor	36	30
Moderate	60	50
Major	75	69
Respondent using mobility aid		
Cane or crutches	67	62
Walker	78	74
Manual wheelchair	82	81
Electric wheelchair	90	82
Scooter	94	91

somebody by showing that I can get through all this," said Brianna Vicks. "You have to accept it first, what happened to you. That's a small hump right there. Then next thing is just to start doing what you gotta do."

At the end of the day, people say they need to go on. Going on assumes its own value. "I can't make the MS go away," said Sally Ann Jones, "and you can't just stop. You've gotta do what you've gotta do." That doesn't mean it's easy. "Of course I whine," Sally Ann admitted, "and feel sorry for myself, and think I'm the Lone Ranger, and think this was a ridiculous thing to happen. Whoever arranged this, I've done my part. Forty years is enough. Give it to somebody else who's younger and stronger. I really resent not being able to walk. Now I'm working on just being able to stand and pivot—you change your priorities. I'm having more and more trouble dealing with it. It makes me nuts, and I don't know what I'm gonna do about it sometimes."

The hardest thing for Sally Ann right now is finding personal assistance at home. She has trouble getting to the bathroom herself, and she lives alone. Her husband, Chet, who died from cancer, had been her helpmate and true partner. "I've said to myself a thousand times that my life would be so much easier if Chet hadn't died. For all the obvious reasons and because he had a creative mind. He would have thought about ways to ease things. The other day I heard about somebody whose husband divorced her twenty minutes post-diagnosis. The scum! It happens all the time. On the other hand, do you know how limiting it is for your partner? Chet was a real prince about it and very accommodating."

Although her loss is incalculable, Sally Ann remembers Chet with tremendous gratitude. "I feel badly for people who have this or any other disease and have no support system, especially if they aren't assertive. I know a bunch of people like that. They get lots of negative input about their lives. People don't talk negatively to me because I won't let them. But I don't know what I'm gonna do about finding help at home. Me and Scarlett O'Hara are going to work on it tomorrow. I have no choice but to figure it out, so eventually I will. It'll come to me, I hope."

6 At Home—with Family and Friends

One night several years ago, a familiar driver picked me up in his wheelchair-accessible taxi at Boston's Logan Airport. He had immigrated from Afghanistan and wore traditional garb—colorful crocheted cap and multilayered thigh-length cotton shirting—despite the biting December cold. The first time he had driven me, he had asked immediately if I was married, then said how happy he was to bring me home to my husband. He had driven me several times since, always asking the same question: "How is your husband?"

"He's fine."

"I remember you. I think about you. I talk about you to my wife."

"Really? What do you tell her?"

"I like to see a man marry a woman in a wheelchair. It's really wonderful that a man would marry a woman in a wheelchair. He will have a special place in heaven. He will get his reward in heaven." The taxi driver seemed genuinely moved, and I didn't want to dampen his enthusiasm for Reed's virtues by revealing that I walked nearly normally when we married fifteen years previously. The driver told me about his brother, still in their homeland, who was "born paralyzed" by cerebral palsy and uses a wheelchair. "No woman will marry him," he said sadly. "He lives with our mother. He is very smart, very charming, but no woman will marry him."

Chapter 5 looked at how people themselves experience their mobility troubles. Yet walking problems often become a family affair. At the most basic level, people may have difficulty performing routine daily activities—dressing, getting to the bathroom, moving around home, preparing meals, housecleaning, shopping. They may rely on those they live with to assist with many tasks, including the most private. Filling emotional needs and expectations is even more complicated. For many people, walking difficulties affect how they see themselves—and how others see them—as spouse, partner, parent, child, or friend. For some, relationships strengthen as the inevitable shifts and redefinitions affect everybody over time. Or, as for the taxi driver's brother, social attitudes can also erect enormous barriers to the most fundamental human connections: gaining the intimacy and friendship of a spouse or partner or the joys and challenges of parenthood. Chapter 6 examines how walking difficulties affect routine daily life and relationships with family and friends.

LIVING DAY-BY-DAY

When examined in detail, daily life is a complex web of recurring tiny tasks, all requiring at least a modicum of mobility. Certain tasks are almost always performed by individuals themselves (like bathing, dressing, going to the toilet), while some may be performed by another (like preparing meals, grocery shopping, cleaning house). All tasks are essential to comfort, if not absolute survival. When mobility problems intrude, alternative strategies become necessary.

Meeting daily needs can demand calculated logistics: every aspect of life is planned. Spontaneity vanishes. Fear creeps in—of falling, of being immobilized, trapped in a fire, burned while cooking, being alone. People parse precious energy carefully. "You have to think of everything, even how you sit down," said Cynthia Walker, the young mother with rheumatoid arthritis. "I have to think of every possible scenario. If I plan poorly at home, that's the scariest. I might not be able to get up." With increasing mobility impairments, people become less and less likely to leave their homes: 11 percent of people reporting major mobility difficulties did not venture out in the prior two weeks (Table 7).

People with mobility problems are more likely to report difficulties with basic activities of daily living (ADLs) than other people.[1] About 31 percent of people with major mobility difficulties report problems with dressing, as do 26 percent with using the toilet. Nevertheless, even with major mobility difficulties, most people perform basic activities without any problem. So-called instrumental activities of daily living (IADLs) present bigger challenges. One-third of people with major mobility difficulties report problems with preparing meals, while over 42 percent note problems with shopping or light housework, and 74 percent acknowledge trouble with heavy chores.

Being unable to perform routine daily tasks is frustrating, sometimes embarrassing, and potentially terrifying. People must concentrate to get through the day. Comments during one focus group exemplify these con-

TABLE 7. Days Out in the Last Two Weeks

	Number of Days Out of House (%)			
Mobility Difficulty	*None*	*1 to 7*	*8 to 13*	*Every Day*
Minor	2	28	11	60
Moderate	4	38	12	46
Major	11	46	11	32

cerns. Martha, in her early seventies, had had a heart attack several years earlier, and now "it's hard getting in and out of the bathtub. You've got to be careful not to fall. You're afraid you'll stumble and fall."

"I got stuck in the bathtub once," said Jackie, in her early fifties. "With MS you can't afford to get overheated"—high heat virtually paralyzes some people with MS for minutes or hours. "When I got ready to get out of the bathtub, I couldn't move my legs. Nobody was home. I stayed in the bathtub two and a half hours until my son came home. I will never take a hot shower again, never ever."

"I fell in the bathtub," recounted Annie, in her early seventies. "I stayed there for about two hours. The phone was near me, but I couldn't get it. All I could see was myself like in the coffin, just lying in the bathtub. Then my grandson came 'cause we were going to church."

"I agree about being afraid of falling," nodded Paula, in her early sixties, "not being able to live your life the way you did before. I have eighteen stairs to get to my bedroom. I had to move downstairs on the couch when the first attack of arthritis hit me because I couldn't go up those stairs. My family tried to be very helpful, but there's only so much they can do."

"I have thirteen steps that go inside of my house," said Harriet, in her late sixties. "I grips that banister. One Sunday, on my way to church, I broke the banister. My pastor said that was the death grip. By holding it, I didn't fall down."

"In other words," Jackie stated, "you have to concentrate on what you're doing every minute of the day."

"That's right," said Harriet. "If I go to the grocery, I have to have somebody carry the things up for me. When I get upstairs, I say, Lord have mercy, and I have to sit down before I can put things away."

"When I go to the grocery store, I get the cart to hold onto," said Martha. "Pushing the cart helps keep me steady. But when you get home, you're pooped out. A lot of times I have to leave the food in the car." Later,

Martha summed up the feelings of the group. "You just can't do what you're used to doing, and it frustrates you a little bit. That may have a lot to do with the anxiety inside—wanting to do things that you used to do and realizing that you can't. You get tired of waiting to ask somebody or just waiting. It's agony."

The interviewees know well the speed propelling society at large. But for them, as suggested by Martha, the pace of life literally slows, without volition. Almost everything takes longer to do. Haste carries consequences of falling or becoming overly tired. Some things just can't be rushed. Esther and Harry Halpern, the isolated older couple, offer a prime example. "It takes me two and a half hours to get dressed and have breakfast," said Esther, "so the morning's gone. And then I usually get some kind of sandwich ready for him."

"I want to help her," interjected Harry.

"Then it takes me another hour, an hour and a half, to get dinner ready."

"There are things that are harder for her, so I want to do them."

"He does."

"We always think we can do certain things for other people."

"For each other," said Esther.

"Yeah, for each other," nodded Harry.

Esther and Harry Halpern have few scheduled activities beyond frequent doctor visits. This doesn't mean their time isn't valuable, but they face little external pressure on their days. For many others, meeting external demands requires careful planning, with the clock ticking. They must arise earlier to perform mundane morning routines; at the end of the day, reverse activities also take longer. For people used to moving fast, spending considerable time and energy on routine tasks can become profoundly frustrating and stressful. Tina DiNatale, in her mid forties, feels that her husband, Joe, often wants to help her just to expedite matters.

> I used to be quite quick. Things had to be done right then, and it's pretty frustrating when they're not. In today's society, which is so fast paced, no one has time to do anything. It bothers me that somebody won't wait five or ten minutes for me, or can't understand that, for me to take a shower, it takes five or ten minutes more than it takes a healthy person.
>
> I don't expect people to know all about MS. But I do care that those who are closest to me be patient, always. I would rather, much rather, that Joe wait the two minutes it takes to go down the steps than have him say, "Tina, I'll pick you up and carry you." Even though he wants to help me, I think that he really doesn't want to waste the two minutes. We have friends we go out with, and the wife always says, "Tina, take the wheelchair." She knows it would be

faster, but I want to walk. So I walk very slowly, and they walk behind me. And I'm like, "Please, this isn't mourning. We're not on a
date. You don't have to do the old Italian tradition where you're es-
corted and watched."

Sometimes the time required for routine tasks gets out of hand. Arnis
Balodis admitted, "Small things do get you irritated. Like if you have a ceiling light, how the heck do you get up there to change the light bulb?"
"How do you do it?"
"Go down to the lumberyard and get some plywood pieces. Build a scaf-
folding, one step, second step. Make them wide. Then I nail a couple of two-
by-fours to grab hold and then up I go. What should be a five-minute job
turns out to be a two-day job." Perhaps Arnis was atypical, but how should
people with mobility problems change light bulbs in ceiling fixtures? Or
turn off blaring, overhead smoke detectors when they burn the toast, as
does Mildred Stanberg?

Some call this extra time "crip time"—always longer than the time
needed by people without "crippling" impairments (Olkin 1999). "Crip
time" can have benefits. For instance, parents who spend longer walking
their child to school have more time together. But the end result is that the
people most likely to be exhausted by effort can find their days consumed
by mundane routine tasks. They need to be late to bed but early to rise.

Broadly speaking, the interviewees use two basic strategies for conducting daily activities: rearranging their physical environments to facilitate
independence and getting human help.

IMPROVING ACCESSIBILITY

Most private homes and smaller apartment buildings pose inconveniences,
outright impediments, and dangers for people with mobility problems—
stairs, insubstantial railings, narrow doorways and halls, inadequate supports (such as grab bars), and cramped bathrooms. In Boston and surrounding towns, many buildings date from the mid 1800s through early
1900s, when people had shorter life spans and before accessibility became
topical. As Lester Goodall put it, Boston's architecture offers "vertical living" while he prefers horizontal. Regions with newer housing offer more
accessible styles. Houses built in areas with many retirees accommodate
limited mobility. But nationwide, relatively few private houses and small
apartment buildings are truly accessible. A 1995 federal housing survey
found that only 20 percent of 20.6 million privately owned multifamily
rental properties had at least one "handicapped accessible" unit (U.S. Cen-

sus Bureau 1999a), as did 12 percent of 8.8 million privately owned single-family rental properties (U.S. Census Bureau 1999b).[2]

Only 51 to 56 percent of people with mobility problems own their homes, compared to over 68 percent of those without mobility difficulties.[3] Over 67 percent of people with mobility problems must use stairs to enter their homes, and around 40 percent of homes have more than one story. Almost 20 percent of people with major mobility problems say they have difficulties using their bathrooms.

None of the homes I visited during the interviews were completely and easily accessible, even in buildings specifically adapted for occupants using wheelchairs. One wheelchair user lives in an old mansion, elegant with ornamental plasterwork, which had been renovated by the neighborhood housing authority explicitly for accessibility. After a chilly, damp ride over in my scooter, I was therefore surprised when the wheelchair entrance, down a ramp to the basement, was locked tight and had no bell or intercom. The only window was well above wheelchair height. I (fortunately) could stand up. Waving at two men dressed as janitors, who tensed cautiously, I gesticulated downward, hoping to convince them that my verticality was temporary. The older man reluctantly let me in. I was bedraggled, wet, a woman, and in a wheelchair—probably not a threat.

Although several people live in one-story houses, these homes had one or two entry stairs without railings, actually a daunting barrier. Esther Halpern performs a complicated ballet getting into and out of her house:

> I hold onto the door. Well, actually, I can use the walker, too, as long as somebody holds the door open. Or if I have to do it myself, I could push that door open, hold on, and then push the door to where it would stay open, and then I can get the walker up onto the first step. And then I can lift it and get onto the second step, and then I would release the door. . . .
>
> Every morning, they drop the newspaper right outside the door, beyond the step. But instead of going down the step, I use my grabber to pick it up so I don't have to go up and down the step.

Esther's "grabber" is a rodlike device with pinchers to reach inconveniently placed items.

Many people resist changing their houses or decor, living with inconveniences—and safety risks (chapter 10). One woman with severe back pain has "three stairs to get into my house, but that's all right. I go up on all fours and come down better." Renovations *are* costly and, according to a 1990 federal survey, people themselves pay for almost 78 percent of home accessibility improvements (LaPlante, Hendershot, and Moss 1992, 9). Some admit concerns about symbolism. Tina DiNatale installed a grab bar in her bathroom but told the workman, " 'I don't want anything to look too handicapped.' I had him put the railing in horizontally so that I can use it for a towel rack."

Nevertheless, almost all interviewees described some adaptation to facilitate independent functioning at home. A few wealthy people built new houses or performed substantial renovations. But for renters, finding existing and accessible housing with reasonable rents is hard. Lonnie Carter, the disability activist, worried, "Landlords want to rent their apartments at market value. They don't want to put in ramps. It's bad news about accessible housing—its getting cut for minorities, for whoever you are." Public housing can also be problematic, as Erna Dodd found:

> I did have a handicap apartment before. We got a house with a rent-to-own. But mice was all on the table, the stove, all over the furniture they crawled. And boys beat up my grandson, so we moved away. Then I live in the basement floor, which was like a handicap unit, and it was easy for me. But it was not really nice. After they start to broke into my house, I got this house where I'm right now. I can't go in the front of my house because the step is too high. I get very short of breath. So I go through the back. I get very scare sometime because I slip coming out of the bathroom, nothing to hold onto, and I hit my head. But I don't have nowhere else to go.

Joe Warren, a wheelchair user, had been in his mid twenties when he moved into a public apartment complex constructed specifically for the "elderly and handicapped." Initially he was pleased. "It was brand new, and it was my first apartment just to see if I could do it on my own. But the elderly and handicapped do not belong together."

"What happened?"

"A lot of rumors started. I'd have friends over and play music. Then the older people'd say I had guns in my apartment. I never even held a gun in my life! The older people that didn't have anything to do saw me come in with friends and just made up stories. So I finally moved out." A real estate developer confirmed Joe's impression, telling me that his housing projects for elderly and younger persons with disabilities just had not worked out—the two groups didn't get along.

Without accessible housing, many make other significant adjustments. A half-dozen interviewees temporarily or permanently moved their bedrooms from an upper floor to the ground level. Two put in lifts along staircases, although one didn't use his because he was "insecure getting on and off." Sally Ann and Chet Jones widened doorways, installed ramps, and built a shower with a "slanted floor" so she can roll in unimpeded. Sometimes costly changes don't work. Tina DiNatale replaced her wall-to-wall carpets with highly polished hardwood floors, which she viewed as both elegant and functional, but they proved too slippery. Tina wonders how to tell Joe that she wants to reinstall carpets.

According to a 1990 nationwide survey, the most common home adaptation is installing grab bars or special railings, followed by ramps, making extrawide doors, and raised toilet seats (LaPlante, Hendershot, and Moss 1992, 3). Grab bars must be affixed firmly into sturdy supports. "Now I grab the towel rack, which I pulled out and broke a couple of times," complained one woman. "They're chintzy things!" Other people use shower chairs when it becomes unsafe or too painful to stand. Some men start using a urinal at night rather than getting to the bathroom. "I cannot see the point of struggling to do something that can be handled in a different way," said one man's wife, "though I realize the urinal is not necessarily what he wants."

Many strategies can improve independence and safety at home (chapter 10). "Grabbers" or "reachers" like Esther's help pluck items from inconvenient places. People carry portable or cellular telephones. Some use "lifeline" services that summon emergency assistance if they press the button on a pendant worn around the neck. Several "carry" (i.e., push) items around home in the basket of a rolling walker, for example moving cans from the cupboards to the stove while cooking. Tom Norton replaced a picturesque but irregular flagstone walkway with smooth pavement. "Give him time," noted Nelda Norton, an avid gardener, "and the whole yard will be concrete." "At least I wouldn't stub my toe," Tom retorted.

Interviewees who still walk frequently rearrange household items for "furniture surfing"—placing objects strategically to grab for balance. This tactic won't work unless furnishings are tall enough to be within easy reach. Many people, especially those with arthritis, avoid low furniture altogether. As Jimmy Howard admitted,

> I can't deal with these low couches no more because it's really hard
> for me to get up. I will take a big, hard chair and sit in it. Before the
> arthritis, I could spring up like it wasn't nothing. When I was
> younger, we had them beanbag chairs that you just plop down on
> the floor, stretch out, and watch TV. That was my favorite thing. But
> let me get down there now, and it takes me an hour to get up!

GETTING HELP

Oftentimes, environmental adaptations are not enough, and interviewees need human help with daily activities. The dynamics of who provides this assistance—and its effects on interpersonal relationships—are complicated. Some people hire professional "personal-care attendants," home-health aides, housekeepers, "Meals on Wheels," grocery delivery services, or other services among the expanding industry aimed at facilitating independent living at home.[4] The likelihood of a person paying for help with daily activities rises with increasing impairments: 12 percent for people with minor, 19 percent with moderate, and 33 percent with major mobility difficulties.[5]

Most interviewees turn first to family. Admittedly, people don't want to "burden" their spouse, partner, or children. Nevertheless, they also don't want to leave home, to be institutionalized. Some feel uncomfortable having "strangers" address daily needs. Among people with minor mobility problems, 60 percent get help *only* from their spouse, parents, or children, as do 48 percent with moderate and 38 percent with major difficulties.[6] This help carries complex nuances and consequences for everybody.

The vast majority of "informal caregivers"—relatives, friends, and neighbors who provide unpaid assistance (Kleinman 1988; Kane, Kane, and Ladd 1998; Roszak 1998; Pipher 1999; Stone 2000; Levine 2000)—are female family, primarily wives or daughters. However, people with mobility problems are more likely to live alone than others: 10 percent of people without mobility difficulties compared to 16 percent of those with minor and moderate and 14 percent of those with major difficulties.[7] In all age ranges people with mobility difficulties are less likely than those without difficulties to be married and more likely to be divorced.[8] People with mobility problems are also much more likely to be poor, uneducated, and unemployed (chapter 7)—additional sources of stress that could damage relationships.

Not surprisingly, therefore, increasing mobility difficulties are associated with suggestions of social isolation (Table 8). While 70 percent of people with minor difficulties got together with friends during the preceding two weeks, only 55 percent of persons with major problems did. Rates of seeing relatives, talking on the telephone with friends, and attending various activities are lower in people with major versus minor mobility difficulties. Almost 49 percent of people reporting major mobility difficulties want more social contacts compared to 31 percent of those with minor problems.

Routine daily activities virtually define grown-up self-sufficiency. Within families, giving and receiving such help blurs the boundaries delineating independence from dependence, privacy from exposure, and being in or out of control. When partners begin performing routine tasks, "this can create inequity, conflict, blame, guilt, dependence, resentment"—a rebalancing becomes necessary (Olkin 1999, 117). Four snippets from my in-

TABLE 8. Social Encounters in the Last Two Weeks

	Social Encounter (%)		
Mobility Difficulty	*Visited Friends*	*Ate Out*	*Attended Church or Temple*
Mild	70	60	46
Moderate	62	52	39
Major	55	44	30

terviews illustrate these diverse dynamics. The first finds Joe DiNatale cradling his wife, Tina, in his arms, carrying her to the basement bathroom of a North End restaurant, to surfside at the seashore, up the two steps of their garage entryway. Joe has the power literally to sweep her off her feet, despite Tina's protestations that she'd rather walk, albeit slowly.

The second shows Gerald Bernadine recognizing that his MS not only partially redefines his sense of self but also shapes his interactions with others.

> I was used to being very self-reliant, independent. And so, when I got MS, I finally just had to accept that I was ill; I had to accept limitations; I had to accept a helping hand from people. One thing that I've learned is that, when somebody reaches out to help you—even if you can help yourself, even if you don't need that help—it's really nice to accept it. Because it does something for them, too. It creates that bond which is really special. I think they get as much out of it as I do.

The third is Walter Masterson's pained recognition of his progressive debility and the "proper role" for his wife, Nancy:

> We are beginning to think about and verbalize some of the things that will be problems. Eventually I'm not going to be able to bathe myself. I'm not going to be able to do much about going to the toilet. In fact, I won't be able to feed myself. I won't be able to do much of anything by myself. So that means that what you see before you, in a slightly reduced form, will have to be manhandled for various things. And that's not something Nancy should be doing.

The fourth comes from Charles Everest, his wife, Doris, and son, Seth. During the early moments of the interview, before his powerful Parkinson's disease medications precipitated their characteristic writhing dyskinesias (abnormal body movements), Mr. Everest sat frozen in his wheelchair, commenting rarely.

"We all had frustrations," Seth confessed. "Dad was very reluctant to ask for help. It was all new to us. We didn't know how much to let him be who he had to be and struggle to get around. But at the same time, we knew there were easier ways—just by us helping him or by getting a wheelchair."

"Charles was not aware for several years, until we did family counseling, of our frustration," said Doris. "We all had been very much affected. I certainly have. He was completely surprised."

"I thought I could deal with it myself," Charles said haltingly. "When I was first diagnosed, I said it'll go away, and I'll get along with my life. I didn't need help from anybody else, which was true for a long time. Again, things have changed. Sometimes I have to admit that the whole family has the disease."

SPOUSES AND PARTNERS

All marriages—and partnerships with significant others—are complicated works in progress. This is especially true for people with progressive chronic conditions. Over the long haul, few marriages are truly one-sided. The psychotherapist Olkin (1999, 116) warns, "When disability joins a couple, predisability marital issues will be reflected and accentuated." Nonetheless, firmly rooted societal stereotypes hold that, when one partner cannot walk, marriages become one-way streets—the walking partner does all the giving, with uniformly negative consequences. The interviewees expressed diverse sentiments, which may not apply to persons from different cultures and social backgrounds. Several themes did emerge.

Finding a Balance

Natalie Strong, in her early thirties and a recent wheelchair user, debated before marrying Patrick, who is able-bodied (sometimes he *does* have a bad back). "I had this independence struggle. We lived together for a year before we got married because I had that problem—I didn't want to feel dependent on Patrick. But I've since come to see where the balance is, and it doesn't bother me anymore."

"Do you let Patrick do things for you?"

"The things that are easier, that are just less energy-intensive for him. But there are enough things that he either doesn't like to do or that I'm simply better at and more willing to take on, so there's balance. The laundry is a good example. The laundry room's in the kitchen. We've set it up so that he moves the clothes around, and I do what needs to be done with them. You know, guys have a wonderful way of putting the black in with the white!" Many interviewees of all ages voiced Natalie's discovery—that partners find a balance.

"I" Becomes "We"

When talking about "dealing with" mobility problems, people often abandoned the first person singular pronoun—instead of "I," they spoke of "we." They and their spouse or partner are in it together. While both cannot share the illness experience, they confront its consequences as a team. The shift in language is subtle, but the implications are profound. For Sally Ann and Chet Jones, this shift happened the day of her diagnosis: "Chet said to me, 'What did the doctor say?' And I said to him, 'That I have MS.' He sort of sighed, then he said, 'At least we know what it is. Now we can deal with it.' "

This doesn't mean that couples agree on everything, but they generally share ultimate goals, love, and respect. Especially in lengthy marriages, they recognize give and take. Mike and Betty Campbell disagreed early on about his using a cane—Betty for it, Mike against. But they confronted his debilitating arthritis together. "I figure it's payback time," smiled Betty as Mike laughed. "The first ten years we were married, I was in and out of the hospital, and he was always there taking care of me. So now it's my turn. We do for each other what needs to be done, and after forty-five years, I guess it gets to be a habit."

Before his MS, Gerald Bernadine and his wife both had busy jobs but found time to talk. They cherished walking together. "For twenty years, we did just about everything together. Skiing. Long walks. It took us a whole hour to walk this circle in our neighborhood, and it was wonderful. We'd take the dog, and we'd talk. We used to do a lot of things together that I can't do now. She misses that. She tells me that she misses her pal."

Communication between partners—in its myriad manifestations—often changes with progressive chronic disease and mobility problems. It requires shared moments, as for Gerald Bernadine and his wife. But good communication is complicated. Some interviewees don't want to talk about their mobility problem, saying it's "depressing," "unhelpful," "talking won't make it go away," "why bother," "what's the use?" One partner may say things the other doesn't hear. Research suggests that talking about disability generally improves family function, although discussing every detail of experiences and feelings is not always helpful (Olkin 1999, 124). Deciding what to say and when to say it, even within a marriage, is a balancing act.

One happy footnote. When Gerald Bernadine got his motorized scooter, he and his wife resumed their long walks and talks. She walks; he rolls.

Intimacy

Sexual closeness remains just as important as before the mobility problems, in some ways even more so. "Physical love is, particularly when you have a physical disability, very important," said one man who uses a wheelchair. "That kind of intimacy is very reassuring. The only thing that's really changed is the technique. My wife has to make up for my disability. But it's therapeutic for me. I think it's beautiful and wonderful." When sexual bonds diminish, "other aspects of physical closeness, such as cuddling, kissing, or holding hands, also decline, resulting in less emotional intimacy" (Olkin 1999, 122). Bodies and people feel unloved.

Misconceptions abound about technical sexual competence among people with mobility problems, perpetuating false stereotypes about whether people still "have sex," even affecting physicians' behavior (e.g., neglected birth control counseling or screening for sexually transmitted diseases, chapter 9). Erroneous assumptions are perhaps most pronounced for people with spinal cord injuries. The reporter John Hockenberry, married with children, recounted a conversation with an airline flight attendant exemplifying these prejudices. Having seen Hockenberry transfer effortlessly into his seat, the flight attendant expressed admiration then added, "I guess you are the first handicapped person I have ever seen up close. . . . Can you, I mean, can your body, I mean are you able to do it with a woman?" (1995, 97). Hockenberry's simple answer would have been "yes," but he was understandably stumped by how to respond.

Sometimes physical aspects of progressive chronic illnesses (e.g., problems with bladder and bowel control in MS, impotence resulting from diabetes) present special challenges to physical intimacy. Irving Zola, who had polio, observed, "There is the absence of a certain spontaneity in my courting. . . . There's simply no sexy, subtle, or even fast way for me to remove my leg braces and get undressed" (1982, 149). Obesity also often accompanies mobility limitations—as a cause or effect. People's body images can suffer, making them shy or embarrassed about physical closeness. Michael Sexton, a gay man, is ashamed of his body.

> My mate, Gerry, and I have been living together for thirty-three years, which is a long time, half my life. I'm taking a shower, and I need help, but I'll say to Gerry, "Don't look!" And he'll say, "I can't help you without looking, dummy!" I've changed so much. I never weighed more than 150 pounds in my life until the arthritis. So, yeah, this is a problem with intimacy.

"It's a Hard Job"

Many interviewees spoke of the burdens their mobility problems foist on their partners, especially in running the household. The reality is undeniable. As one wheelchair user said of his wife's labors, "It's a hard job."

Everybody quickly assured me—and themselves—that they help out as much as they can. They recounted numerous, less physically demanding activities, and their heartfelt desire to contribute. But one man ruefully acknowledged, "There's some things I can't do on my own." In this situation, the role of gratitude becomes complicated. Expressing thanks for every helpful act—day in and day out—reinforces people's sense of dependence and potential inequity in relationships. Without the proper contrition, however, they may feel selfish or afraid that their partner will abandon them. Some people make self-sacrifices, not asking for something they really want or need. Jeanette Spencer's husband, Bertram, led lengthy hikes in the surrounding hills, leaving Jeanette alone. "Can you do much physically nowadays?" I asked Mrs. Spencer.

"No. I can do a few things, very little. That puts a terrible burden on Bertram."

"Does he do all the housekeeping?"

"Everything that gets done he does."

"How do you feel about that?"

"I think he does a great job. I feel sorry for poor Bertram because he has everything to do. I feel that I shouldn't ask him to do too much, taking me out to places, because he has so much else to do. When he goes off hiking, I wait for him. I just take out my little chair, sit down, and wait." Mrs. Spencer rarely left her home except for doctor's appointments, although her three grown sons lived nearby.

"Life Works Around It"

"For five years, no one, not anyone in the family except myself, could know that he had been diagnosed with a disease," Nelda Norton said about her husband, Tom. Finally, Mr. Norton told his children, then, gradually, his friends. "Now life works around it," Nelda observed.

Dynamics often differ depending on whether the husband or the wife has the mobility problem, especially among older couples. Husbands more than wives will hire outside help to perform tasks vacated by the disabled spouse, so husbands typically "experience less role strain" (Olkin 1999, 119). Some husbands, in particular, learn as much as possible about their wife's disease to help devise mechanical solutions. Sally Ann Jones was an early scooter user because of Chet's research.

He wrote to the MS Society. He got all this information about MS and made himself as well-versed as he could. Then he heard about these scooters. I was getting to the point where, if I wanted to go shop in a mall, I got really tired. I was still doing all the grocery shopping because I had the grocery cart to hang onto. So he said, "Let's get a scooter." We had a station wagon. He built this ramp, a lift gizmo, so that the scooter would go in. That's how I went to the mall.

Chet aimed to make Sally Ann as independent as possible. But for Nelda Norton, things are different. Tom insists that daily life revolve around his needs. He forbids anyone other than Nelda to assist with his routine activities or pick him up when he falls. "We don't go out to dinner anymore," Nelda complained to Tom. "We have people here instead, and I have to cook. I think it's nice to go out for dinner once in a while." As Mr. Norton remained silent, Nelda described a recent vacation cruise. "I couldn't push his wheelchair anymore the whole length of that boat. He finally said, 'I'll just stay in my room.' He'd get to feeling sorry for himself, which upsets everybody else. Either I left him and felt bad about leaving him, or I'd stay in the room, too."

"I still do a lot of things," Tom countered. "I go to Mass every Sunday. Walking in and walking out."

A few interviewees hinted that perhaps their spouse could be more sensitive to their preferences and experiences. Certainly, Tina DiNatale lamented being carried by Joe, apparently to save himself time. "My wife is sixteen years younger than I am," said Lester Goodall, "and she's not sensitive to a lot of little things. Like whenever we go to the mall, my wife will get out of the car and start walking toward the entrance. She doesn't wait for me. Sometimes I wish she would offer to help even though I'd refuse; it's just nice to be offered. She does the laundry, does the house cleaning, but I do things, too. If she cooks, I'll clean, wash the dishes. We do share things like that." But Mr. Goodall was obviously uncomfortable about his criticism. "I don't mean to make her sound insensitive," he added quickly.

Clearly, such complaints carry risks, of appearing ungrateful, selfish, entitled, although some are probably valid. "We don't talk too much about the whole thing," said Lester. "I don't ever want to be a burden."

"Some Kind of a Life for Myself"

Finally, nondisabled partners need some space. Doris Everest cares deeply for her husband, Charles. She overcame her personal terrors—agoraphobia or fear of the outdoors—to accompany him to doctor's appointments, visits with friends, and cross-country medical quests. She admits having grown tremendously from the experience. Yet she needs time for herself:

I work at a women's shelter that I don't want to give up. I take a granddaughter once a week. I found that if I can't keep doing these things, that I'm really going to get angry and bitter, and I don't want to. I bark when I'm losing patience. I know I need to keep some kind of a life for myself.

Paradoxically, forgoing one's private space can heighten loneliness. After Tom's retirement, the Nortons retreated to a stone bungalow on a bluff overlooking the northern Atlantic coast. A thick canopy of trees and rhododendrons cloisters their house. Life now centers around Tom, but Nelda Norton had once kept time for herself. "I used to go on a retreat once a year with friends and spend maybe five days. Then I started feeling guilty, like I was unfair. He doesn't even know how to make soup, to open a can. I felt it was my fault for never showing him how. I showed him where the pots and pans were, where the cans were, the can opener. He got very angry. He didn't want to know. While I was gone, he was going to take his daughters out to dinner anyway. He always wanted someone to take care of him. He's fortunate in that."

"The way I look at it is, don't fix it if it ain't broken," said Mr. Norton.

"But it is broken," Nelda replied. Tom said he would hire professional assistants when necessary, but Mrs. Norton disagreed. "The times that he needs me and the things that he needs me for, no one else is going to do. You have to have someone who will sit by your bed, so that when you wake up about three in the morning and say, 'I cannot move my leg,' they will move it for you. I get up and I lift or pull. No one else is going to be here to do that."

After the interview, Nelda followed me to the car. "I'm terrified that Tom will come out alone someday and get injured. When he is out in the yard, I'm always wondering where he is, whether he's fallen and hurt himself. I am so scared of that." For all her bravado, Nelda obviously felt responsible for Tom's safety, comfort, and well-being. She also seemed isolated and alone.

PARENTS AND CHILDREN

Mobility problems can complicate intergenerational relationships at two points. The first happens early, in choosing parenthood and raising children. The second generally arrives later, with concerns about whether and how children should help out. Studies have examined families with disabled young children (Curry 1995; Olkin 1999, 92–111), but few have looked at how chronic diseases and disability affect adult filial relationships. Obviously, complex issues arise, and here, I only scratch the surface.

"Don't Get Pregnant"

According to the federal survey, only 9 percent of people age eighteen to forty-four with major mobility problems have at least one living child, as do about 17 percent of those with mild and moderate impairments.[9] When mobility problems coincide with child-bearing years, decisions about parenthood precipitate not only the usual angst (e.g., am I really ready to have a kid?) but also societal ambivalence if not outright condemnation. Society seemingly views fully functioning legs as essential prerequisites to meaningful parenting, despite scant evidence that children of disabled parents suffer (Olkin 1999). Public consternation reflects two erroneous expectations: unless fully ambulatory, parents cannot care effectively for children; and when parents fail (as seems inevitable), responsibility will devolve to the state.

Given these concerns, mothers with mobility problems attract the greatest hostility; fathers presumably have wives who do what's needed. Many women cannot even find physicians willing to counsel them on birth control, pregnancy, or childbirth (Fine and Asch 1988, 21). Six obstetricians turned away one woman wheelchair user before a seventh agreed to deliver her baby. Most hurtful was the censure of her now-former best friend, who asserted that her pregnancy was selfish and she would "ruin" her child's life. Her baby is now one year old, and she acknowledges the usual ups and downs of new parenthood. But she glows when speaking of her daughter.

Certain progressive chronic diseases affecting mobility, like diabetes, do heighten pregnancy risks, for mother and child. Some, as did the DiNatales, decide not to have children. Candy Stoops worried about how her newly diagnosed neurologic disease would affect her pregnancy.

> I was having the final test to confirm my diagnosis. The last words out of my neurologist's mouth were, "Don't get pregnant." Well, a little too late! I found out I was pregnant with my son that following Friday. "We have to make some decisions here," my neurologist said. I said that I didn't want to abort unless I absolutely had to—if it meant danger to the baby as well as me, we might consider it. My neurologist called a specialist in New York to talk it over, and he said, "Go for it!"
>
> For people with my disease, once pregnant, you either stay the same, get better, or get worse. Obviously I had gotten worse. But my neurologist felt that we could keep things under control enough for

me to at least have this baby. Actually, I had a fantastic pregnancy except I was extremely tired. I worked until my eighth month.

Candy said she had "a natural delivery because they had no idea how I was going to react under anesthesia," but then for seven years she took medications with significant side effects. She and her husband decided not to have other children, worried that it might worsen her disease. Plus, "I didn't feel that was fair to my son. I wasn't able to go bike riding with him or skating—my husband did that. But if I got worse, what am I taking away from him?" Mrs. Stoops feels her disease had some good consequences for her son. Instead of working as she would have done, she stayed home with her boy. Admittedly, she couldn't carry him, so when he was fourteen months old, "he could climb up and down the stairs because he had to." But her husband and their extended family pitched in. "Do I think he missed out? No. We've done a lot. We're very close."

Other mothers of young children did raise concerns and regrets. Mattie Harris wishes she could play ball in the park with her kids. One woman feels badly that she cannot pick up and carry a child tugging at her sleeve. Another woman spends hours playing cards and board games with her children in lieu of trips to the playground. Divorced women fear losing custody of their child. Bonnie Winfield was six when her thirty-year-old father, a third-generation dairy farmer, developed polio from a rare vaccine reaction. Afterward, he first used a wheelchair but worked his way onto crutches.

My parents didn't really sit my brothers and me down—we were all under eight—and try to explain what is going on with Dad. We just knew, all of sudden, we had this stuff in the house, from the portable commode to shower curtains on bathroom doors because Dad's wheelchair couldn't get through with the door there. We had a long hallway that connected our bedrooms, and my dad used to take his walker and practice walking going up and down. You knew Dad's legs didn't work, and you knew he was trying to get them to work again. But you didn't really understand the full dynamics. It was a bit confusing, but you muddled through. We had a normal house- hold as far as we were concerned. You know, that's Dad.

It was a real team effort between juggling all of us kids and the farm. We had to pick up some of the slack. Us kids had to go out and round up the cows, and we learned to milk, and my mom and my grandmother milked. But he was just a real trooper. It's funny, I never thought of him as handicapped. He wasn't. When people would hold open doors for Dad, we kids would just walk through. We wouldn't hold it for him. But that was what he wanted because he didn't want to be treated any differently than anybody else. That was very important to him. I mean, he dances up a storm. You should see him at weddings!

In contrast to Bonnie, many children have grown and left home by the time their parents develop mobility problems. So the long-standing relationships between parents and children shape the impact of mobility difficulties. Walking per se isn't the issue, although it may catalyze changes in the dynamics of relationships. One woman with severe back pain lives with her daughter, and she's losing patience. "She's no help. It's the same as living alone except sometimes I have someone to talk to. I really wish she'd go out and find a husband. She'll be thirty-seven in March. I wish she'd just leave me. It's time now for me to be alone. I'm in pain. I want to live my life in peace." Bonnie Winfield is now in her early thirties and her father, in his mid fifties, is becoming more physically limited:

> As we get older, my Dad and I have actually grown a lot closer. We talk about a range of topics that obviously you don't talk to kids about. I would describe myself as my Dad's confidante. My parents are divorced, so he talks to me a lot about what he's thinking inside. He's slowly starting to realize that his body just can't take some things anymore. . . . "If I go back to a wheelchair or using my crutches full time, who would want me?" You're perceived as a "broken man," which is something I really have a hard time with. If people can't value the person, respect him, you don't want them. So mostly I'm the listener, someone he can vent his concerns to: "What happens if I can't walk again?" . . . I give as much emotional support as I can. He's taught me so many lessons in life and was always there for me. For all of us children, no matter what. It's the least I can do. It's not payback—not that you ever pay it back. It's just that he's a marvel.

"My Daughter Cooks Most of the Time Now"

Almost uniformly, parents protest that they don't want to burden their children. Whether they will accept their children's help is a slightly different question. Sometimes this assistance is essential to getting through the day. "I used to go in the kitchen and cook a big meal," said Mattie Harris. "I still cook some, but not like I used to cook. It's terrible, 'cause I just can't stand at the stove. I gotta sit down and do most of the preparations or get the girls to do it. My daughter, she cooks most of the time now."

Daughters typically help out more than sons (Stone 2000, 50), despite also caring for their own children. "Theirs has been called the 'sandwiched' life. No sooner do they finish raising their children than their ailing parents move in for care" (Roszak 1998, 93). Some women spend more years caring for their parents than for their children. Daughters and sons generally do different things. Daughters assist with cooking, household chores, even personal care, such as bathing and dressing. As in Mattie Harris's family, older daughters sometimes help care for younger siblings. Daughters also take parents shopping, to doctor's appointments, to visit friends, and to church. Sons typically perform activities outside the home, picking up groceries, and doing other errands. Exceptions to these stereotypes obviously exist: Arnis Balodis looked after his mother's every need. Proximity helps. Children living in the same building or neighborhood stop by more easily. Tensions among children can erupt, when siblings perceive responsibilities—or "burdens"—are inequitably distributed. But different children typically play different roles reflecting lifelong patterns, as in Charles Everest's family.

"I was home for one or two years when he first had Parkinson's," said his son Seth, "then I went to college."

"Our younger daughter Posie suggested the wheelchair," said Mrs. Everest. "She was around longer than the other kids."

"Posie would have been home more and seen Dad's decline," agreed Seth, who lives 3,000 miles away. "In the past five years when I visit, I've become more aware of demands that Dad puts on the person taking care of him. I'm much more aware of what my mother has to go through. You have to be pretty physically strong to take care of Dad. And it does cross my mind quite often that she constantly has to find a way to balance it out. It's very difficult with me being at a great distance. There's not much that I can do."

"All my children play a role," said Mrs. Everest, "and they have their own roles. Seth's role is to listen to his mother when she calls and she's upset, which is very important because he's a good listener. The other children do other things for me."

Depending on who's around, other family members also help—parents, grandchildren, siblings (especially sisters), nieces, nephews, cousins. Parents caring for their adult children raise particularly poignant and complex emotions. Children often feel guilty for dependency they had seemingly relinquished years ago; parents can become bewildered and despondent witnessing their child's physical decline. Especially as children reach middle age, parents may be ill or impaired themselves. Among people age forty-five to sixty-four years with mobility difficulties, only around 40 percent have at least one living parent, and the fraction falls to about 4 percent for people age sixty-five or older.[10]

"My mother basically takes care of me," said Marianne Bickford. "She likes to do the cooking. It's hard for me to watch, but I don't say that to her."

Marianne's widowed mother had cancer and was physically frail. "It's hard when your mother's crying because she can't help you get up when you fall down. I don't want her to help me because she could hurt herself. She has fractured ribs. I always fight and struggle and get up myself. By the end of this year, I feel like I'm going to lose my mother. I know it's up to God," Marianne said softly as the tears finally came. Her mother did die soon afterward.

Some people have no living relative and reside alone. These people most likely must pay for assistance. "Baby boomers," on average, have smaller families than their parent's generation, and relatively fewer children will therefore be available to help out. Even when children are around, the historian Theodore Roszak warns that relying on relatives as caregivers could "destroy even the best-intentioned families by burdening them—especially the woman of the house—beyond endurance" (1998, 94). To relieve families, many are thinking of new ways to organize needed assistance at home (Kane, Kane, and Ladd 1998; Roszak 1998; Pipher 1999; Stone 2000; Benjamin 2001).

FRIENDS

Finally, friends play diverse roles. On one level, people try to keep friendships as they once were—balancing expectations, the give and take—but now one friend may need help. Defining the boundaries of these new roles is sometimes complicated. Many friends do not have the implicit sense of obligation or lifelong responsibility linking family members. But friends often still want to assist yet hesitate to offer, afraid of intruding, overstepping their bounds. The person with mobility problems is similarly sometimes shy to ask, worried about imposing, demanding too much, embarrassed about admitting basic needs. In examining friendships between women with and without mobility problems, Fisher and Galler found that friends, in an unspoken bargain, often trade physical help for emotional support.

> Recognizing that friendship requires a certain special accommodation (if not direct physical help) by non-disabled friends, the disabled women attempted to balance the scale by being especially attentive and supportive in the emotional sphere, being extragood listeners, comforters, and so forth. Such an attempt, however, needs to be understood in the context of the strong investment in physical autonomy. . . . All of [the disabled women] resented being given help they did not need or want. (1988, 180)

Finding that new balance between friends can be challenging, but sometimes it happens without words. Fundamentals can remain unchanged, especially with old friends. Sally Ann Jones said her many friends often forget she is "handicapped" and suggest doing "something like skiing. But that's been good. That's how I like people to feel about it." Sometimes friendships offer support with privacy that family relationships don't allow. "I have a very dear friend who comes over on Friday and takes me shopping," said one older woman, admitting this keeps her from becoming "house-bound." People urge her to move in with her children, with whom she has loving relationships, but she likes her privacy.

Friends may not see people day in and day out, so they cannot appreciate fully the realities of limited mobility. A seventy-year-old woman with osteoarthritis observed,

> I had friends in Boston, and we used to walk all over the Back Bay. But I can't do it now. I can walk for maybe ten minutes and then I sit awhile. Almost more trouble for me is standing still. . . . If I meet friends outside and they want to stand and talk, it's difficult. But I really miss walking, and I feel as though my friends in Boston perhaps don't quite understand. They keep saying, "Come in and have lunch with us. Take the train." Well, getting up and down the steps on the train is not a good idea for me, and once I get to Back Bay Station, I've got to walk all over the place. Even though they know I have the arthritis, I don't think they really understand.

On the other side, sometimes friends want to help but don't know how. Charles Everest's co-workers "would approach me," recounted his wife, Doris, "and they would say, 'What should I do when I see Charles in the lunch line? Should I offer to take his tray?' And I got so that I would say, 'Just ask him. I can't tell you.' He finally let this man who he was close to help him on with his coat. That was a big deal."

"It *was* a big deal," agreed Mr. Everest.

Certainly friends, acquaintances, and family sometimes don't know what to say. But even tentative interactions can convey warmth. Near the end of my first year of medical school, I was hospitalized briefly when I became completely unable to walk. Although I had tried keeping my situation secret, a classmate I barely knew came to my bedside one night. "Gosh," he said reverentially, "I hear you have a really serious disease." The class had just learned about MS in neuropathophysiology lectures.

"I guess so," I replied, uncertain what to add.

"Gosh," he paused again, obviously lost for words. After a minute, he rallied. "I brought you a cheesecake." He handed me a big box, then retreated hastily. Even awkward gestures can be wonderful.

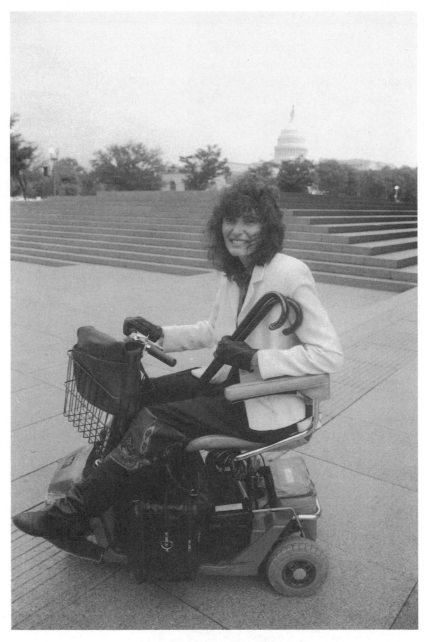

Plate 1. I got from Boston to the Capitol by wheelchair-accessible taxi, airplane, and Washington's subway, the Metro. I have canes for walking and a suitcase rides below my legs. (Photo by Mark L. Rosenberg, M.D.)

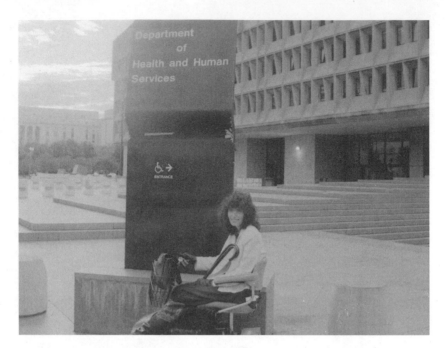

Plate 2. Barriers surround me: zigzagging stairs and concrete blocks. The wheelchair-accessible route into the U.S. Department of Health and Human Services building (which the sign points out) leads to a side entrance. (Photo by Mark L. Rosenberg, M.D.)

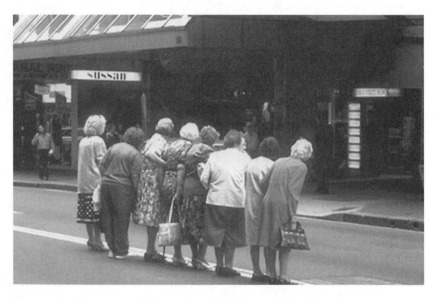

Plate 3. Linking arms and hoping for safety in numbers offer scant protection against anxiety, fears, or cars when people walk slowly. (Photo by Fred Kent, Project for Public Spaces)

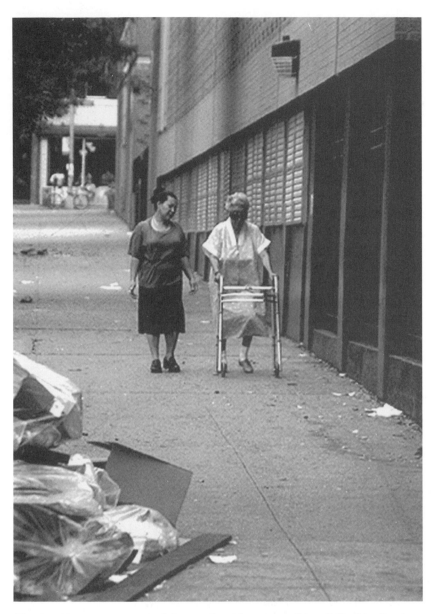

Plate 4. About one quarter of the people with major walking difficulties live in poverty. Trash-strewn or poorly maintained walkways, physical isolation, fears of injury or violence present other barriers. Many people with mobility problems live alone and cannot easily find walking partners. (Photo by Fred Kent)

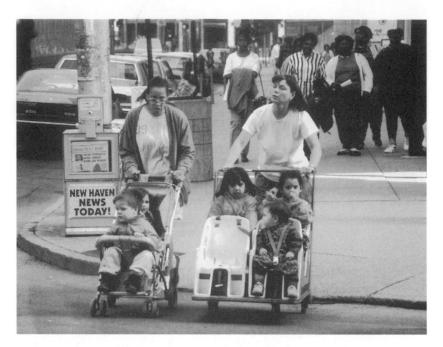

Plate 5. Curb cuts make it easier for everybody to get around. (Photo by Fred Kent)

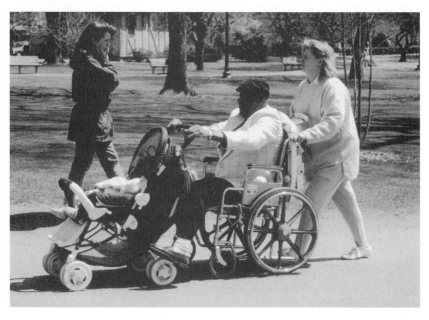

Plate 6. One woman moves all three people. The man's wheelchair appears heavy, institutional, hard to self-propel, with no seat cushion or back support to maximize safety and comfort. (Photo by Fred Kent)

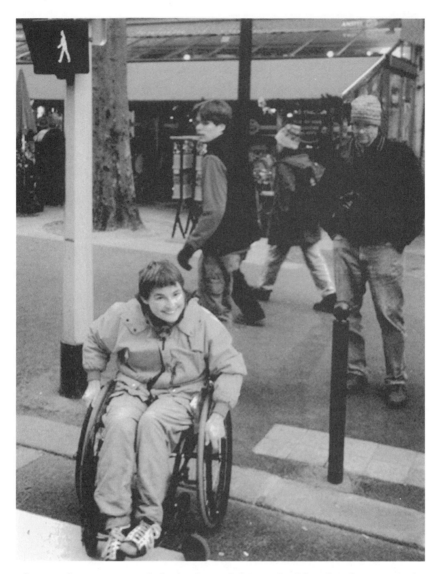

Plate 7. This woman in a lightweight rigid-frame wheelchair has the upper body strength to self-propel; she also has curb cuts. Even so, she moves below the gaze of most walkers. (Photo by Fred Kent)

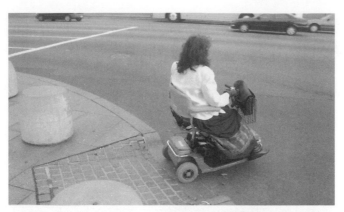

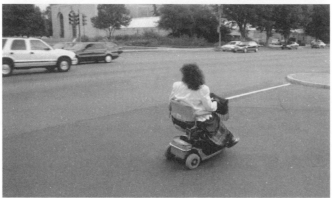

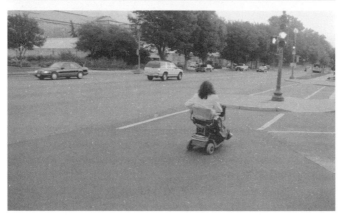

Plate 8. Waiting at a corner with curb cuts but without clearly marked crosswalks, I hope—as always—that my scooter won't fail and that the drivers will see me as I pass their way. Nonetheless it feels terrific to be on wheels, powered by batteries, after having had so much trouble walking. I often feel I'm grinning like a fool as I buzz along. (Photo by Mark L. Rosenberg, M.D.)

7   Outside Home—at Work and in Communities

The possibility of experiencing discrimination had never occurred to me—of course not, given my demographics. I am white, upper middle class, well educated, from a family of girls taught we could achieve whatever we wanted if we worked hard enough. I therefore didn't recognize the warning signs until they almost literally knocked me over.

As I noted in the preface, the uncertainty and physical consequences of MS consumed most of my psychic energy during my years at Harvard Medical School. And people's reactions to the "me" they equated with MS were equally daunting. Though the medical school made necessary academic accommodations (absolving me from staying up all night on clinical rotations, fearing that excessive fatigue could exacerbate MS), hints of trouble started immediately. During a critical clerkship, the chief resident peered around corners as I sat at nurses' stations writing notes on patients. Later I learned that the clerkship director had requested his surveillance to confirm that yes, indeed, I was "working up" patients. An attending physician had complained that I was lazy and not doing my job.

Over the two years of clinical rotations, such episodes recurred countless times. I became inured to them. I didn't fight back—I was bewildered and overwhelmed more than angry, and my immediate goal was slogging through. Why did the elite of this caring profession persist so doggedly in marginalizing and excluding me? But was this discrimination? Medical school *is* physically arduous: was my exclusion justified by some Darwinian imperative that only the physically "fittest" should become doctors? Even if it were, I was startled by the hospital leader's pronouncement recounted in the preface: "There are too many doctors in the country right now for us to worry about training handicapped physicians. If that means certain people get left by the wayside, that's too bad."

As I looked for post–medical school jobs, two incidents solidified fears that my career—any career—was in jeopardy. One potential employer, an academic researcher, asserted, "Even if you work full-time, we couldn't give you a full-time salary. Full-time here is eighty hours per week, and I'm sure you'd only work forty hours. So we'll pay you half a salary." A second possible employer, a medical educator, mused aloud: "I see three options. I could hire you because I feel sorry for you; or I could not hire you because I don't want to deal with your disease; or I could try pretending you're not sick and look at your qualifications." I rejected his job offer.

Finally an influential friend from my Harvard School of Public Health days stepped in and pulled a few strings. With his generous recommendation and assurances, Boston University hired me for a research job that, over the next six years, offered many opportunities. A few weeks after I started work, a senior physician did ask me to fetch him a cup of coffee. By that point I had become irremediably feisty. Openly incredulous, I refused—I couldn't have carried it anyway. And I thought disability always trumped gender in workplace dynamics!

As does everybody, people with mobility problems need an income to live, if not a career to thrive. To participate fully in their communities, they also need to enter buildings; use public restrooms; board buses, trains, and airplanes; reach pay phones and checkout counters; wander through parks; stay at hotels; attend theaters, movies, and sporting events. All aspects of American communities—from public spaces to employment policies to transportation networks—were designed primarily for walking people. This context has changed somewhat over the last three decades, as suggested in chapter 4. Cataloging these efforts is beyond my scope here. Chapter 7 focuses on two topics, both reaching outside the home: having an income to live and getting around the community.

MONEY AND JOBS

Mike Campbell kept working in building maintenance long after painful arthritis invaded his knees: "You gotta make a living! And I had a hard job doing that." Mr. Campbell had a high school education and had worked since childhood. "When we started raising a family, I didn't have any real profession; I was just a common laborer. If you wanted the kids to eat, be dressed right, you didn't have much extra money to spend." The interviewees amply and repeatedly confirmed what we already know: richer people have more opportunities to compensate for mobility difficulties than poorer people. They can buy stair lifts, customize mobility aids, hire drivers, and renovate homes, for example, whereas persons with little money cannot.

Progressive mobility limitations threaten incomes and careers, risking both subsistence and self-esteem. "Handicapped is a 'gotcha,' " said one older man. "You have nowhere else to go, and they get you. Everything for the handicapped is exorbitant." He can't do heavy chores around the house, so he must hire someone from his fixed income. Medicare refused reimbursement for essential home modifications and his scooter—he inherited one when somebody died. The only bargain he sees is the local public wheelchair van service, the RIDE.

Gracie Brown, an older woman, has a seventh-grade education and had been a housekeeper. "Retirement and Social Security—that's all I get to pay rent, light bill, grocery, telephone bill. There's no way I'd be able to pay anything more. I don't get enough money to pay the doctor bill."

"What about your cane?" I asked. She had the standard, no-frills, wooden cane with a crook handle, $10 to $15 at neighborhood drug stores.

"They gave it to me after my hip operation. I didn't buy it." She could not afford to pay for it herself.

Serious illnesses of one family member, especially debilitating diseases, can decimate family savings. One study found that 31 percent of families lost most or all of their savings when a family member developed a life-threatening illness; families also moved to cheaper housing, delayed education, or postponed medical care for healthier family members (Covinsky et al. 1994, 1841). Mobility problems can similarly affect not only familial relationships, but also family finances and potentially the careers and plans of others. Because of health problems of people reporting major mobility difficulties, about 7 percent of family members changed or reduced their working hours; 6 percent quit their jobs or retired early; and 5 percent did not take a job.[1] Mrs. Campbell resumed her former job, from which she had retired after twenty years, when her husband left work—they needed the money. Her employer was accommodating, letting her schedule her work hours around Mike's medical appointments.

Martha Daigle, who was in her early sixties, wanted desperately to quit her job as a hospital housekeeper to care for her husband, Fred, but she was terrified of losing her work-related health insurance, which supplemented Fred's coverage. His medical bills were enormous; Medicare only paid 80 percent of his hospitalization costs. "If I don't work, it isn't the money I'd lose as much as the health insurance. If I lose it, there's no way of taking care of him. I don't want to go on welfare. We never had to live on that; we're not going to start now."

"It costs me close to $100 in pills a month," said Mr. Daigle. "Whatever couple bucks you got in the bank, you got to blow it. Then they'll turn around and tell you to sell your house. Where could you go?"

As physical limitations increase, people face realities about their jobs. Persons with mobility difficulties have, on average, less education than people without impairments, so their job opportunities are more limited from the outset (Table 9). About 70 percent of working-age people reporting major mobility difficulties cannot work because of their health conditions, compared to only 3 percent among those without mobility problems.[2] Even among those with jobs, people with mobility difficulties often work fewer hours per week.[3] Not surprisingly, therefore, people with mobility difficulties are much more likely to live below the poverty level, especially if younger (Table 10). Over 26 percent of all adults reporting major and moderate mobility difficulties have incomes below the poverty level, compared to 21 percent with minor mobility problems and only 9 percent without impairments.[4] The percentage with high incomes falls as impairments increase.

Walter Masterson modified his job to match his diminishing physical abilities. These changes carried costs:

> I've really not done any company traveling in a year and a half,
> and that's beginning to restrict my effectiveness in strategic plan-
> ning. . . . I don't have enough stamina to put in the time required.
> So, all of those things are cutting back on what I can be effective in.
> My means of communication is being eroded. The time to back off
> entirely, well, I'm not going to actually retire. Those aren't the
> words being used, but that, in effect, is what is about to occur.

Dr. Jody Farr began falling when she was a medical resident. "I used to make up for any inability to perform physically by knowing more than the other people around me."

"That was a conscious strategy?"

"Yes, and it worked, at the time. Attending physicians would say I was doing really well and that I would find a great job. Then I became friendly with another doctor who has muscular dystrophy, and he said, 'What you're doing is wrong.' "

"What did he mean?"

"He meant that I had all these evaluations saying nice things, but they are skirting the issue—they don't say I am disabled. He wanted me to use some mobility device, like a scooter, before I was ready to do it." Dr. Farr did have a difficult time getting a job. At one interview, "I had to ask the person's assistance in getting up from the chair. I thought, 'If I don't ask her for assistance, I can't get up!' Then the second person I saw said to me, 'We

TABLE 9. Education and Employment Among
Working-Age People

| | Education (%) | | Employment (%) | |
Mobility Difficulty	High School or Less	Beyond College	Employed/ Attending School	Unemployed Because of Health
None	14	10	82	3
Minor	27	5	55	32
Moderate	34	3	40	56
Major	31	4	29	70

have a lot of people applying, and we just can't take someone like you.' "
Dr. Farr now has a job but has made compromises—not taking the more
prestigious but rigorous tenure-track academic position with its employment assurance, instead working under contract, year-to-year.

Many interviewees no longer work because of mobility problems,
sometimes compounded by their underlying medical conditions. Older
interviewees had often retired early from their jobs. None spoke happily
about this. Stella Richards, an accountant formerly anticipating a generous
governmental pension, was matter-of-fact about her losses.

> I think my mind is leaving me now. I haven't been working—it's
> been a long time. . . . On April 1st, April Fool's Day, I went shopping
> with my friend. When we came home, I had such awful back pain.
> My friend took me to the emergency ward. There was this young,
> black doctor, a surgeon, there. I kept asking him to give me some-
> thing for the pain because I couldn't even lie down to take X rays. I
> told him I had to work Monday, and he said, "I'll give you some-
> thing for the pain, but I'm afraid you won't be able to go to work for
> at least two or three weeks." I said "Weeks? Oh no, I have to go to
> work!" I've never been to work since. That was April 1, and my op-
> eration was in early December. I lay in the fetal position in my bed,
> except for my hospital appointments, until the operation. . . .
>
> When I had to retire, I lost half of my pension because of my age.
> I retired too young. I think I was fifty-six. It never entered my mind
> that anything like this would ever happen to me. No. When I re-
> tired, I planned to be traveling, not walking around here on a walker.

Stella Richards is now over sixty-five, receiving Social Security. She feels
she has enough money to live comfortably. How do other people support
themselves when they can no longer work? Some interviewees have private,

TABLE 10. Annual Income

Mobility Difficulty	Below Poverty Level (%)		Income $50,000 or More (%)	
	Age 18–64 years	Age 65+	Age 18–64 years	Age 65+
None	9	6	34	14
Minor	23	10	16	9
Moderate	29	13	13	8
Major	29	15	14	7

long-term disability pensions or insurance, purchased individually or through their employers.[5] Some are wealthy, live off savings from prior well-paying jobs, or are supported by spouses. Other unemployed working-age people receive incomes through the federal "safety-net"—Social Security.

INCOME SUPPORT

Western societies have long provided some financial support to "deserving" and "needy" disabled people unable to work, founded on presumptions of innocence and suffering:

> Innocence means that the condition of being disabled is beyond individual control. Society helps disabled people because they find themselves in bad circumstances through no fault of their own. . . . People who are unemployed because of disability have a higher moral claim because (it is assumed) they really wish to work. (Stone 1984, 172)

While the Social Security Act of 1935 covered elderly people, federal disability insurance arrived only in the 1950s, coming in spurts.[6] Anxious to prevent abuses, Congress structured Social Security as the "last resort" for people who absolutely cannot work because of long-term impairments.[7] Today, the Social Security Administration (SSA) oversees two programs covering almost 6.7 million people with disabilities: Social Security Disability Insurance (SSDI, Title II of the Social Security Act); and Supplemental Security Income (SSI, Title XVI).

Title II authorizes payment of SSDI benefits to persons who have worked and contributed to the Social Security trust fund through taxes on their earnings. Workers injured on the job who receive cash through state-run, employer-financed workers' compensation programs generally have their Social Security benefits reduced by the workers' compensation amount. People who have received SSDI cash benefits for two years become eligible for Medicare (in 2001, the two-year wait was waived for people with ALS). Title XVI provides SSI payments to disabled persons, including children, who have passed a means test documenting limited income and resources. Some states add dollars to federal SSI payments, and persons receiving SSI get Medicaid coverage. Poor people qualifying for SSDI can also receive SSI after passing the means test.

For both SSDI and SSI, the SSA "defines disability as the inability to engage in any substantial gainful activity by reason of any medically determinable physical or mental impairment(s) which can be expected to result in death or which has lasted or can be expected to last for a continuous period of not less than 12 months" (SSA 1998, 2). Disorders "markedly limiting ability to walk and stand" feature prominently among the lists of qualifying impairments. The SSA makes yes/no decisions—either people can or cannot work.

Although the SSA's judgments about employability supposedly use objective medical evidence, boundaries blur: "the scientific link between [complete] work incapacity and medical condition is a weak one" (U.S. General Accounting Office 1996a, 35). Disability determinations generate substantial disagreement, and denials are often disputed vigorously. Applications rise during recessions and fall during boom times (Chirikos 1991, 165): in 2000, the SSA processed approximately 1.3 million SSDI applications, approving almost 47 percent; musculoskeletal disorders were the most common medical condition (Martin, Chin, and Harrison 2001).[8] Among working-age people with major mobility difficulties, 30 percent have applied at least once for SSA disability, with 20 percent applying three or more times.[9] Roughly 24 percent of people reporting major impairments receive SSDI and 34 percent receive SSI, compared to 1 percent for people without mobility difficulties.[10]

Social Security was never intended to guarantee lifetime support for most people. Congress clearly aimed to move persons off Social Security and back into the labor force. However, for complex reasons, this happens relatively rarely (U.S. General Accounting Office 1996a, 1997a). Concerns about losing Medicare and Medicaid, in particular, pose significant disincentives to leaving SSDI or SSI. The SSA neither funds assistive technology nor mandates workplace accommodations. The Ticket to Work and Work Incentives Improvement Act of 1999 offers incremental reforms, especially addressing health insurance coverage and vocational training.[11] Whether this new initiative will move significant numbers of disabled people from Social Security into the work force is as yet unknown (Batavia 2000).

Jimmy Howard, in his late forties, exemplifies the complexities of income support programs. He has painful arthritis, but he claims he was fired from his ManuCo (a pseudonym) warehouse job because of a work-related foot injury. Mr. Howard has received SSDI payments for less than two years, so he is not yet eligible for Medicare. He pays $400 per month for private health insurance under COBRA provisions; sometimes he and his wife, who also doesn't work, can barely make this payment.[12]

Mr. Howard hired an attorney to contest ManuCo's claim that he was fired because of arthritis, not a work-related injury, and tried to win corporate long-term disability payments to supplement SSDI. Mr. Howard feels that ManuCo, a multinational manufacturing company, did little to find him a less physically demanding job so he could keep working—even though, to qualify for SSDI, he had to assert that he was incapable of gainful employment in any capacity.

During our afternoon meeting, Mr. Howard was animated, jocular, and articulate, with an infectious laugh. Over 6 feet tall, he is big all around. He walked firmly and purposefully, without flinching, using an aluminum cane. Mr. Howard's arthritis does, however, sometimes precipitate sudden falls, he has incapacitating stiffness each morning, and he met the clinical criteria for "arthritis of a major weight-bearing joint" specified in *Disability Evaluation Under Social Security:*

> With history of persistent joint pain and stiffness with signs of marked limitation of motion or abnormal motion of the affected joint on current physical examination. With
>   A. Gross anatomical deformity of hip or knee . . . supported by X-ray evidence . . . and markedly limiting ability to walk and stand; or
>   B. Reconstructive surgery . . . of a major weight-bearing joint and return to full weight-bearing status did not occur, or is not expected to occur, within 12 months of onset. (SSA 1998, 22)

These criteria do not consider use of mobility aids or helpful workplace accommodations, since they are not covered by the Social Security Act. For instance, Mr. Howard could zip easily throughout the cavernous ManuCo warehouse on a motorized scooter. Even if he no longer lifts heavy boxes, he could perhaps deliver mail or handle smaller items. Mr. Howard spoke at length about his dispute with ManuCo:

> My case is pending right now. My lawyers are fighting to get me long-term disability from ManuCo. They say I didn't get hurt at the job, but this is what happened. My foot got hurt at ManuCo, and I went out on [workers'] compensation. I missed days, OK? So

ManuCo says to me, "Mr. Howard, we got plenty of work for you." I said OK, and I went back to work on crutches. I went to work every day, on crutches, never missed one day. . . .

Then the ManuCo doctor said that the plant is so big and huge, the walking distances are so long. So he put me on four hours a day because he said the walking was too much. We did that for maybe about a month, then I went back on full-time floor duty. . . . But my foot swelled up so bad, I couldn't get my sneakers on, so the doctor told the bosses I couldn't do that job no more. He said I could do something if I could sit down—that I would work as much time as they want. . . .

Then one day, they met with me at the office, and they told me they didn't have nothing else for me to do. They was letting me go. So, I says, "After all this time, you firing me?" They said, "Oh, no, we're not firing you. We're just letting you go." Well, what's the difference? I'm calling it firing; he's calling it letting me go. So, they gave me what they called short-term disability. They paid me for maybe a month and half, and then they cut me off. For about two months, I didn't have no money coming in. So my lawyers fought that. . . .

I didn't ask to be let go. I don't think that's fair to me. They said, "Mr. Howard, we just got nothing for you to do." Well, they got plenty for me to do. OK? They said, "You can go somewhere else to get another job." I said, "Let me ask you a question. If I tell you I worked for another company and they let me go, would you hire me? You let me go. Who else is going to hire me?"

The majority of working-age people with mobility problems do not receive SSDI or SSI. As they and other people with disabilities venture into the labor market—and as SSDI and SSI recipients consider entering the work force—they face three major barriers: discrimination and inadequate workplace accommodations; inadequate training; and perverse incentives built into the system, such as the threat of losing health insurance. These issues are complex and in discussing them here, I do not touch on vocational rehabilitation, which is infrequently offered to people with progressive chronic diseases.[13]

WORKPLACE RIGHTS AND ACCOMMODATIONS

Employment discrimination related to disability differs in fundamental ways from other causes.

> Seldom do race, sex, or national origin present any obstacle to an individual when performing a job or participating in a program. Disabilities by their very nature, however, may make certain jobs or

types of participation impossible. Compounding this difficulty is the fact that both disabilities and jobs vary widely. Although an individual . . . may not be able to perform one type of job, he or she may be eminently qualified for another. In addition, unlike discrimination on the basis of race, sex, or national origin, discrimination against persons with disabilities is more often motivated, not by ill will, but rather by thoughtlessness or by ignorance of an individual's abilities. (Jones 1991, 30)

Mobility difficulties preclude some occupations, and they are generally impossible to hide. So employers' first impressions of prospective employees with mobility problems must compete with long-standing stereotypes about what is possible (McCarthy 1988). Early in his career, John Hockenberry was a freelance reporter for National Public Radio (NPR). Since he lived across the country from NPR's headquarters in Washington, D.C., nobody knew he used a wheelchair until he missed a deadline. Hockenberry needed to file a story by 5:00 P.M., but "there were no pay phones anywhere other than the old-style phone booths. I tried to get into one and failed. The only way would be to get out of the chair, but then I would be far too low to reach the phone" (1995, 168). By the time he found a telephone, Hockenberry was too late, and his editor was unhappy.

> When I returned home the next day he telephoned and wanted to know why I hadn't called; why, he asked, had I let him down?
> Up until that moment I was just a voice on the phone to him; now he would have a picture. . . . "I missed my deadline because I couldn't get my wheelchair into the phone booth to file." I blinked at the ceiling and paused. There was no response, so I continued, "I looked everywhere for a pay phone I could use. When I found one, it was too late. I'm really sorry." My editor said something about not letting it happen again, then rang off.
> The cat was out of the bag. . . . Because of a phone booth I had come out of the closet, and I no longer knew what to expect. In the little logistical details of countless assignments I was the inventor of what was possible. . . . Until I missed that deadline, those truths were known by me alone. (169–70)

Hockenberry made his own accommodations to do his job. Recognized for the quality of his work, not his means of doing it, his career took off. Most wheelchair users, however, do not go incognito into their workplace, and typical jobs have more set routines and requirements than does freelance journalism. Even Hockenberry could have benefited from workplace accommodations. When he moved to Washington, D.C., the men's room at

NPR "was narrow and small. The door was difficult to get through, there was no wide stall, and getting back out the door was most challenging of all" (176). In the office, "there was no room for even one person to turn around in a wheelchair" (174). He could only roll forward and backward.

Title I of the ADA bars discrimination against persons with disabilities in employment—hiring and firing, advancement, compensation, training, and benefits (Jones 1991).[14] The law applies to commercial entities with at least fifteen employees, requiring employers to provide "reasonable accommodations" that do not cause them "undue hardship" (Illingworth and Parmet 2000). Necessary accommodations vary by the nature of the disability. Progressive chronic conditions that wax and wane over time (such as rheumatoid arthritis or MS) pose different challenges than those with fixed functional deficits (such as an amputation). Arthritis, the most common cause of work loss, typically causes "morning stiffness, which makes getting up and out very difficult. During a flare, the person with arthritis may have to reduce work activities both to garner rest and to visit the doctor" (Yelin 1991, 142). As for Jimmy Howard, flexible schedules can substantially assist people with arthritis or other chronic conditions to work.

To help employers and others identify potential accommodations, the President's Committee on Employment of People with Disabilities sponsors the Job Accommodations Network (JAN).[15] The JAN's Internet web site contains over 250 links to disability-related information sources, as well as "accommodation ideas" for specific conditions, like arthritis, back problems, heart conditions, and wheelchair use. The MS page lists dozens of potential accommodations, such as those requested by Sally Ann Jones, whose pre-ADA employer was very accommodating:

> I worked in an old building. The parking lot would fill up with people. I made them designate a parking spot for me so I wouldn't have to walk so far, which they did cheerfully. There were no other designated spots back then. The first year I worked there, my office was on the second floor, and the women's toilet was on the first floor. I said, "Guys, we have to reverse these toilets," which they did in a second and didn't complain about it. Then the building had half a dozen stairs at the front, but there was no handrail. So I went to the dean and said, "You got to put a handrail up. I have to haul myself up these stairs." So they did that for me. Then, my doctor insisted I had to have an air-conditioned office, so they bought a little air conditioner. I was the only person who had air conditioning, so everybody was in my office all the time. And the last thing was, I couldn't do the damn stairs to the second floor anymore. So I moved my office to the first floor, then they reversed the bathroom again.

In the mid 1990s Lester Goodall's Fortune 500 company finally made minor changes to improve access to their building in Boston's financial district: they installed an automatic opener on the heavy front door. When I visited, it didn't work—a common occurrence, according to Lester. Disputes continue about the costliness of reasonable accommodations and whether these expenses affect an employer's willingness to hire workers needing accommodation (Young 2000).[16] Lonnie Carter, the disability activist, was convinced that "companies don't want to take us because they've got this idea that they've got to build something. For me, all they have to do is give me a chair." According to the JAN, accommodation costs average $200 (Stein 2000, 198). Improving physical access for wheelchair users *is* generally the most expensive accommodation (Chirikos 1991), but it is not always costly. Wooden ramps to surmount one or two stairs can cost only a few hundred dollars.

Despite the ADA's lofty aspirations, its moral authority, and the booming economy of the late 1990s, unemployment among persons with disabilities remained high ten years after the law's passage (Batavia 2000; Blanck 2000; Stein 2000). Why is unclear. Numerous studies from the past fifty years have found comparable overall productivity among workers regardless of disability, and disabled workers are more likely than others to stay with their jobs. The law professor Andrew Batavia knew that Title I of the ADA does not require affirmative action in hiring disabled workers.

> An employer who is intent upon rejecting an applicant with a disability is likely to find ways in which to do so without being subjected to the substantial risk of a lawsuit. It is difficult to conceive of a law that would be politically feasible and would induce an otherwise recalcitrant employer to hire such an applicant. (2000, 289)

Hints of discrimination are often subtle, leaving no tangible trace. A few years ago, a colleague at a large university asked me to consider a senior academic position. I agreed and was invited to visit by the surgeon leading the recruitment. A few days before the visit, I called the surgeon's secretary to remind her that my meeting locations must be wheelchair accessible. Embarrassed silence ensued: the secretary and surgeon hadn't known; my colleague hadn't told them. The visit was scheduled, and I came—the university's brochure asserted prominently that they are an equal opportunity employer. But from the outset, the surgeon barely looked me in the eye, he did not seriously discuss details of the job, and he hurried from our last encounter without saying good-bye. I never heard from him again. I know that I was qualified for that job, and I know that my wheelchair rattled the surgeon. But how could I prove this? "The surgeon didn't look me in the eye or say good-bye?" Hardly definitive—and I'd sound silly saying it.

Gerald Bernadine's case was more obvious. In the early 1990s, he was managing a large law firm when he was diagnosed with MS. His walking difficulties were already apparent.

> I went to the people at my law firm and said, "Look, I'm telling you right up front that I have MS. This is a major league illness, and before we go any further, I am authorizing you to talk to my physician to find out the full extent of this illness and how it may affect my job. After you do that, let's sit down and talk about where we go from here." So they talked to my doctor—he was one of their clients.
>
> They came back to me and said, "Gerald, we're going to do whatever you need. Any problems, anything we can do to make it easier for you, just let us know." That all sounded great; I felt great. I went back to my work with renewed energy, positive attitude. And what happened over those next six months was that I kept getting more and more work piled on me. No accommodations. They made me supervise four floors of office space in another building downtown. They could have had somebody else do that—it wasn't even in my job description. They were not doing things to make it easier. The firm was going through tough times, and because I was a manager, I had to go through the tough times with them. Of course, my walking kept getting worse. . . . They called me one Monday morning and told me it wasn't working out, and that I was fired. . . .
>
> They gave me these release papers to sign because I had an employment contract with a severance clause. They would pay my severance pay, but only on the condition that I sign the release of liability—that I'd promise I would never sue them. . . . I said, "Let me tell you something, if I was on my death bed, I wouldn't sign those papers." And so, within a week, I was out of there.

Mr. Bernadine sued the firm for "failure to offer accommodation. It wasn't like I couldn't do things. I just needed them to make it easier for me. Put my office closer to the men's room, give me a more flexible schedule. They wouldn't do a thing." In court, the employers argued extenuating financial distress, but Gerald's accommodation requests required minimal, if any, expenditures. "It all came out in court. One guy basically told the jury, 'Hey look, our butts were up against the wall. We were losing money. Our company was in trouble. We didn't have time to screw around with this accommodation stuff.' " The firm offered Mr. Bernadine $3 million to settle; on principle, he refused. Although the court awarded him slightly less, that didn't faze him. He had proven his point: people with disabilities have rights.

WELFARE, WORK, AND MOBILITY AIDS

Several interviewees worried that disability-related income might be welfare—something they don't like. But if they can't work, for whatever reason, they need the money. Myrtle Johnson articulated her ambivalence:

> When I grew up, my parents always taught us you don't take welfare and you don't take charity. You work for what you get. It was a different world. I grew up feeling that you can manage if you know what to do. This country is here for you, but you have to know what to do.

Mrs. Johnson feels she's paid her dues and programs exist for people like her to use.

At one focus group, participants expressed few concerns about accepting income support. "We're all independent and we like our independence for as long as possible," Jackie stated. "I don't feel that we should put the burden on the family. I think we should put it on the system, which should be there to help us. We are U.S. citizens, we pay our taxes, we have a disability. It is out there. There shouldn't be no question about people with disabilities." Others nodded.

"When it came to my disability, I filled out the papers," said Eva, referring to her SSA application. "I went to a hearing. I went before a judge, and they denied me. Then my doctor went, and I got disability right away."

"People say that if you're on disability, you're really poor, you don't deserve it," observed Salvador. "I felt the same way, but then I thought about it. I said, look, I started working at sixteen years old and didn't stop until a couple of years ago. Even the rich get disabled. People in Wellesley get Social Security, too." Salvador referred to an affluent suburb. He's probably right—Wellesley residents get SSDI, too.

Although I did not perform formal assessments, some interviewees receiving SSDI, SSI, or private disability pensions seemed willing and able to work, albeit not using their legs. Once people obtain SSDI or SSI, however, substantial disincentives conspire against their returning to work (U.S. General Accounting Office 1996a, 1996b, 1997a). Fear of losing health insurance (Medicare or Medicaid) predominates. The yes/no disability determination process (either you can or you cannot work) forces people to accentuate their debilities and minimize their abilities. Over the years, various incentive programs have aimed to motivate work by maintaining cash payments, medical benefits, and program eligibility during work attempts (U.S. General Accounting Office 1996a, 1996b). But overall, these programs have failed to return large numbers of people to work.

For people with impaired walking, mobility aids can help. Scooter-less, I would be unable to work and would easily qualify as disabled under current SSA (1998) criteria. Nevertheless, as noted earlier, Social Security does not fund purchases of wheelchairs or other assistive technologies.[17] Medicare coverage for assistive technology is limited; Medicaid coverage varies and is state-specific, but it is typically more generous than Medicare. While vocational rehabilitation programs supposedly assess clients for assistive devices that could restore employment, SSDI and SSI recipients are not systematically evaluated for technological fixes, such as power wheelchairs. Very few people receive special aids or technologies for vocational rehabilitation: 8 percent of persons with major mobility problems; and 2 percent of those with minor and moderate difficulties.[18]

After Gerald Bernadine was fired from his job, he found part-time work as a teaching assistant at a local college. "It takes a lot of energy to get ready to teach, to get in here. This place is really big. By the time I got home, I was dead." Gerald wanted a scooter, but couldn't afford one. He and his wife lived on her earnings, awaiting the verdict in his lawsuit. "It was just a question of money—I had limited funds. So I waited till we had some dough, and I ended up with this scooter. And now that I have it, I love it." These days, Gerald cruises the campus with few complaints.

GETTING AROUND

Harry Halpern's wife, daughter, and physician decreed that he should no longer drive because of his physical frailty and, perhaps, growing concerns about his mental acuity (chapter 5). The precipitating incident was Harry's fall out of bed: "I didn't even realize I had fallen! My wife got the police to come down, as they always do, and put me back in bed." Esther Halpern doesn't drive because of her painful back: "I will drive again. I used to drive all the time, but I just don't feel safe—yet!" So the Halperns now stay at home, isolated, except when their daughter takes them out or when a volunteer from the local cancer support network drives them to medical appointments. Shortly after our interview, Mr. Halpern ended his long-term relationship with his oncologist because the volunteer could no longer drive him into Boston. He switched to a physician nearer home.

For almost a century, cars and driving have been national obsessions. While walking symbolizes independence within our personal microenvironments, cars extend independence beyond distant horizons. Driving represents control and mastery, the ultimate in mobility. Beyond its symbolic import, driving also has immediate practical utility. Increasing physical distances separating shops, work, home, friends, and family complicate daily life for people who do not drive. Harry Halpern couldn't get his hair cut, and now he has changed his physician.

> Patients who forgo driving often lose independence, compromise their ability to work and provide for their dependents, and have difficulty maintaining social contacts, continuing involvement in personal interests, and participating in community activities. These losses have profound implications for many patients in terms of emotional and physical well-being, quality of life, and evaluation of self-worth. (Berger et al. 2000, 667)

No hard and fast rules delineate when people should stop driving, although this question increasingly vexes local governments and physicians as the population ages. Crash rates for drivers 15 to 19 years old exceed those for persons 85 and older (2,000 versus 1,500 per 100 million miles). Because of their physical frailty, however, drivers over age 85 have 2.5 times higher death rates per mile driven than the youngest drivers (Berger et al. 2000, 667). Physician organizations, such as the American Medical Association, have tried specifying legal and ethical obligations of physicians to report persons who should no longer drive, but these efforts have proved controversial. Physicians fear breaching patients' confidentiality, and medical contraindications to driving (apart from severe dementia, like Alzheimer's disease, and very low vision) are not clear-cut. Only a few states require physicians to report impaired drivers.

Driving ability relating to progressive chronic conditions varies widely from person to person. One study of older persons found walking speed and distance had no effect on motor vehicle incidents, although limited neck rotation significantly heightened risks (Marottoli et al. 1998). Another study assessed driving abilities of people with arthritis and back problems (Jones, McCann, and Lasser 1991). Almost everybody could drive safely and comfortably after making simple adaptations, such as moving from manual to automatic transmissions and using special seating cushions. Older people who stop driving often become depressed (Marottoli et al. 1997).

Among people with major mobility difficulties, 48 percent say they never drive, compared to 32 percent with mild problems.[19] Of those who never drive, 67 percent of people with major mobility difficulties attribute this to their health condition, as do 42 percent with moderate and 35 percent with mild mobility impairments. Some interviewees had completely abandoned driving, although several older women had never learned. ("I always depended on other people," admitted Mildred Stanberg, a widow. "I baked a lot and people came over for my baking. I would ask if they minded taking me one place or another.") Those who had stopped worried about safety, as does Esther Halpern. "When I drove that car," observed one woman with arthritis, "my legs hurt so bad I wasn't paying attention to the driving." Sometimes people only take a hiatus from driving. Now chauffeured by their wives, several men asserted that they will someday reclaim the driver's seat. In most instances, however, interviewees devise ways to make driving easier and safer, and they still drive.

Still Driving . . . and Parking

Tina DiNatale, whose MS causes profound fatigue, knows her physical limits. When I made the appointment to visit, she inquired about my beverage and food preferences, anxious to be a good hostess. I urged her not to prepare refreshments, but she was embarrassed to offer nothing.

> If I feel I can drive, I will drive, if I have to. For example, today, I really would have liked to have pastry. I would have to make a mental decision as to what the trade-off would have been. Did I feel like driving? Today I could have, because I've been up since 6:30. So I could have done it. What I would have done, since I have trouble walking, is call the bakery and have them make an assortment of Italian pastries, because I'm of Italian descent. You know, the little miniatures. Most stores have been pretty accommodating. They would bring the pastries out to me.

People time their trips, driving off–peak traffic hours or only during daylight or good weather. They parse their trips, doing a little each day. Irene Foster, the oldest interviewee, is ninety-three; she uses a four-point cane because of arthritis and neuropathy: "Fortunately, even at this age, I can drive a car. But I limit myself. I'll go, for instance, to the bank and that's it. And then another day I might go to the hairdresser. So I am limited, but on the other hand, I can still get around."

Some people find technological solutions, such as vans with wheelchair lifts and hand controls for acceleration and braking (Scherer 2000; Karp 1999), although these are relatively rare. Even among people reporting major mobility difficulties, only 6 percent say their cars have special equipment.[20] Heavy-duty large vans or trucks are necessary to transport massive power wheelchairs, but scooters and smaller power wheelchairs fit readily into trunks of mid-size sedans or minivans. Various companies adapt minivans for wheelchair access, such as installing kneeling systems that lower vans toward the ground and reduce the slope of ramps. Walter Masterson still drove: "The van has manual controls. The driver's seat

backs up and pivots, so I can drive the wheelchair into the van, line up beside the driver's seat, transfer and then pull the driver's seat forward to the
wheel." Sally Ann Jones has a van but she cannot drive herself because of
equipment incompatibility: the scooter's configuration, with its steering
column up front, blocks access to the car's steering wheel. Someone else
drives her van for her.

When people arrive at their destinations, convenient parking becomes
paramount. All states issue permits—special license plates or placards that
hang from rearview mirrors or are placed on dashboards—which entitle
people to park in special spots designated by the stick-figure wheelchair
logo. Typically, physicians must complete applications for these permits,
certifying the medical conditions that impair mobility. The decision even to
apply for the permit is often complicated. Jimmy Howard voiced commonly held reservations:

> I never thought about myself as a handicapped. Never did. None of
> that in my blood. Then Dr. Barton says to me, "Do you have a hand-
> icapped plate?" I says, "For what? I'm not no handicapped." He says,
> "Yes, you are. You have arthritis." I didn't make no comment on it at
> that time. Then I thought about it and told my wife about it. She
> said I should get a handicapped plate, but I still didn't want to. Then
> one day I got frustrated and couldn't find a place to park. The next
> day, I had the appointment with Dr. Barton, and I got the applica-
> tion. It took maybe a month, and then I got my handicapped plate.

At one focus group, participants wondered whether their mobility problems are severe enough to warrant handicapped parking permits, even
though they feel they need them. They see others who are worse off, but
they also find people abuse the privilege. Cynthia Walker wonders how
strangers would view her:

> I don't have a handicapped plate on my car. Some days I don't need
> one; other days I would love to have one. . . . To look at me some-
> body would say, "Oh, yeah. You're really a cripple, aren't you?" You
> don't see me at night. My day begins and ends on crutches, quite lit-
> erally. Most of the time, I don't feel I deserve one because I see
> many people far worse off than myself. But once in awhile, on a
> flare day, when my husband's traveling and the baby needs formula,
> and I just can't maneuver the crutches and the child at the same
> time, I would love to have it.

Sometimes physicians urge people to get a permit, even if they balk. "I
have a handicapped license plate," said Arnis Balodis. "Mitch made me get
one."

"Your doctor made you? Didn't you want one?"

"No. I had a very fast Chevrolet with a souped-up engine. If you drive at night, it's a clear sign you're somebody to pick on. You have no defense."

"Then why did you get the handicapped plate?"

"It started getting to me in the wintertime." Arnis had trouble walking on the snow on his bilateral leg prostheses.

Once people have plates or placards, the search begins for designated parking spots. Typically, parking marked by the wheelchair logo is close to buildings, and sometimes it is extrawide to accommodate vans and wheelchair lifts. But, "there are far more permits issued in many cities than there are reserved parking spots. The competition for space has become fierce" (Karp 1999, 459). Some worry that placards, in particular, are given to people with relatively minimal mobility problems. Regardless of the definition of those deserving handicapped parking spots, few disagree there are rarely enough. "When I didn't have a handicapped plate, the spot was always empty," laughed Jimmy Howard. "Now they're always full. I think it's very selfish of people to park in them if they aren't authorized to do it." Only a few interviewees reported confronting interlopers, restrained by endemic fears about approaching strangers. Walter Masterson wryly observed, "You compete for parking spots, and the closer into the center of Boston, the more you compete. There's not much respect for the handicapped parking spot."

"Why do you think that is?"

"Because, for one thing, there's not much parking in Boston anyway. Secondly, Boston drivers are anarchists, for which I admire them."

Getting On and Off the Bus

People who don't own cars often rely on public transportation. Over the last several decades, policies relating to public transportation for people with disabilities have flipped between two notions: "effective mobility" (providing transportation by varying means, even if separate from main systems) and "full accessibility" (creating a fully integrated transportation system for everybody).[21] The ADA extended the full accessibility concept beyond the public to the private sector, while aiming not to impose an "undue financial burden" (Katzmann 1991). Localities and companies need not retrofit existing buses with lifts, but all new buses purchased or leased must be accessible.

Transportation systems obviously reflect local terrains, policies, and populations, so each is unique. Around 55 percent of people report having accessible transportation services available in their areas, but far fewer have used it in the last year: 11 percent of people reporting mild, 16 percent with moderate, and 17 percent with major mobility difficulties.[22] However, about 11 percent of people with major and moderate mobility problems use public transportation almost every day.

Difficulty walking is the major impediment to using public transportation, followed by needing assistance from another person and problems boarding with wheelchairs or scooters.[23] Several interviewees said they no longer take buses because the drivers are impatient at their slowness getting on and off. Arnis Balodis found, "Everybody's rushing. Somebody wants to get off, so you have to jump. I can do it, but older people or weaker people—there's no way they'll get off the bus." One woman with arthritis observed that, on certain buses, drivers can lower the steps, but "some of them won't, even if they see you scuffling, trying to get up." Brianna Vicks, who uses a power wheelchair, finds that wheelchair lifts on buses are unreliable—sometimes they work, sometimes not. Similarly, elevators to underground subway stops periodically break down. Brianna therefore tries to ride her wheelchair where she needs to go—she doesn't want to get stuck.

Metropolitan Boston's demand-responsive, public system, the RIDE, generates strong emotions. With its fleets of large, heavy vans with automatic wheelchair lifts, the RIDE serves people who cannot manage the fixed route systems (buses, subways) alone, or who need to go someplace the fixed route systems do not reach. Applicants for the RIDE must submit medical justifications from their physicians. For efficiency, the RIDE picks up multiple riders at the same time, so people often take numerous detours before reaching their final destinations. Not surprisingly, therefore, the major complaint about the RIDE involves delays, perceived as disrespect for people's time, compounded by the rudeness of drivers. Eleanor Peters uses a power wheelchair.

> There have been times when I have actually had to miss a doctor's appointment because of the RIDE. It may look bad on the patient, but it's definitely not our fault. The RIDE is a horrendous company to have to use, and I have to use it every day, so I'm talking experience. I always tell them that I have to be places a half hour earlier than I really do, and they still sometimes either get me there late or they don't get me there at all. So the RIDE can be a real nightmare if you have to rely on it for medical appointments or school or work. And I use it for all three.

Other interviewees are more forgiving. "The RIDE's been very good for me," said Myrtle Johnson, who does have fewer fixed obligations than Eleanor Peters. "A lot of people complain about it, but there's thousands of people that use it. Sometimes people have big heavy wheelchairs that take forever to hook up and strap down. So the RIDE comes late! If you don't complain and are nice to them, they're very good to you. They get me places late a lot of times, but I'm not going to yell at the driver. He's not out there having a good time."

ACCESSING PUBLIC SPACES

Finally, many of our nation's public spaces remain inaccessible, with absent curb cuts, inoperative or missing automatic door openers, stairs without elevators or lifts, and other physical impediments. Years will elapse before spaces become as accessible as they can be, spurred by the ADA, state and local laws, and other public initiatives. Describing the full extent of physical barriers and ongoing efforts to remove them is beyond my scope here. But before moving on, I must emphasize that all health-care settings are not yet fully and easily accessible, even those built after the ADA. Justice Department investigations have found persistent problems with physical access to health-care facilities (President's Advisory Commission 1997).

Eleanor Peters and her fellow focus group participants Michael and Jamie and Bobby (all wheelchair users) go to the same academic hospital-based outpatient center, which opened in the mid 1990s. The architect and builders complied with the letter of the ADA, but even for hospital facilities, the ADA requires only that access be technically feasible—not necessarily easy. "The doors to the clinic are crazy," said Eleanor, referring to large plate-glass doors with shiny chrome handles but without automatic door openers. "They are so heavy, I can't open them."

"I went to the bathroom, and like you say, the doors are so heavy," Bobby reported. "I couldn't get out of the bathroom. I thought, oh my God, I'm going to have to stay here until somebody comes in."

"We're just disabled people, and we need to be at home in our houses," Eleanor parodied public views. "We don't need to be going out and having fun and traveling in the community."

Stella Richards goes to the same outpatient center, and she did not mince words: "That new clinic is too much. It's not handicapped accessible. The doors are too narrow, about this wide," Stella gestured with her hands, "and my chair just barely fits through it. You can't even get into the Starbuck's coffee shop if you're in a wheelchair. All you can do is sit there and smell it. They could have put a window there that people in wheelchairs and on walkers could walk up to and get a cup of coffee. . . .

"They need to do that building over again. They've left out a lot of things, like railings on the wall you can hold onto. They're supposed to cater to handicapped people. Handicapped people don't need special privileges, but the hospital should make it easy for them to get around. They've made it so hard. If I didn't have good doctors, I'd go somewhere else, somewhere they cater to sick people." Since then the hospital has tried hard to patch some of these problems, which thoughtful design in the first place could have prevented.

8   People Talking to Their Physicians

"Everyone who is born holds dual citizenship, in the kingdom of the well and in the kingdom of the sick," wrote Susan Sontag (1990, 3). "Although we all prefer to use only the good passport, sooner or later each of us is obliged, at least for a spell, to identify ourselves as citizens of that other place." Sontag argues that, when ill, we should remain unencumbered by "punitive or sentimental fantasies concocted" about living with illness. Her advice certainly applies when walking fails. Preconceptions about using wheelchairs, for example, typically convey dismal dependence and limited lives. Actual experiences often differ significantly from these unhappy expectations.

For people with progressive chronic impairments, Sontag's term "illness" holds layered meanings. According to Dr. Melinda Whittier, a physiatrist, "By and large, people with walking problems have some disease process. Trouble with walking is not normal." Yet "illness" suggests active disease. In contrast, for people with chronic conditions, physical function can decline slowly over years or decades. Some people rarely feel acutely ill, as they would with a high fever or asthma attack. Depending on the underlying cause, conditions can wax and wane, with flares and remissions. Nevertheless, at some point, almost everybody seeks medical attention, having their passports stamped by the gatekeeper of the kingdom of the sick—the physician.

Sally Ann Jones, now in her mid fifties, traces early MS symptoms to age nineteen. Over the decades, her MS has periodically flared, confining her to bed and hospitalizing her once or twice. Between times, she doesn't feel ill. She has physical difficulties, not illness: "I just can't stand up." Mrs. Jones has popped back and forth across the borders of Sontag's kingdoms, with physicians' pronouncements marking major transitions. The first and arguably most important was being diagnosed with MS in her early thirties. Mrs. Jones had visited her general practitioner complaining of weakness and numbness in her legs. "He said I was working and had two children. I was exhausting myself. If I would just change my lifestyle a bit, I would get better." When she returned three years later still symptomatic, the general practitioner "threw up his hands" and sent her to a neurologist.

"The neurologist looked me over—he was a very cold and clinical man—and he said, 'I don't think you have MS.' Now I hardly knew what MS was—it was one of those poster diseases, somebody sitting in a wheelchair. I was so elated that I didn't have MS." Four months later, symptoms persisting, she returned to the neurologist. "The doctor spent about a minute and a half with me, and then he said, 'The bad news is, Mrs. Jones, you have MS. The good news is, when I saw you before, I wrote down three potential diagnoses in my notes. If you'd had either of the other two diagnoses, you'd be dead by now.' . . . And with that, he left. He didn't talk to me about what to do. He didn't say, 'Do X.' He didn't say, 'Come back in six weeks.' He just left. Period. He spent about ten minutes, beginning to end."

This happened almost thirty years ago, when little was available medically to treat MS. Today's immunologic therapies, which slow disease progression for some patients, were years away. Nevertheless, those first encounters shaped Mrs. Jones's opinion of physicians: "General doctors don't want to bother with MS. Even though MS affects your whole body, general doctors don't know what to do about it. They don't have the expertise." Focused on clinical technicalities, neurologists have never initiated conversations about her walking. Sally Ann herself requested physical therapy, and Chet researched scooters. "I have this thing about neurologists. I don't expect them to be people people, so I cut them a lot of slack. . . . The neurologist I go to now is a sweet man. I'm on him relentlessly—I call, I fax." Since she fell, Mrs. Jones has had trouble standing and pivoting; she needs assistance using the toilet and has hired home help. "The neurologist says, 'You've still got help at home? God! That's expensive and must make you crazy.' He didn't say another word. Now if I can't stand and pivot, how the hell can I go to the bathroom? Actually, he doesn't think, not about the practical things."

People with progressive chronic diseases need physicians to diagnose and treat their underlying disorders and secondary conditions. Effective, even if not curative, medical and surgical therapies now exist for many people with impaired mobility, including new pain medications and joint replacement surgery for arthritis. Treatment, such as clot-dissolving drugs administered soon after strokes, can lessen or prevent debility. For diabetes or heart or lung diseases, medical interventions can acutely save, prolong, and improve the quality of lives. People must tell physicians about signs and symptoms of their diseases to benefit from medical knowledge.

Should people talk to physicians about their physical limitations and the consequences for daily life? How can physicians help? These two questions may seem odd. Of course, physicians should work to improve physical functioning and appreciate how diseases affect people's daily routines. After all, "the purpose of the health care system must be to continuously reduce the impact and burden of disease, injury and disability, and to improve the health and functioning of the people of the United States" (President's Advisory Commission 1998, 60). Admittedly, no cures or long-term effective treatments exist for MS, ALS, Parkinson's disease, intractable pain, and numerous chronic conditions that impair mobility. But reducing the burden of disease should remain a viable goal.[1]

Many physicians view the paucity of medical options as a hopeless situation. "Chronically ill or disabled people being cared for by action-oriented professionals who thrive on dramatic results may be at special risk for this reaction" (Barnard 1995, 54). Medicine cannot reverse established physical debilities or cure MS, for example, and physicians grow frustrated because they can't make people with MS "normal." However, "when we insist that every human problem can be solved, and normalcy restored, failure is inevitable. The result is usually fear, anger, or the pretense that the differences do not exist or do not matter" (Douard 1995, 172). Many physicians do not think about the end goal—safe, independent movement, regardless of whether people use their own legs—and options outside standard medical and surgical interventions. Even when they cannot walk, people need not be immobilized. Ambulation aids and wheeled mobility technologies can effectively reopen the world when walking fails (chapters 11 and 12).

Chapters 8 through 10 present competing viewpoints and expectations complicating relationships between people with mobility difficulties and their physicians and other health-care professionals. I do not describe specific clinical treatments but focus instead on roles, expectations, and communication around mobility.

WHAT PEOPLE EXPECT FROM PHYSICIANS

Eleanor Peters had polio as a small child and now uses a power wheelchair. She knows what she wants from physicians.

> They have to listen to us. We may not know every little intricate thing about medicines and different diseases. But I know my body. I know when there's something that's not right. I know when some-

thing's hurting; I know where the pain is. If something's not right, I'm going to go to the doctor, and I expect them to listen to me and tell me something to do. If they don't listen to us, then we're not going to get the quality of services that we should. We don't need to be intimidated by a doctor or a nurse. They're just people, too.

Eleanor says that her physicians "are fine. They listen to me." But as described in chapter 12, despite her frequent falls, Eleanor's physician initially opposed prescribing a power wheelchair, approving the equipment only after "a little bit of fighting." Although Eleanor is an exemplary "empowered consumer," her satisfaction with her doctors highlights their help on urgent issues. Perhaps Eleanor has low expectations of physicians assisting with daily mobility, so she momentarily forgot the tussle over the wheelchair. Certainly, she doesn't ask her doctors for a cure: "I love my wheelchair. I wouldn't trade my life for anything."

Most people do expect their physicians to treat their chronic diseases. Expectations around mobility, however, fall into several categories—some high, others low.

"I Wanted X Rays"

For four years, Harry Halpern was frustrated that physicians could not diagnose why Esther "wasn't walking right." Mr. Halpern joined actively in his wife's many appointments, often describing them in the first person, as if he were the patient. When Esther finally saw a specialist at a Boston teaching hospital, "I spoke to his secretary and said exactly what I wanted."

"What did you want, Mr. Halpern?"

"I wanted an explanation of what has transpired. I wanted X rays. Any jerk can come along and pull the fingers." Mr. Halpern obviously found neurologic examinations unhelpful. "I've had that done several times, and I don't want to see it anymore. They should have had X rays. It was a fiasco." Nonetheless, the physician did diagnose Esther's spinal condition.

People need an explanation—a medical explanation—for why they have trouble walking. It validates that the problem is "real," not "all in their head" or a fundamental character flaw, like laziness. Preferably the explanation involves pictures: people literally see exactly what is wrong. Myrtle Johnson insisted on viewing the degeneration in her knee before agreeing to joint replacement. During arthroscopy, a fiberoptic scope enters the knee joint and transmits pictures on a screen in the operating room.

I had an arthroscopy, and the pictures showed all the deterioration. It showed me everything that was happening. I wouldn't have it any other way: I have to see the whole thing. After I saw it, I understood it. That leg wasn't gonna hold; it really wasn't. My weight didn't help. So the surgeon put in a total knee replacement, but then all the pain came back again. So I had a second arthroscopy, and it showed that something was out of line where they put in the prosthesis. They had to open it and fix it again. Now it's getting better. I don't have that intense pain anymore.

"I Didn't Feel the Doctor Was Going to Help Me"

"Have you talked to Dr. Rich about your walking difficulties?" I asked Margaret Freemont, the emeritus professor.

"Not really. It never occurred to me."

"Why not?"

"I guess they don't know much about it. Dr. Rich is very good about medications. That's something I can talk to her about. She seems very up-to-date on what is happening in MS research, the latest articles in medical journals. She's very nice, very sweet. But she's a neurologist. She's interested in what she can do for me." Based on Dr. Rich's perceived interest and expertise, Dr. Freemont raised standard medical topics (although no medical therapies could actually improve her relatively severe MS), while ignoring mobility (her most important daily concern). As another woman explained, "I just didn't feel the doctor was going to help me."

The corollary problem is that many physicians don't raise the issue either. One woman with arthritis who uses a cane said that her primary care physician never seems to notice it: "He ain't said nothing to me about my cane. Never." Mary Sanderson described her new primary care doctor:

> I started with a new doctor last summer, and I forgot at first to tell him about the arthritis. I've lived with it for so long, I just didn't even think of it. He told me to get up on the examining table, and I looked at him and said, "I may need help. I have arthritis in my knees." He didn't ask anything about the arthritis. I think if I had pushed it, he would send me to a specialist. But I feel as though, at this point, a doctor isn't really going to do anything for me that I want. With the exercise I'm doing, I'm probably as well off as I could be.

Nelda Norton feels that Tom's neurologist neglects key questions: "Tom goes to a neurologist maybe once a year, and the neurologist always says, 'You're just the same as you were. You're still doing just fine.' But Tom's walking has deteriorated a great deal." Nelda turned to Tom, "Has he seen you walk? Has he ever asked you: 'Did you come in by yourself? Did you drive by yourself?' He keeps saying, 'You're doing just fine.' I'm not saying they're purposely not doing anything. I don't think they have anything else to offer." Nelda shook her head with frustration, "Zilch!"

Some physicians do raise the walking topic and try to help. Mildred Stanberg, in her late eighties and afraid of falling, never broached walking with her physician. After she bought a cane at a local drug store and carried it to her next appointment, the physician noticed it—he adjusted the cane's height and told her how best to use it. Stella Richards insisted that Dr. Johnny Baker, her primary care physician, circle the clinic with her as she pushed her walker. He went willingly, and Mrs. Richards felt it "opened his eyes" to the difficulties she faced. Nevertheless, Mrs. Richards remained in terrible pain, still using the walker two years later. "Do you talk to Dr. Baker about walking these days?" I asked.

"Oh, not much. Not much at all."

"Why not?"

"Because really there's nothing to talk about. I'm not getting too much help with the walking."

"Not Sympathy, But Empathy"

"What do you expect from your doctors?" I asked.

"Empathy," responded Michael, a scooter user with arthritis. "Not sympathy, but empathy, understanding, and asking me questions." Interviewees want their physicians to listen, respect, believe, and understand their problems, even if no medical treatment exists. For Cynthia Walker, listening is only a first step; understanding must follow. Mrs. Walker recently changed physicians, and she worries about her new rheumatologist.

> I don't feel heard as a patient sometimes. I'm not one to just scream and complain. I want to work with this doctor and make my situation better. My insurance is set up that I am forced to work with this doctor. . . . [And] our conditions are so incredibly emotionally draining. Unless you have a similar experience, a doctor that hasn't, if you forgive the expression, "walked in our shoes," can't have the sensation of sympathy or understanding on that level. In order to instill the power of positive thinking to go on, you have to be listened to first. I mean, we're all children at heart. We need a little praise; we need a little understanding—an ear, if you will. And sometimes a person in the medical profession is more interested with moving the cattle through.

Lester Goodall believes that physicians feel they are failing people with chronic, incurable conditions, prompting some doctors to build barriers between themselves and their patients. "My neurologist is one of the best doctors I've dealt with," Mr. Goodall asserted. "She's heavily involved in research on MS. I feel sometimes that she keeps herself at arm's length. When I ask her how I can get better, she can't tell me any more than the man on the street. She doesn't have the answers. They can give you the clinical diagnosis, but they can't make you better." Mr. Goodall senses that physicians feel this way when "there's no magic bullet. There's no pill they can give us to stop the pain. Sometimes we start transferring our aggression toward them. They feel for us, but they can't do anything. If she could push a button and make me better, I'm sure she would. But she's not a magician."

"We Learn That Nobody's Normal"

Many people hold onto hopes of getting better, of not getting worse. Few interviewees, however, expect their physicians to raise or sustain these hopes. Perhaps it's a question of timing. Most interviewees had had their chronic conditions for years. Around the time of diagnosis, especially for diseases with widely varying clinical courses (some people do well, others do poorly), hopeful physicians can buoy spirits and help people confront the new uncertainty of their lives. Candy Stoops was diagnosed with myasthenia gravis in her late twenties, and she asked Dr. Gold, her neurologist, many questions. "You know the old saying, 'Will I be normal?' We learn that nobody's normal. You look at what you're going to be able to do. Dr. Gold said, 'You'll have more kids. You're going to do this; you're going to do that.' She was very, very supportive."

Now ten years later, her hopes and desires have evolved, along with her sense of self. Candy knows her disease, and she no longer relies on her neurologist to predict her future. "There are days when I think, that's it! Can't do this. Can't walk this far. I'm tired. But I'm stronger than I thought. I have a really good attitude about everything that's happened to me. There are people who are worse off, much worse off, and they're doing it."

ACCESS TO PHYSICIANS

The vast majority of people with mobility difficulties have a physician. Among people age sixty-five and older, about 95 percent (regardless of mobility difficulties) have a source of care they usually visit when sick. So do roughly 90 percent of persons age eighteen to sixty-four years with mobility difficulties, compared to only 81 percent without mobility impairments.[2] Very few people with mobility difficulties have not seen a physician in the last year (Table 11). Older people are more likely than younger people to see physicians, and rates of doctor visits increase as mobility dif-

TABLE 11. Use of Health-Care Services

Mobility Difficulty	No Physician Visits in Last Year (%)		At Least One Hospitalization (%)	
	Age 18–64	Age 65+	Age 18–64	Age 65+
None	30	14	5	11
Minor	11	8	17	21
Moderate	8	6	23	26
Major	7	5	32	37

ficulties worsen.[3] Rates of hospitalizations also rise with increasing mobility problems, probably reflecting surgery (such as joint replacements) or treatment of underlying medical diseases or secondary conditions, like injuries from falls.[4]

Most people visit general medical doctors as their usual source of care.[5] As mobility problems worsen, however, more people use specialists as their usual source of care. Among persons age eighteen to sixty-four years with major mobility difficulties, 22 percent use specialists as their usual caregiver, compared to 4 percent of younger persons without impaired mobility.[6] Among persons under age sixty-five, being uninsured and unable to afford it is the major reason for not having a usual source of care (Table 12). Almost everybody at least sixty-five years old has Medicare insurance, so lacking coverage is rarely a problem for them.[7]

One provocative finding here involves people's attitudes toward physicians. Among persons age sixty-five and older, over 20 percent with major mobility difficulties report they don't like, trust, or believe in doctors, compared to 7 percent of persons without impaired mobility. Perhaps this gap reflects prior experiences and expectations—from patients' perspectives, physicians may have provided little help.

EXPERIENCES WITH PHYSICIANS

People visit their physicians with high expectations, seeking understanding, empathy, and respect; a listening ear that will hear what patients say no matter how long it takes; and a good communicator who will inform patients what can or cannot be done to address the problems they raise (Edgman-Levitan 1993; Gerteis et al. 1993; Kaplan and Sullivan 1996). Sicker

TABLE 12. Reason for Having No Usual Source
of Health Care

Mobility Difficulty	No Insurance/ Can't Afford It (%)		Doesn't Like, Trust, or Believe in Doctors (%)	
	Age 18–64	*Age 65+*	*Age 18–64*	*Age 65+*
None	19	3	3	7
Minor	39	5	7	9
Moderate	40	5	5	8
Major	27	6	10	20

people are often less satisfied with their physicians than healthier persons (Hall et al. 1996, 1998). Some people develop wonderful relationships with their physicians. "I really give Dr. Baker and Nurse Fyffe thanks," said Erna Dodd of Dr. Johnny Baker, her primary care physician, and his nurse practitioner colleague. "They always sit down and listen to me, and they always help me when I'm sick. I have my confidence in them. They've done more for me than some family."

Others are less positive. As Lester Goodall anticipated, perhaps part of the dynamic involves conflicting expectations between physicians and patients around chronic disease. Acute exacerbations of illness are straightforward. Physicians believe their job is to cure disease—or at least significantly improve its course—and, for many acute problems, they succeed. For chronic conditions, they frequently fail. Most patients, however, don't expect cures—they have often lived with diseases for years and are realistic. They'd like help dealing with the daily, physical, functional consequences, but many physicians don't know how to help. Consequently, people learn not to expect assistance from their physicians.

Ironically, however, health insurers typically require prescriptions from primary care or other physicians before paying for physical or occupational therapy or mobility aids (chapters 13 and 14). Therefore, the professional who is often least knowledgeable about improving mobility determines access to important services. Several common themes emerged as interviewees described experiences talking to physicians about mobility problems.

"They Just Didn't Listen"

Natalie Strong has cerebral palsy affecting only her legs. Since childhood she has walked, first without any assistance, then using crutches. A few years ago she began falling, injuring her knees, and her walking steadily worsened: she had developed a progressive chronic condition. The final fall—the one making her a wheelchair user for the foreseeable future—happened at work. Her boss deposited Natalie at the local emergency room (ER). Although her orthopedist was based at that hospital, the ER wouldn't call him. "The ER doctor didn't listen to the fact that I have CP and put me in an immobilizer," a device that straightened Natalie's knee and held it rigidly in place. "My knees are never straight! I'm sure that worsened the tear—I ended up going home with this immobilizer on my leg. They just didn't listen. I was in pain and panic-stricken. My boss dropped me off and ran. I had no one there to advocate for me."

Natalie concedes that "going to the emergency room was the wrong thing." By definition, ERs practice the ultimate in acute-care medicine and are appropriately preoccupied with saving lives. In ER calculus, Natalie's knee injury was low risk—of death. The ER doctor assumed he knew the right intervention, acted quickly, and moved Natalie out the door. By not listening to Natalie, however, the ER physician likely worsened her knee injury, perhaps increasing the possibility of permanent impairment.

Some interviewees equate not listening with arrogance. "Listening is incredibly important," observed Cynthia Walker. "Doctors shouldn't assume they know the whole story without listening. Every patient is unique and should be treated as such. Every doctor is also unique in their capabilities, too. However, they'd be far more capable if they'd be open to learning." Cynthia feels her rheumatologist didn't fully listen to her for years. "The doctor says, 'This is how it is. I know this because I'm a specialist, and I've learned this.' Your situation is not heard because he doesn't have time for you." Cynthia feels that her rheumatologist did little as rheumatoid arthritis destroyed her ankle joint. "It's three and a half years, and my ankle joint's gone."

"Actually, He Doesn't Think"

Sally Ann Jones's neurologist knew that she couldn't stand or pivot—maneuvers essential to using the toilet independently. Nevertheless, he professed surprise that she needs personal assistance at home. To Sally Ann, this was another example of physicians not considering the practical consequences of the impairments they carefully quantify during physical examinations. "Actually," said Sally Ann, "he doesn't think."

Sometimes physicians' pronouncements make little sense within people's daily experiences. S. Kay Toombs recounts: "My neurologist, in discussing the pros and cons of estrogen therapy to prevent osteoporosis, tells me that I do not need to worry about falling and breaking bones—because

I will not be able to stand up" (1995, 22). Without thinking, her neurologist may see Toombs as literally "confined" to her wheelchair, but of course she is not. Falls happen as people move in and out of wheelchairs to chairs, to beds, to toilets, to shower seats, to cars, and so on. Toombs probably now takes this neurologist's observations with circumspection.

Cynthia Walker concluded that, "You have to get information and learn as much about your own condition as you can. You can't expect your doctor to do it for you." Cynthia finds helpful information through the Internet. She doesn't always follow her physician's advice, particularly when it ignores practical realities. Her rheumatologist prescribed an orthotic or ankle brace: "It's an artificial way to fuse my joint to find relief when I'm walking." He told her to wear it twelve hours daily, but she wears it only six, afraid that longer use might cause her leg muscles to wither or atrophy. "Once those muscles are gone, they never come back. The doctor said to do exercises in bed at night to prevent atrophy. Well, the rheumatoid also affects your blood with anemia. You're very tired. I can't stay awake to do exercises for a half hour every night." Nonetheless, Cynthia worries about her decisions. "I force myself to use the foot and ankle. Now I have anxiety about losing my knee too quickly. In short, sometimes I feel that I am the doctor in practice, and he's the patient who's learning."

"You Just Have to Live with It"

Older people, in particular, can feel that physicians pay little heed to physical function problems generally associated with aging. Physicians minimize the difficulties and make few efforts to help. Gracie Brown, now in her mid seventies, had a knee that used to "ache, ache, ache all day, and all I did was rub it, rub it, rub it. So I told Dr. Greenberg [her primary care physician] about it. He says, ain't nothin' but artheritis in your knees." Gracie returned later, still in pain. "He told me to take Tylenol. That didn't help. So he said, 'Do you want it operated on?' I said, 'Would it help?' " She had her knee replaced. "See, it don't ache at all."

Mary Sanderson's primary care physician also dismissed her pain, attributing it to age although she was only fifty years old at the time.

> My joints started getting sore—probably twenty years ago. The doctor that I went to then passed it off for a few years: "Oh, it's just a little arthritis. You're getting older, and everybody has that. You just have to live with it." But after a few years, I thought there might be some more comfortable way to live with the arthritis. A friend at a Boston hospital gave me a recommendation for a doctor over there. I went, and he sent me to a physical therapist and gave me exercises and things that really helped me. He did as much as he needed to do

in two visits. Doctors really need to listen to the patients in the beginning. They shouldn't say, "Oh, that's nothing."

Mrs. Sanderson underscored something emphasized by many interviewees: that physicians should refer patients to specialists for problems outside
their expertise. People do not see referrals as admissions of inadequacy; they
know medical knowledge is vast and continually expanding. Referrals to
specialists show respect, concern, and a desire to do everything possible.
Some people are reluctant to ask for referrals, afraid of offending the doctor.
Mrs. Sanderson hadn't asked her physician for a referral—she just didn't
want to: "He was very upset when he found I had gone to another doctor.
He said, 'I would have sent you to someone.' I said, 'I know, but you didn't
offer so I found someone.' . . . I left that doctor because I didn't like that
kind of attitude."

"They Rush You In and Rush You Out"

Finally, almost everybody noted that clocks tick loudly in today's medical
encounters. Visits to physicians grow shorter and shorter as financial pressures mount. "I don't think they give you as much time as they should,"
said Anna. "They rush you. For most [other] black people I've seen, they
rush you in and rush you out. But I tell them what I'm feeling. I ask as
many questions as I can. I ask, but they seem to want to get away from me.
I ask them questions anyway."

This problem affects everybody, but people with progressive disabling
conditions and multiple ailments are especially vulnerable (Burns et al.
1990; Gans, Mann, and Becker 1993). People like Erna Dodd, who had emphysema, diabetes requiring insulin, congestive heart failure, seizures,
obesity, and arthritis, need considerable attention to manage active illness
(e.g., review medications, check for side effects and complications), let
alone talk about functioning daily at home. Ironically, addressing the full
range of health-related concerns may require multiple office visits for the
people least able to get around.

Beyond limited discussion times, shortened appointments have physical
consequences. Some people simply cannot move as quickly as the physician wants, for example, climbing onto examining tables. Andrea Banks, a
primary care physician, told me about a young man with cerebral palsy
whose aunt brings him to appointments in his wheelchair. The first few
visits Dr. Banks examined the patient in his wheelchair, thinking it would
be easier for him. She never asked the patient if he preferred to get onto the
examining table. The aunt complained to the nurse: "Dr. Banks never even
watches my nephew walk." Concerned about his worsening walking, they

wondered how Dr. Banks could evaluate it. Dr. Banks vowed to observe her patients walking, even if briefly. She ruefully acknowledged needing additional assistance to help people with mobility problems onto the examining table—assistance that consumes precious minutes.

Interviewees feel that being rushed can defeat the purpose of what's supposed to be a therapeutic interaction. "Just give the client a chance," said Nan, who has arthritis. "Be patient and understanding. Don't rush us: 'Hurry up, hurry up. Come on, come on. I'm watching the clock.' But we can't rush, so we get upset. If you stress the client out, then nothing's going to work. So be patient and be careful, be careful."

WHEN PAIN IS THE PROBLEM

Pain is the sentinel and steadfast symptom for perhaps the plurality of people with mobility problems (chapter 3). Talking about one's pain is difficult, whether with family, friends, co-workers, or physicians. Pain is a popular public topic much in the news recently, with highly publicized releases of new drugs, such as the controversial COX-2 (type 2 cyclooxygenase) inhibitors.[8] Controlling pain is a touchstone of the "death with dignity" movement. Drugs *do* exist to control even excruciating pain, drugs as old as the hills—narcotics, the descendants of opium.

The dark side of pain control involves complex societal and personal fears of addiction and its myriad, destructive consequences. People can feel trapped by societal and personal prejudices and misconceptions. "I need some pain pills," said Stella Richards. "Nobody wants to prescribe pain pills for you. If they do, they regulate them so you don't become addicted. I'm not one who abuses medicine. But nobody wants to give me any pain pills except silly things like Motrin, naprosyn. Those things don't help me. I don't want them anymore." Mrs. Richards visited a specialized pain clinic but got no relief.

Because of conflicting emotions, people find pain particularly difficult to discuss with physicians. "Sadly, pain continues to be one of the most feared and debilitating aspects of illness and medical treatment" (Walker 1993, 120). Mattie Harris is a case in point. Her arthritis pain feels like "bone rubbing against bone." I asked Ms. Harris to recount her conversations with her physicians about the pain.

"I went to my arthritis doctor about two weeks ago, and he told me, 'Mrs. Harris, I can't do anything else for you. I gave you all kinds of medicine.' I know from the way he's sitting there, just looking, that he doesn't believe me. I said, 'You think this is all in my mind? You think I'm crazy or something, that I'm not really in pain?' He said, 'No, I didn't say that. I believe you. But we can't do nothing else for you.' " Her primary care physician, Dr. Johnny Baker, sent her to the Pain Clinic, but nothing worked.

"So what are you going to do about the pain?"

"When you got kids, you got a house, things have to be done. I put up with it."

Some time later, I ran into Dr. Baker and asked him how Ms. Harris was doing. He looked at me sadly, "Not so well." Her pain was no better; there seemed nothing he could do. I could tell there was more, but I didn't ask, respecting her privacy. Ms. Harris had told me about many complexities in her life, including alcoholism. Yet part of her story and resultant anger seemed easy to read—Ms. Harris fits one oft-held stereotype of the "drug seeker," medical slang for people who want narcotics, presumably to feed addictions. She is black, poor, and alcoholic. And she knows these views well: "You gotta understand, where we live at, so many people is prejudiced, and they don't want no black people." Ms. Harris sees herself as a survivor.

Controlling pain is clearly complicated. For Mattie Harris, as for millions of others, no quick solution exists. Pain is a lonely state, outside the preferred medical paradigm of being easily quantified, measured objectively (by an outsider), visualized, or scanned. "Because I'm in pain," Ms. Harris said, "there's nobody knows what I go through and how I feel."

TAKING CONTROL

Lonnie Carter had lived with many medical conditions, starting with congenital hip disorders and extending through severe diabetes with numerous complications. Over the years, she learned to take charge of her body, teaching numerous physicians that she was in control. "Doctors have been wanting to grab me for years, and I refuse to let them touch my hip," said Lonnie. Her original hip operations occurred in childhood, over thirty years ago. Surgeons wanted to redo her hips with new technologies, but Lonnie refused "because they cannot give me 100 percent that I'll never be in a hospital again.

"Doctors don't like people who know something. I learned that I could go into a hospital and tell the doctor, 'You ain't doing this to me unless I say. It's my body. You don't touch it unless I give you permission.' I'm not a doctor's next statistic. They don't want that. They want people to say, 'Yes, Doctor; anything, Doctor.' " Lonnie finally found physicians she liked, well trained to ask her permission. She also arranged for her physicians—diabetes specialist, gynecologist, orthopedist, ophthalmologist—to talk to one another, coordinating her care. In particular, Lonnie liked and trusted her gynecologist: "She's excellent. She doesn't do anything unless she calls me, and we talk about it. That's what she does. My doctors call me; they let me know. It's my body."

Lonnie and other interviewees like Eleanor Peters, Cynthia Walker, and Mary Sanderson have taken control of managing their chronic conditions. They make daily decisions, investigate options, and participate fully in choices of specific medical interventions. They fit into the self-care or self-management movements (Ellers 1993; Holman 1996), where people with chronic conditions and physicians negotiate as "therapeutic allies," each bearing different but reciprocal responsibilities (Kleinman 1988, 4). These interviewees were probably unaware they had adopted a new care paradigm—it simply works for them. The rheumatologist Bevra Hahn (Manning and Barondess 1996, 68) warns against creating "one size fits all . . . strictly Caucasian" self-management programs: "A lot of ethnic groups that we deal with in Los Angeles are not interested in self-management and are much more interested in being directed." Guidelines for the relative roles of patients and physicians in self-management programs do exist (Holman 1996), but almost by definition, the ultimate design is crafted individually, fitting each person's circumstances and preferences.

The African-American women in one focus group see self-management as necessary to protect themselves. A woman with arthritis had an allergic reaction to a drug administered despite clear warnings in her medical record—an all-too-common medical error (Institute of Medicine 1999, 2001a). That acute event was her wake-up call. "It shows you the ignorance of some doctors. They feel they know more than the patient, and he didn't even listen to me. I read my records and knew the allergy was there."

"And you know your body."

"Exactly. Exactly."

"Doctors don't want you to speak up for yourself."

"Exactly. One doctor comes in telling me what I need. I said I know my body. You got to learn your body."

"They don't have that in the medical books—where a doctor should sit down and have a one-on-one with a patient and listen to the patient before they diagnose what they think is wrong with you."

"That's what I'm saying. Everybody's an individual. I deal with my back problem every day. It's my life. I know how to deal with it. Doctors can't link everybody with back problems all together. It's an individual thing. It's what each person wants to do for themselves."

9 Physicians Talking to Their Patients

> Addressing walking is outside of those things that you view as doing doctoring. . . . [It's] social worker-type stuff. It's useful, but it's not really internal medicine.
>
> DR. JOEL MILLER, general internist in his early forties

Medicine is not monolithic. As in other professions, some physicians, generalists and specialists alike, are more knowledgeable, technically skilled, and interested than others. I interviewed wonderful physicians who seemingly do the "right" things for people with mobility problems. Nevertheless, as mentioned repeatedly by physician interviewees, especially those in primary care: physicians receive little training about addressing mobility; they wonder if it's really their job; and general medical publications provide little information about assessing mobility or physical functioning, in general. No wonder people sometimes question the utility of talking to physicians about walking problems.

Ironically, however, physicians are the anointed arbiters for many decisions that have critical consequences for peoples' lives. Physicians determine whether people meet medical criteria for disability from Social Security, the state, or private insurance, and for workers' compensation (chapter 7). To ensure health insurance coverage, physicians oversee physical and occupational therapy; doctors write prescriptions for mobility aids, attesting to their medical necessity (chapters 13 and 14). Doctors diagnose people's underlying diseases, providing socially "legitimate" reasons for walking difficulties as well as treatment and prognoses about future functioning.

Chapter 9 examines how physicians assess and address impaired mobility. These activities require time—skill in questioning patients and families, patience to watch patients walk, however slowly, and willingness to work with other clinical professionals. The only diagnostic technology required is often a clock with a second hand. In today's medical marketplace, however, physicians are paid more for technological services than for spending time talking with patients. Financial disincentives reduce physicians' ability and willingness to perform comprehensive functional evaluations, adding to substantial educational and attitudinal barriers. This chapter touches only lightly on specific clinical specialties—neurology, rheumatology, geriatrics, orthopedic surgery, and physiatry—which assert expertise in mobility problems. I concentrate primarily on outpatient care provided by general medical doctors—often people's first contact with the medical system.

FORMAL TRAINING ABOUT MOBILITY

The remarkable thing to me when I reflect on it—and I've been a doctor for twenty years—I've learned virtually nothing of whatever little I know about this from my training—medical school, residency. Even what I learned outside of training, I learned about on the fly.

DR. JOHNNY BAKER, general internist in his early fifties

In organizing this chapter, I vacillated between beginning with physicians' training versus their attitudes about mobility. Attitudes clearly influence actions: after all, physicians are people too. Like others, they grew up within a society that historically marginalized people with difficulty walking and may themselves, consciously or unconsciously, share these views. "My upbringing was like everybody else's—not to talk about it," Dr. Baker observed. "The message from parents or teachers is that it's not polite to ask people about it, it's somehow hurtful, you're not supposed to stare."

Educators debate whether medical schools can teach empathy and compassion, touchstones of the physician's art, or must seek students born with these traits. The medical profession generally sees education as key to all knowledge and skills: "By the content of his education the student is 'socialized' to become a physician. . . . In the course of such an education a new kind of person is created" (Friedson 1970, 84). Therefore, I start with education, concentrating on general medical training.

In Medical School

Medical schools emphasize the diagnosis and treatment of acute problems (Pope and Tarlov 1991; Cassell 1997). Chronic progressive conditions that cause most mobility impairments are not ignored, but students learn primarily about their acute manifestations and technical therapeutic interventions, such as surgeries and treatments for acute exacerbations. Most clinical education still happens in hospitals, so students gain little insight into how patients function at home or rebound from acute short-term debilities. Because students see patients with chronic illness only during these acute episodes, trainees may erroneously undervalue their functional capabilities and usual quality of life, absorbing "the impression that the chronically ill are problem patients for their failure to improve and for their frequent need of physicians' services" (Kleinman 1988, 257).

"Heart, lung, kidneys, liver, blood," Dr. Patrick O'Reilley, a general internist in his late thirties, described his medicine student clerkship. "Nobody paid attention to gait. You could go through a whole rotation and never watch a patient walk. Nobody ever questioned it. It just doesn't come up." Mobility is missing from formal didactics at most medical schools.[1] So is the broader topic of assessing people's physical, cognitive, and emotional abilities to function in daily life (Brandt and Pope 1997; Cassell 1997). Medical schools rarely require clinical rotations in rehabilitation medicine or training with interdisciplinary clinical teams to address functional impairments (Pope and Tarlov 1991, 231).[2] "Rehabilitation has been one of the major advances in American medicine since World War II, yet it remains peripheral in the education process" (Cassell 1997, 166).

Almost every physician interviewee denied having formal training about mobility in medical school, with modest exceptions. Several physicians had attended a medical school that requires a home-care clerkship. Although mobility is not explicitly addressed, students inevitably meet persons who have trouble walking. "We saw patients with functional impairments and what it does to quality of life," remembered one physician in his mid forties. "There was never any formal discussion of how to evaluate gait. But the home-care physicians were very tuned into safety and how you can improve functioning."

The vast majority of physicians, however, responded as did Dr. Stanley Nathan, a primary care physician in his late forties, who denied having learned anything about mobility in medical school. "In fact, I still find it a puzzle," admitted Dr. Nathan, "how to actually evaluate function. I certainly ask people what it's like to be at home, but I don't know what to do other than that. I wouldn't know how to begin an actual evaluation." Dr. Johnny Baker, a medical educator, suggested why medical schools neglect evaluations of functional ability:

> It doesn't fit the paradigm of the people who run medical schools: the job is cure. If you find out what's happening on the most molecular level, you can figure out how to fix it. That's the ultimate goal of this human genome project, right? Just put in some new DNA, and all the problems of society go away. That simplistic, reductionist view is, I think, the fantasy of why people went to medical school. To cure, to be the hero. That's what everybody wants. To be thanked, right?

In Residency

General medical postgraduate training programs (internships followed by residencies) also offer little formal teaching about mobility or general functional evaluations. Beyond specific functional assessments (e.g., vision testing, neurologic exams), "primary care providers are not typically trained to recognize the general health care needs of people with disabling conditions" (Brandt and Pope 1997, 181). Most programs nowadays require residents to receive some outpatient training, for example by having a "continuity" clinic in which they follow patients over time. Residents therefore have greater opportunities for seeing how functional impairments affect people's daily lives.[3]

During residency young physicians begin defining their roles, the perimeters of their practice and expertise. Physician interviewees repeatedly described crafting such boundaries during residency, with most deciding that evaluating and improving function is another professional's responsibility, not the job of primary care doctors. "I did a geriatrics rotation," recounted Dr. Janet Posner, a general internist in her late thirties. "I recall interdisciplinary meetings, physical therapists being present. My take-home message was that there was a useful interdisciplinary group process focusing on the functional abilities of the elders. Others were doing that, and I was dealing with the medical problems. Functional issues weren't on my radar screen."

"You must be joking," laughed Dr. Alan Magaziner, a general internist in his early forties, when asked if he was trained about functional evaluations. He felt swamped as a resident. "I had about two hundred patients that I built up and followed over the three years. I was trying to figure out how to order mammograms and handle cholesterol and hypertension and cardiac arrest. It was virtually impossible to think too much about falls or gait at the same time." His clinic preceptors also never raised the topic.

Dr. Patrick O'Reilley admits that his limited training means he could miss important clinical problems. "As a resident, we focused on internal medicine. If a person got hospitalized for something with their gait, we thought it through for triage. We'd say, yeah, there's a problem here; let's get neurology or some other specialty involved. We never really analyzed the problems." Now in practice, he continues first to determine whether patients have difficulty walking, then refers to specialists when he has questions.

Learning Later

After finishing formal training, physicians often claim that they learn constantly, that each patient brings new insight.[4] Many general medical doctors do eventually learn something about assessing mobility. After all, roughly 10 percent of their adult patients have some difficulty getting around. Some physicians find special mentors or role models who teach them; others learn with experience. Dr. Patrick O'Reilley takes "bits and pieces of different patients and fits them together to learn about functional impairments. I have a lady now with a dense peripheral neuropathy and cataracts. . . . She falls all the time and grabs onto anything. As her vision gets worse and worse, her gait gets worse and worse. There's a good chance her gait and vision are related. I don't think I would have made that connection when I first got out of medical school or residency. I didn't realize how these different pieces connected or how big a problem walking is for people."

Some physicians like Alan Magaziner "continue to struggle with patients with gait problems, with falls and balance problems and dizziness. There's a sort of haphazard, random interaction between me, my nurse practitioner, and home-care nurses—my eyes and ears on the ground at home. It's not a satisfying process. I don't have a strategy with defined goals." Dr. Magaziner regrets that he has no one to teach him about evaluating and improving mobility, functioning, and quality of life. "I'm not growing in this area."

HOW PHYSICIANS VIEW THEIR PATIENTS

Physicians share society's attitudes about walking: whenever possible, they want their patients to walk. Dr. Arnie Hawn, a general internist in his mid forties with an academic practice, described one patient who stands out in his mind.

> She is a woman from Southie who was probably in her mid fifties when she was turned over to me. She hadn't left her house for who knows how long. Her former doctor sent her Valium whenever she wanted. When she got into my practice, I declined to give her any Valium. That really riled her, but I insisted I couldn't give her drugs unless I saw her. She explained that she couldn't walk so she couldn't come in. I said, "You're going to have to get here somehow, or I'll send someone to get you. If I must, I will." And I did. I got her in. What she really had was a bad case of fibromyalgia and a lot of psychiatric problems. Over the years, I worked with her. Now she swims daily in the ocean; she sings; she's out doing all sorts of things; she walks miles every day.

Physicians want what they view as best for their patients—doctors are accustomed to being in control. In hospitals, their orders are typically obeyed to the letter, by clinical colleagues and patients alike. Outside hospitals, their control erodes. Physicians can write prescriptions, for example, but patients must purchase medications and follow instructions. Most people understand the rationale for prescription drugs and generally trade off potential side effects for explicit, anticipated benefits. But when therapies ask people to alter daily routines—to exercise, lose weight, use a cane, rearrange their home—physicians wield only the power of persuasion. Dr. Hawn's story exemplifies this situation, with hints of confrontation, a battle of wills, physicians forcing reluctant patients to pull themselves up by their bootstraps and march onward. Of course, this is often for the good: the woman from Southie is probably much happier now than before Dr. Hawn's ultimatum.

Many physicians recognize that, with progressive chronic conditions, patients make the important daily decisions about managing their health (Ellers 1993; Holman 1996). In these circumstances, an important role for physicians is defining expectations. Although doctors are critical guides, patients are generally in control. "This means that central to *medical* considerations are the patients' motivations, values, purposes, concerns, and relationships to self, others, body, and (maybe above all) the doctor," wrote the physician-educator Eric J. Cassell, elevating physicians to perhaps a higher height than many patients might accord. Nevertheless, "All these things that in acute disease seemed peripheral have now become central. We see the difficulty for medicine. If chronic disease is overwhelmingly personal, than [*sic*] the person is central. This means that the body of knowledge of medical science that has served medicine so well in acute disease, is only part, albeit a crucial part, of the story in chronic disease" (1997, 25).

"I've noticed that there's a group of people who are disabled and never get into trouble," said Dr. Ron Einstein, a busy primary care doctor in his mid fifties. "They are in total charge of their disease and are remarkably independent. Then there are others with even less disability who get decubitus ulcers. They don't take care of themselves as well, don't turn their bodies, and don't initiate what they need to do."

"What do you think explains the differences?" I asked.

"I don't know. I have people of all economic circumstances without any obvious pattern. I have one guy who was high-level corporate—rich. He's lost both his legs because of decubitus ulcers that didn't really need to develop. I have another fellow with polio. Not rich. He gets all over town in his wheelchair, going down the street real fast. Very independent guy. He has a personal-care assistant, and he's got the whole system down pat. He knows every form I'm supposed to fill out, researched the Internet. He's the world's expert on how to get everything that you need to live successfully. If you really want to take care of yourself, you take care of yourself."

Denial and Depression

Some interviewees observed that their patients, especially older people, are stoic and won't complain about difficulty walking. Or they suggest another possibility—"denial," refusal to admit or acknowledge that anything is wrong. In doctors' minds, denial hinders care on two levels: patients withhold important data that could inform their care, then reject actions to "improve" their situations. Dr. Patrick O'Reilley practices in a poor neighborhood where many elderly people live alone. He worries that people hide their walking difficulties:

> Let's be honest. The patients who come to see me want the doctor to be happy. They don't want to get him upset. People minimize what's going on. I'm not blaming anybody. I'm just saying that happens a lot of the time. People won't reveal information. I've got this patient now. If you ask, "Mrs. Smith, how's your walking?" she says it's OK. Everybody around her says she's falling all over the place. "Oh, it's all right. I'm OK. I hold onto the wall, and it's OK." She's practically on her face constantly, and everything's fine. She doesn't want to upset me. She's happy. She wants to talk about my kids. She doesn't want to talk about her walking. It might be a generational thing. Older people—some of them—don't want to complain.

Physicians are not surprised that walking difficulties can precipitate depression. While primary care physicians often miss depression among their patients in general, some physicians expect this problem for people with difficulty walking. According to Dr. Ron Einstein,

> You have to be very attentive to people's psychological needs—how depressed you can become when you're not able to do things that should be routine. I've learned the most from a couple of cases. One doctor who had Parkinson's disease said that the simplest things could become the most horribly humiliating experience that you can imagine. Like on a bus, he wasn't able to move out of the way quick enough. Then another patient—the most horrible thing. He was a young guy who was a diver and broke his neck, was quadriplegic. As best as you could tell, he did everything perfectly right, but he got so depressed that he killed himself.

One young internist feels that she can't do anything to improve walking problems, but at least she can treat depression "with pills or counseling." Nevertheless, vigilance to depression treads a fine line: physicians, acceding to prevailing societal views, can see depression as a reasonable response to a "lesser life." As Cassell wrote,

> The basic struggle in chronic disease *is not against death; it is against disability*. . . . Of course, people die from chronic disease, but disability—the loss of function and independence—has always come first and marked their lives. Keep in mind multiple sclerosis, severe strokes, Tay Sachs disease, many cancers, and Alzheimer's disease. In considering these diseases personally and professionally, it is not the deaths of these patients that we find so awful but their lives. . . . There has been a natural presumption since antiquity that death is the worst fate. In the modern era we know more awful futures than death, and they are all related to disability. (1997, 22–23)

Such views can lead down a slippery slope, as suggested by the disability rights activist Jenny Morris. She interviewed a woman named Ruth Moore whose spine was "crumbling," risking complete paralysis. Moore worried about her physicians' attitudes, observing,

> The neurosurgeon told me that he was only interested in quality of life and that in no way would he be looking to prolong my life if he didn't feel the quality would be acceptable. However, neither he nor anyone else has asked me what criteria *I* would use in judging what was an acceptable quality of life. I am very worried that if I get admitted unconscious or without the power of speech, he will take a decision based on *his* judgment and *his* criteria about what is an acceptable quality of life. (1996a, 62)

Malingering

Every once in a while—most doctors said "rarely," a few said "all the time"—patients report being physically impaired when other evidence suggests they are not. "Malingering," or feigning difficulties, riles physicians. "It's a big problem," said Dr. Magaziner. "You see your patients on the street, and they're bee-bopping along. Then you see them up in the office, and they're hunched over and just barely moving."

Several years ago, Dr. Johnny Baker's office looked directly onto the handicapped parking places outside his building. "One of my patients was a former nun who had been to Lourdes to get cured," Dr. Baker recalled. "She used to drive into a handicapped space, get out of her car, walk to the back and take the wheelchair out of her trunk with no difficulty, and then get into the wheelchair and visit me."

"What was going on?" I asked.

"There seemed to be a lot of secondary gain for her from being in a wheelchair. I'd point out that I'd watched her through the window, but she wouldn't address the situation." These instances obviously reflect complicated psychological or interpersonal factors that defy easy understanding. Whether and how physicians should address underlying concerns is often unclear.

Sometimes relationships between patients and physicians become polarized around whether walking problems are "legitimate"—in physicians' minds, whether patients have a measurable, observable physical cause. Several interviewees described physical examination strategies to test, from their viewpoints, the veracity of patients' claims. Dr. Jina Saleh, a general internist in her early thirties, practices in a working-class neighborhood and says malingering is common:

> There's ways to pick up when people are faking their physical exams. They know a little too much medicine; they know a little too much anatomy; they know how to answer the questions a little too well. They're subtle. You can tell when people are trying to use the system. I just had a woman come in with a limp. I made her do a couple of things, and she tried to fake part of the exam, but it didn't work. I didn't tell her what I was doing. She was able to do the physical exam pretty well aside from when I had her move to different positions. All of a sudden she had a lot of pain. Then she thought I wasn't looking, and I watched her walk away. She walked pretty well. That limp was all of a sudden not that bad. I was taught really well how to check for people who are cheating.

Dr. Saleh had trained at an inner-city public hospital where she recounted seeing many patients who sought narcotics. She remains on guard against being deceived. Dr. Baker suggests that, throughout training and practice, physicians are "socialized *medically* around this issue of malingering. Doctors hate to be duped. Even though malingerers are a tiny fraction of patients, there's always this fear that people want something and that somehow society deems us to be the guardians of what people get— handicapped parking, the RIDE, financial assistance, whatever it is. But we weren't trained to be the public's guardian. We don't think about it clearly. That makes all this tension and confusion between doctors and patients."

Dr. Ron Einstein refuses to play the role as arbiter in administrative decisions about disability: "There's often a sense that more is being made of a disability than is obvious to your physical exam," said Dr. Einstein emphatically. "I've made it a policy: I don't get involved in any workman's compensation cases. If a lawyer asks me to testify or write a letter in support of a patient, I say, 'You can look at my records. I'm not an expert on disability, and I won't comment on it.' I'll take care of the medical problems and refer them, but I won't get involved in financial rewards for anybody. I don't study it, I'm not interested in it, and I'm not an expert on it.'"

Both the public and private sectors have put physicians in charge of determining, with "objective" medical evidence, who qualifies for disability-related benefits, like SSDI, SSI, and workers' compensation payments (chapter 7).[5] Almost all interviewees raised this issue, saying it made them uncomfortable. Doctors feel their allegiances are torn between advocating for their patients versus protecting the public purse (Geiringer 1998; Rondinelli et al. 1998). The Social Security Administration explicitly prefers that the person's own physician, the so-called "treating source," perform disability evaluations, seeing them as "likely to be the medical professionals most able to provide a detailed longitudinal picture of the claimant's impairments and may bring a unique perspective to the medical evidence that cannot be obtained from the medical findings alone or from reports of individual examinations or brief hospitalizations" (SSA 1998, 13).

This role makes some "treating sources" nervous. "Doctors are put into this incredibly awkward, poorly conceived situation," said Dr. Johnny Baker. "It makes us uncomfortable; we resent the position we're in. People come to us with a form. Doctors hate that—most doctors do—because they're confused about their role. Usually the doctor is the advocate for the patient, and the doctor counts on patients to be open and honest. With these disability forms, all of a sudden, you're not the patient's doctor. You're the doctor for Social Security, for the insurance company. Patients want the form filled out a certain way and might not give the exact same history as they would otherwise. So the rug is pulled out from under the usual doctor-patient interaction. Doctors are thrown for a loop by that."

Outright confrontations can erupt when doctors feel patients are bilking the system. "Don't get me started," laughed Dr. Eva Patel, who practices in a neighborhood health center in a poor community. "I've had quite a few patients like that. One woman in her thirties came in complaining of excruciating pain. I couldn't find anything objective on exam. I accidentally spotted her in the parking lot looking quite nimble one day. She insisted that I send in the disability forms. I wrote a letter explaining five or six objective reasons why she shouldn't get disability. I mailed it to her and asked her if she would like me to mail it to the agency." Such interactions certainly can't enhance patient-physician relationships.

MOBILITY AND ROUTINE CLINICAL PRACTICE

Despite feeling unqualified, Dr. Baker believes that assessing mobility is central to his medical mission:

> If we don't pay attention to people's function in the face of their illnesses, then we have really cut ourselves off from the biggest opportunity we have to help as doctors. We have violated the social contract of why society gives us so much, puts so much faith in us, allows us to set our own agenda, and pays us better than most people. . . . We all went into medicine, despite fantasies of cure, wanting to be helpful. Doctors feel frustrated when they don't know how to be helpful. They feel inadequate, overwhelmed, befuddled and not sure what to do.

Major primary care textbooks say little about evaluating gait (Goroll, May, and Mulley 1995; Barker, Burton, and Zieve 1999; Noble 2001; *Up-to-Date* 2001).[6] *Office Practice of Medicine* (Branch 1994) addresses gait within "Neurologic Disorders," beginning, "The office evaluation of the patient with impaired gait is one of the more troublesome problems in medical practice" (Sudarsky 1994, 766).

As Dr. Baker suggests, the value of performing functional evaluations seems self-evident. At a minimum, assessments show how people function now, the baseline for tracking progressive impairments and predicting prognoses (American Medical Association 1996; Pearson 2000). Mobility evaluations are essential for planning interventions, like rehabilitation or physical or occupational therapy, and considering mobility aids. Evaluations also serve administrative purposes, supporting documentation required to ensure payment for professional services or assistive devices (chapters 13 and 14). Tools exist to evaluate walking, requiring nothing more sophisticated than just a hallway, chair, and stopwatch (Tinetti 1986; Tinetti and Ginter 1988; Mathias, Nayak, and Isaacs 1986). Yet little "hard evidence" supports the value of functional evaluations. Few randomized, controlled trials have examined the benefits (or risks) of assessing function. "I think there are still holes in the literature," said Dr. Janet Posner, a general internist, "and those holes make it hard to convince other people. . . . I think it would be easier to sell functional evaluations if we really had hard outcomes data." Not surprisingly, primary care physicians often fail to recognize fully patients' functional deficits (Stewart and Buck 1977; Wartman et al. 1983; Nelson et al. 1983; Calkins et al. 1991, 1994) and are uncertain about when to refer to rehabilitation specialists (Hoenig 1993).

No large studies have examined whether and how physicians assess mobility or other functional abilities. The 1994 NHIS did ask whether healthcare providers inquire about problems with daily activities. People with mobility difficulties are much more likely than others to have been asked: just over 25 percent of persons with major mobility problems.[7] Admittedly, respondents may have forgotten being asked about ADL or IADL difficulties, but even if doubled to compensate for faulty recall, these percentages are too low.

Unlike medication errors that can be dramatic and life-threatening, lapses in evaluating patients' functional abilities are unlikely to attract public attention. "When people do quality monitoring," Dr. Magaziner observed, "they're not going to care if you asked about someone's gait." According to Dr. Joel Miller, being good at evaluating walking is "not something that is solidly, unquestionably, part of a doctor's competence responsibility in the same way as skill in breast exams. If I do a breast exam and miss the mass, that's incompetence. On the other hand, if I relate to my patients in a relatively mechanical, biomedical, purely medical kind of way and don't ask about functioning, then that's style. That's not incompetence."

Most primary care physicians reported trying to observe patients as they walk into examining rooms or climb onto examining tables. These efforts are neither rigorous nor consistent. Only a few ask their patients to walk down the corridor and formally evaluate their gait. Most rely instead on the "history," the accounts people give of their recent symptoms and physical difficulties, to identify mobility problems. "In the busy clinical practice setting, assessment of physical function is often based on verbal report of symptoms without observational data being systematically collected" (Pearson 2000, 17). Such assessments differ from other aspects of medical evaluations where histories are only the starting point: physicians then insist on observing or exploring potential problems themselves.

People with major medical illnesses compromising endurance, like heart or lung disease, are a special case. Physicians have long used patients' abilities to walk or perform other physical activities as explicit clinical indicators of the severity of these illnesses. The physician interviewees report carefully questioning patients with congestive heart failure or chronic obstructive pulmonary disease about how far they can walk before becoming short of breath or unable to go on. "We'll walk them around the office," said one general internist. "We take them with an oximeter on a little track to see how far they can go"—the oximeter is a small device clipped onto the patient's finger that monitors oxygen levels in the blood. "We measure their pulse, oxygen, and the distance, but we don't do any formal gait evaluation."

Some physicians remain skeptical about patients' descriptions of their difficulties and adjust their questions accordingly. One physician reported that patients hate to admit having fallen, so he asks, "Have you found yourself on the floor unexpectedly?" and believes he elicits accurate responses. Physicians recognize that patients may not reveal the whole story, as recalls Dr. Lawrence Jen, both an internist and rheumatologist:

> We were doing home visits for 400 frail elderly in East Boston, Jamaica Plain, and Dorchester. One of the first patients I saw was someone with "arthritis." His name was Mike. His wife had died many years earlier. Seventeen years ago, he got admitted to hospital with a urinary tract infection. When he came out and went back to his apartment, he was weak and he stumbled. He was convinced that something bad had happened and he'd never be able to walk again. When I saw him seventeen years later, he had 90 degree flexion contractures of his knees and couldn't walk. He never had arthritis, just the contractures of soft tissues. We administered a questionnaire about functional status, and he didn't list any functional problems. His support system had sort of enveloped him. His kids would bring him food. At Christmas, people came in from charitable groups. He sponge bathed. His whole apartment was denuded except for this cockpit around his couch. That's where he spent all of his time.

Dr. Jen learned the full story only from going to Mike's home.

For some people with mobility problems, their chronic diseases demand immediate and constant attention, preoccupying both patient and physician (Burns et al. 1990). Other people, however, are not all-consumed by their clinical conditions and reasonably anticipate long lives ahead. They need good basic medical care, just like everybody else, including routine screening and preventive services (Bockenek et al. 1998; Gans, Mann, and Becker 1993; DeJong 1997).

> Practices that promote general well-being and good health are as critical to people with disabling conditions as they are to those who are free of limitations. In fact, available evidence suggests that health-promoting behaviors may be more important to the population of people with disabling conditions, given their elevated risk for secondary conditions and, consequently, for negative effects on the quality of their lives. (Pope and Tarlov 1991, 223)

Efforts to promote general health fall squarely within the purview of primary care physicians. However, time pressures, misunderstandings, and anxieties can lead physicians to concentrate narrowly on the underlying debilitating disorder to the exclusion of other health-related concerns (Gans, Mann, and Becker 1993; Chan et al. 1999). Physicians' attitudes may

TABLE 13. Routine Screening Questions and Tests

Mobility Difficulty	Screening Questions (%)[a]			Screening Tests (%)[b]	
	Tobacco	Exercise	Contraception[c]	Pap Smear	Mammogram
None	57	50	41	81	64
Minor	41	49	30	80	58
Moderate	51	44	27	80	52
Major	35	43	13	63	45

[a]Questions asked only of persons reporting having had a routine physical examination within the last 3 years: during this last check-up, were you asked about whether you smoke cigarettes or use other forms of tobacco?; were you asked about the amount of physical activity or exercise you get?; or (asked only of persons < age 50) were you asked about the use of contraceptives?

[b]Rates for women age 18–75 who had a Pap smear within the last 3 years and who do not report having had a hysterectomy; rates for women ≥ age 50 who had a mammogram within the past two years.

[c]Results are for women only.

affect their practices, as is the case for reproductive health. Women of childbearing age with major mobility problems are asked about contraception 70 percent less often than other women (Table 13).[8] Perhaps physicians share general views of women with impaired mobility as asexual or uninterested in sexual activity.

Routine screening and preventive services, such as those recommended by the U.S. Preventive Services Task Force (1996) and Healthy People 2010 (U.S. Department of Health and Human Services 2000), are therefore important (Iezzoni et al. 2000a). Regardless of whether people have mobility difficulties, however, many receive screening and preventive services at lower-than-desirable rates (see Table 13). Women with major mobility problems are much less likely to receive important screening tests: 30 percent less likely for mammograms and 40 percent for Papanicolaou smears.[9] Smokers with major mobility problems are 20 percent less likely to be asked about tobacco use.

Also worrisome are low rates of vision tests. Among persons age sixty-five and older, 23 percent report having vision tests, regardless of mobility difficulties. However, for persons in this older age group, 26 percent with major mobility problems have serious difficulty seeing, even using glasses or contact lenses, compared to 5 percent without impaired mobility.[10] Poor vision is a major risk factor for falls and further functional declines, so it should be addressed aggressively for people with mobility problems.

Lower rates of screening and preventive services probably relate to many factors, including patients' clinical status and preferences and physicians' attitudes and actions. One significant barrier is the paucity of automatically adjustable examining tables and wheelchair-height mammography machines (Welner 1998, 1999; Welner et al. 1999). One internist joined a Medicaid health maintenance organization (HMO), where she encountered many patients with disabilities (Andriacchi 1997, S17). However, the practice did not have adjustable examining tables: tables that lower (to wheelchair height) and rise (to examination height) when physicians press a foot pedal. One new patient, a forty-five-year-old woman with MS, had never had a Pap smear because physicians had not offered her one. When the internist and her assistants tried to move the woman onto the high unadjustable examining table, they failed. The patient's daughter, familiar with transferring her mother, lifted her up. The internist ordered a mammogram, but the HMO's approved facility required women to stand for the test: "Then I had to get approval from the HMO system for her to go outside of their usual place" (Andriacchi 1997, S18).

Most physician interviewees do not practice in settings with automatically adjustable examination tables. Even those who do, such as Drs. Nathan and Posner, admit being unsure how to use the equipment. In addition, scheduling specific patients for a particular room is often logistically complex in a busy practice. One internist admitted she dislikes the adjustable table: it rises and lowers too slowly for her quick practice pace. Because of physicians' protests, the clinic considered removing the automatic tables but kept them because some patients do need them.

REFERRALS TO MEDICAL SPECIALISTS

"Let me make a radical statement," proposed Dr. Alan Magaziner. "I'm a primary care doctor, and I'm overwhelmed. Too goddamn much to do. Lots of stuff gets plopped in the lap of primary care doctors, and it's literally impossible to do everything. . . . I'm not saying that walking isn't part of the doctor's job—it interacts with too many things that are definitely part of the doctor's job. But walking and gait evaluations could easily be done by people trained in this, not necessarily even M.D.'s. Just a thought."

Referring patients is the answer for many primary care physicians, as for Dr. Magaziner. Granted, they must first recognize that patients have difficulty walking, then decide which professional would best diagnose and handle the problem. Often they send patients directly to physical therapists with the open-ended request "evaluate and treat." Referrals to physical therapists seem easy: physical therapists clearly have a different "skill set" than most physicians. Some doctors resist referring patients to other physicians because of the implied challenge to their capabilities and authority. But most primary care interviewees openly admit their limitations in addressing mobility and welcome expert advice, typically from specialists in neurology, rheumatology, geriatrics, and orthopedics. I describe their roles briefly below; extensively describing each specialty is beyond my scope here.

Physician Specialists

Orthopedists generally perform surgery, aiming to ease pain and improve function. Primary care physicians typically refer patients to orthopedists to evaluate whether surgery is warranted, although some patients independently seek orthopedic input. Some orthopedists specialize in replacing hip or knee joints, while others mainly do back operations (in some institutions, neurosurgeons also perform back surgery). A few often avoid operating, recognizing that surgery carries risks and benefits are sometimes uncertain. "There are many people—worthy surgeons—who think you simply put in a replacement and fix up the joint," observed Dr. Stuart Hartman, an orthopedist in his early fifties. "As a society, we want a quick fix, to minimize even minimal discomfort, and sometimes I think patients would do better with rehab, exercises, using a cane, walking more. I give people an idea of their options." He spends considerable time asking people about how walking difficulties affect their daily lives.

Neurologists diagnose and treat many conditions that impair gait, like Parkinson's disease, MS, and ALS—an expertise generally beyond the knowledge of primary care physicians. Nonetheless, many neurologists are not trained explicitly in mobility aids or improving walking per se (as opposed to addressing the underlying illness), so they refer patients to physical or occupational therapists. In fact, until recently, few neurologic diseases had effective treatments; neurologists learned primarily to diagnose disease, leaving day-to-day (often palliative) care to other physicians. "I wanted to do primary care neurology," said Dr. Betty Lacey, a neurologist in her mid fifties who specializes in MS. She likes being the primary physician caring for her patients over time and explicitly addressing mobility needs. "To me, that's the satisfaction. My old professor used to say he could teach anybody to diagnose neurologic diseases, but managing patients separates the men from the boys." She knows volumes about practical aspects of living with MS, while some neurologists continue to act as consultants: "diagnose and adios," as Dr. Lacey says.

Unlike orthopedics and neurology, geriatrics and rheumatology are subspecialties of internal medicine. Many primary care physicians learn aspects of these disciplines during their training, sometimes complicating decisions about when to refer patients. Both specialties emphasize daily functioning and quality of life. "Being a geriatrician is dealing with functional impairment," said Dr. Jacob Rogers, a geriatrician in his late forties. "Not complete recovery, not cure, but how to deal with functional problems, improve, have a better quality of life." Geriatricians themselves may not be trained explicitly in evaluating gait or addressing walking problems. "Most geriatrics training programs don't go much into the physical medicine side of things," noted another geriatrician. "But they're very good with the internal medicine piece—Alzheimer's, urinary incontinence, multiple illnesses." Geriatricians often lead multidisciplinary teams that consider the whole patient, working "in partnership with primary care physicians who provide the majority of the care for the elderly population" (Urdangarin 2000, 402).[11] Distinctions between roles of geriatricians and primary care physicians sometimes blur.

Rheumatologists, also internal medicine subspecialists, care for people with arthritis and other rheumatic diseases—disorders of connective tissues and joints marked by inflammation, degeneration, and metabolic derangements. Primary care physicians commonly see patients with arthritis, and they know the prevailing medical treatments, so the question becomes when to refer to rheumatologists. Dr. Josh Landau trained as both a primary care physician and rheumatologist. "Primary care folks, including my mentors and preceptors, seemed to feel there wasn't much to help people with arthritis and functional problems," Dr. Landau recalled, describing why he entered rheumatology. "I felt that if I could properly evaluate these patients and their problems that I might help them more."

"What did you learn in your rheumatology fellowship?" I asked.

"I was trained to think about three things: overall quality of life, pain, and function. I was taught a mnemonic—ADEPT, that is ambulation, dressing, eating, personal hygiene, and transfers. A fourth category is more physiologic: blood tests and X rays. If the X rays are worse but all the other things are better—function, pain, quality of life overall—then we put X rays as a lower priority. We don't treat the X ray; we treat the patient."

"How can you help?"

"I used to think about cures. My favorite disease is gout. We don't cure it, but we can treat it so that it is essentially gone. Its treatment is reasonably safe, which is not true for other rheumatic diseases, by and large. We don't have fantastic therapies, safe therapies. Our goals are much more modest, keeping the disease at bay. I try to help patients feel better, move in the right direction. That includes function, activities of daily life, pain, not hurting them with my medicines. I look at nonpharmacologic things. I usually give a speech about podiatrists and occupational therapists, splinting, things that are terrifically safe. They may or may not help, but they're very safe—more than I can say about my medicines. But I have a harder time getting many patients to accept these kinds of maneuvers than medicines."

Dr. Landau worries that primary care physicians "refer patients way too late or not at all, either to a rheumatologist or an orthopedic surgeon. They aren't really aware of the indications for joint replacement surgery or how that can help people. They underutilize rehabilitation services, view it as voodoo, an unproven remedy, which to be honest it is. We don't have randomized control trials of physical therapy with sham physical therapy. On the other hand, rheumatology fellowship taught me a sense of what these different modalities offer in terms of function and quality of life."

Dr. Landau's comments highlight the complexities of referrals, especially when physicians have some knowledge in a field. "In the presence of chronic disease, the role of the specialist changes. The specialist usually does not provide continuous care. . . . The role of the specialist is one of advising the patient and the primary care physician" (Holman 1996, 42). Primary care physicians must coordinate care and bear ultimate responsibility when specialists have no solutions. Dr. Patrick O'Reilley again described his patient with peripheral neuropathy and cataracts.

> It took a year to get her to agree to have cataract surgery. She just didn't want it. She should be having her cataract surgery tomorrow, in fact. It took another whole year to convince her about her gait problem. I referred her to a neurologist who confirmed my suspicions that she has peripheral neuropathy, but he didn't come up with any specific reasons for it. Nothing really can be done. I got physical therapists out to see her in her house, and they say, "We've done as much as we can." So it's me and this woman who's unable to walk. We're going to fix her eyes. That's the only thing I have left in my little bag of tricks. God help me if her eyes get better and she doesn't walk any better.

According to Cassell, "specialists tend to think in terms of their specialty, have less knowledge of contextual or personal factors in the illness, and use technology earlier and more extensively in the diagnostic process than generalists do" (1997, 170). Yet Dr. Landau's comments suggest that important exceptions exist. Certainly, referrals generally aim to benefit from specialized knowledge. But in evaluating walking difficulties, some specialists inquire more about people's daily lives and activities than do their primary care physicians. The most important job for Dr. Hartman (an orthopedist), Dr. Lacey (a neurologist), Dr. Rogers (a geriatrician), and Dr. Landau (a rheumatologist) is enhancing overall quality of life through understanding and improving function. To do so, they learn about their patients' lives. Some specialists thus know more about patients as people than might their primary care physicians.

Physical Medicine and Rehabilitation Specialists

The stated mission of physiatrists, physicians specializing in PM&R, is tailor-made for people with difficulty walking. Over 6,100 physiatrists practice throughout the United States, trained by eighty accredited PM&R residency programs. They assess functional needs and provide nonsurgical interventions, frequently working alongside physical and occupational therapists (DeLisa, Currie, and Martin 1998). According to the American Academy of Physical Medicine and Rehabilitation (2000), whose motto is "physicians adding quality to life,"

> Physiatrists focus on restoring function. They care for patients with acute and chronic pain, and musculoskeletal problems like back and neck pain, tendinitis, pinched nerves and fibromyalgia. They also treat people who have experienced catastrophic events resulting in paraplegia, quadriplegia, or traumatic brain injury; and individuals who have had strokes, orthopedic injuries, or neurologic disorders such as multiple sclerosis, polio, or ALS.

Dr. Melinda Whittier, a physiatrist in her early forties, put it succinctly: "Physiatrists look at the whole patient." She admits that patients with single straightforward problems generally don't need a physiatrist. "We get involved with more complicated problems, when you need someone who can look at the whole patient—what's going on neurologically, the musculoskeletal problem, depression, a little dementia. The physiatrist could help clarify the diagnosis or recognize that something subtle is going on. Meanwhile, we can handle the walking problem. How do you compensate for it? Where might therapy help? Talk directly with the patient about the mobility problems." Dr. Whittier recognizes that physiatry is often the last resort, after patients exhaust other specialists. "You have to deal with that person and his or her family. You don't have an option to send them somewhere else. You're teaching individuals to improve their quality of life, their health status, within their environments. You have to think about their world, where they live. Can you do something in the environment to make things better?"

Yet none of the primary care interviewees recommended referrals to physiatrists. Why? One explanation is ignorance. "Isn't a physiatrist like a physical therapist?" laughed Dr. Posner. "It's a black box," said Dr. Landau. "I don't know much about it." Some interviewees saw physiatrists only within rehabilitation hospitals, caring for patients with functional deficits from strokes, spinal cord injuries, or other acute events. Another explanation is idiosyncratic: for historical reasons, physiatry has been slow to take root in Boston.[12] Nonetheless, with the aging population, demand for PM&R services will certainly grow. The Graduate Medicine Education National Advisory Committee targeted PM&R as one of three medical specialties facing personnel shortages (Pope and Tarlov 1991, 231).

Established medicine came late to rehabilitation (Berkowitz and Fox 1989, 146).[13] Into the early twentieth century, orthopedists, then seen as "the specialists best suited to the care of cripples," were nevertheless denigrated as "sawbones" (Byrom 2001, 134). Treating wounded World War I soldiers gave orthopedics credibility and catalyzed initial medical rehabilitation efforts—designing prosthetics and orthotics to improve mobility of injured veterans. Between world wars, improving function for polio survivors gained attention, although the greatest advances involved nonphysicians in Warm Springs, Georgia: Franklin Delano Roosevelt and the physical therapist Helena Mahoney. In the mid 1920s Roosevelt requested endorsement from the American Orthopedic Association (AOA), but the AOA refused to allow Roosevelt even to address their annual convention in Atlanta: "He was told he was a man without standing. He was not an orthopedist. He was not even a doctor" (Gallagher 1994, 46).[14] With World War II and the massive influx of seriously wounded veterans, rehabilitation professionals extended their goals beyond ambulation and low-energy activities to comprehensive restoration of physical, mental, vocational, emotional, and social abilities (Brandt and Pope 1997, 31).

Nowadays, PM&R can generate controversy. Some disability rights activists argue that rehabilitation specialists further the medicalization of disability, exhorting people to "fit in or cope with 'normal' life and expectations so that they did not become a burden on the rest of society" (Barnes, Mercer, and Shakespeare 1999, 20). Leading PM&R specialists, however, assert their aims of assisting people to find and fulfill their own "desires and life plans. Patients, their families, and their rehabilitation teams work together to determine realistic goals. . . . Rehabilitation is a concept that should permeate the entire health-care system" (DeLisa, Currie, and Martin 1998, 3). If patients can't walk, the physiatrist's job is to help find alternatives. According to Dr. Whittier,

> Mobility is key to everything we do day-to-day. If what's causing [the mobility problem] is not easily reversible, then you've got to face up to the fact: "I've got an irreversible condition here, and I've got to compensate for it." Compensating for it may take money, time, and it's a change, a loss. So trouble with mobility is a very

complicated psychological and physical problem. Despite that, early on in my rehabilitation training, we often said that mobility problems were the easiest things to rehabilitate. Fundamentally, the person still has their mind, they are a human being with their social relationships. It's this nasty problem with physically moving their body from point A to point B. That can be solved with power chairs or scooters. Granted it's not a cure—oh, I wish we had cures. But at least there are ways to compensate that don't mean staying immobile at home, surfing the Internet, or talking on the phone. You can physically get your body and mind out there in the world.

LINGERING CONCERNS

At the end of the day, Dr. Magaziner often wonders what physicians can really do to help people with limited mobility: "I bump up fairly quickly against what feels like the borderline between what's medical and what's social. I often just throw up my hands and say, 'I've done everything I can do.' "

For Dr. Magaziner, "the problem is not so much diagnostic as therapeutic." What treatments can he offer that will really make a difference? "The medical part is generally not complicated. That's what I'm trained to do; that's easy. What's difficult is when you're done with the medical evaluation and you find that this person has rotten social supports, is lucky to have any apartment (never mind the third floor walk-up), and has no financial resources to make things any better." Dr. Magaziner asks a nurse to visit the home, to gather essential information, then feels powerless to affect change even at the most basic level. People don't do—or can't do—what he advises. "I suggest all these nice things, but I don't believe that many of my patients implement any of these things. They don't do the exercises. They won't or can't change their homes. They don't get rid of the damn throw rugs!"

10 Physical and Occupational Therapy and Other Approaches

Dr. Alan Magaziner feels stymied. He hits that "borderline between what's medical and what's social" and can't make the leap. Firmly rooted on the medical side, he recognizes that walking difficulties raise complex issues—physical, psychological, social, environmental—that he is poorly equipped to address. Unsure exactly what they do, Dr. Magaziner nonetheless calls on physical or occupational therapists (PTs or OTs).

These two health professions have roots not only in medicine but also in social perspectives, including the effect of environmental factors on people's daily functioning. Their approach thus "melds two significantly different models of health, illness, and medical care. This duality can lead to significant confusion for traditionally trained physicians" (Hoenig 1993, 884). Physicians' referrals to physical and occupational therapy are often idiosyncratic and highly variable. Despite this, physicians generally control people's access to physical and occupational therapy. Unless people pay out-of-pocket, health insurers demand physicians' orders to cover therapy, then typically set strict limits on the amount of therapy covered, regardless of patients' feelings about its benefits (chapter 13).

Today, physical and occupational therapy are vibrant professions, adjusting—as is medicine—to new financial realities and insights about the causation and course of diseases and physical impairments. Home-based services are expanding rapidly for both professions, prompting concerns about local labor shortages and the certification of lesser-trained aides (Feldman 1997). Most acknowledge that more scientific proof is needed of the effectiveness of physical and occupational therapy, especially to convince health insurers to cover these services. Perhaps because of its stronger medical origins and traditions, physical therapy has generated more research, although occupational therapy studies are now appearing.

These results are rarely packaged for primary care physicians, so it is not surprising that physicians like Dr. Johnny Baker wonder about the scientific evidence that therapy works.

Here, I briefly review how physical and occupational therapists approach people with walking difficulties and judge their success. Other sources examine in depth the philosophy, clinical practices, and research evidence for physical therapy (*Guide to Physical Therapist Practice* 2001; Scully and Barnes 1989) and occupational therapy (Neistadt and Crepeau 1998; Trombly 1995a). I rely heavily on comments from seven physical therapists in one focus group and six occupational therapists in another, recognizing that these practitioners do not represent either field as a whole. Unlike many physical and occupational therapists who work in hospitals or clinics, most of my focus group members practice home care, where virtually all patients have some trouble walking. These therapists see the daily practical consequences of walking difficulties up close.

One warning before I begin this chapter: I cannot delineate clearly between physical and occupational therapy, especially in home care. Some people do etch clean boundaries. "It has to do with which limbs are involved," asserted Dr. Lawrence Jen. "OT is more upper body. Hands to head is OT. If you have a back problem, knee, hip, ankle problem, you'll see PT." The OT focus group rejected this upper-lower body distinction (made, after all, by physicians). In some minds, the difference involves level of focus: impairment (abnormality of an individual body part or anatomical structure) for PT versus activity (ability of the whole person) for OT. But physical and occupational therapists themselves are not always so clear. As Tina Elliott, a physical therapist, commented,

> Fifteen years ago, the disparity was clearer: OTs took a very functional approach; PTs took a very impairment-based approach, strength and range of motion. PT's realm had been: Can you stand up? Can you get from point A to point B? OT's realm was: Can you dress? Can you eat? I think the pendulum has started to swing in the opposite direction for each profession. I think we're realizing that it's not an either/or situation: it's both.

The identities of physical and occupational therapy are evolving.

About 25 percent of persons reporting major mobility difficulties saw a physical therapist within the last year, but only around 6 percent encountered occupational therapists (Table 14). Rates of using each type of therapy increase with worsening mobility impairments, but only about two-thirds of services are for conditions expected to last more than twelve

TABLE 14. Physical or Occupational
Therapy over the Last Year

Mobility Difficulty	PT (%)	OT (%)
None	3	< 1
Minor	16	1
Moderate	22	3
Major	25	6

months.[1] When people do receive physical or occupational therapy, both generally last three or four months, regardless of the extent of mobility difficulties. The average person getting PT has around twenty visits, while those with OT obtain eighteen to twenty-four visits.[2] These survey findings, however, reflect the mid 1990s. The therapist interviewees would argue that the number of allowed visits has plummeted with tightening health insurance.

Substantial fractions of people therefore do not receive physical or occupational therapy. Fifty-four to 70 percent of respondents say they don't need physical therapy, as say 35 to 52 percent about occupational therapy.[3] Around 20 percent of people say occupational therapy is too expensive and they can't afford it; up to 14 percent report their insurance doesn't cover it. Few (up to 2 percent) say they don't like physical or occupational therapists.

PHYSICAL THERAPY

On its Internet web site, the American Physical Therapy Association (APTA 2001) answers the question: who are physical therapists?

Physical therapists, or PTs, are health care professionals who evaluate and treat people with health problems resulting from injury or disease. PTs assess joint motion, muscle strength and endurance, function of heart and lungs, and performance of activities required in daily living, among other responsibilities. Treatment includes therapeutic exercise, cardiovascular endurance training, and training in activities of daily living. More than 120,000 physical therapists are licensed in the U.S. today, treating nearly one million people every day. The median salary for a physical therapist is $51,000 depending on position, years of experience, degree of education, geographic location, and practice setting.

As of 2002, physical therapists must have either master's or doctoral degrees while PT assistants must have two-year associate's degrees from one of over two hundred accredited educational programs nationwide.

Physical therapists have developed an extensive battery of diagnostic assessment tools and therapeutic modalities. According to the 2001 *Guide to Physical Therapist Practice*, over 700 pages with meticulous detail, physical therapists follow "an established theoretical and scientific base" (S13). As did physical medicine and rehabilitation, physical therapy emerged from World War I and efforts to rehabilitate injured veterans. Physical therapy today is organized around the "disablement model": the effect of acute and chronic conditions on specific body systems, on performance of the whole person, and on people's ability to perform desired and expected roles in society. Medical diagnoses connect directly to the disablement model since "disease and injury often may predict the range and severity of impairments at the system level" (S21). The disablement model includes four interacting domains: pathology and pathophysiology (diseases, disorders, or conditions); impairments (abnormalities of tissues, organs, or body systems); functional limitations (difficulties performing physical actions, tasks, or activities); and disability (difficulties with self-care, home management, work or school, and community and leisure roles within the person's social, cultural, and physical environments).

The *Guide to Physical Therapist Practice* organizes evaluations of "gait, locomotion, and balance" around these four domains, defining gait as "the manner in which a person walks, characterized by rhythm, cadence, step, stride, and speed" (S64). In addition to eliciting detailed histories from patients and simply observing them walk (with and without assistive devices), physical therapists employ various tools for measuring gait, such as dynamometers, force platforms, goniometers, motion analysis systems, and videotaping. For arthritis patients, for example, physical therapists would observe gait, assess the mobility and integrity of joints, evaluate range of motion and pain, and query patients about the implications of their physical limitations for daily activities (Cwynar and McNerney 1999).

When asked their goals for a patient's first visit, the seven focus group participants differed somewhat, depending on whether they practice in clinics or do home care. "I do a lot of functional testing," said Donna Hitchcock, who works in a clinic, "like the balance test and the six-minute walk. I try to get primary measurements addressing strength and tone and standing and balance—try to get an idea of what's going on."

"Oftentimes the patient can't identify the exact problem with their walking," said Tina Elliott, who also practices in a clinic. "Is it a distance problem? Is it a speed problem? Is it a strength problem? Is it a range of motion problem? I try to figure that out based on observation, timing, measuring distance, and then looking at strength and range of motion, trying to assess what's limiting their ability to walk fast or far or safely."

"In home care I find that I can do a lot of this very casually," observed Edith Leder. "I see who answers the door, if it's them or a caregiver that gets up, opens the door, lets you in. If somebody's sitting in a chair telling you where things are rather than getting up and showing you, that's a clue that things aren't well. You can pick up a lot of clues without asking. People, especially at home, often like to cover up."

"On a first visit, I focus on determining the patient's impairments and coming up with their goals," said Lois Grant, who practices home care. "What they hope to achieve through physical therapy."

"What's an example?"

"A home-care patient of mine who basically is very debilitated—could walk to and from the bathroom and up and down her hallway. Her big goal is to get down to the hairdresser in the lobby. That would entail getting in and out of the elevator, reaching for the elevator buttons, walking the distance to the hairdresser, getting her hair done, and then walking back. The patient's goal was different from my goals for her."

"What were your goals?"

"Objective things, like ambulate such and such a distance with an assistive device, get in and out of the shower. Anyway, we incorporated the patient's goals into the treatment plan for the long term."

Starting with World War I, physical therapy treatments typically occurred during long hospital stays, following an acute event like a war wound or polio.[4] More recently, rehabilitation hospitals admitted people recovering from strokes, hip fractures, joint replacements, and other major illnesses, giving intensive physical and other therapies for multiple hours each day. Louanne Mawby stayed in a rehabilitation hospital for three months following her stroke in her early forties:

> It was rough. You get up in the morning. You have your breakfast.
> Then you got to work out, just like you go to a job. You work all day
> long. One therapist got you, and then the other one take you. All
> day long. Then you have your lunch and your supper, and you go to
> bed. But you get up early in the morning again. . . . I kept thinking
> about my house and when I would go home. My house has upstairs
> and downstairs. I was very worried: can I get up and down the
> stairs? So I kept pushing myself.

Mrs. Mawby walked when she left the hospital.

Today, less than 5 percent of physical therapists work in rehabilitation hospitals (APTA 2001), and health insurers have cut the length of these hospitalizations dramatically. Today, Mrs. Mawby would stay in hospital much less than three months. She would probably be discharged with physical therapy home visits. "Patients no longer have the luxury of leaving the hospital when they are close to resuming a normal daily routine" (Rimmer 1999, 497).

Decreasing reimbursement has stimulated interest in interventions that help people care for themselves. Certainly, physical therapists still actively administer some therapies, with patients as largely passive recipients: for instance, treatment for low-back pain includes ultrasound or microwave diathermy for deep heating, ice massage or vapocoolant sprays for therapeutic cold, and even low-power cold laser treatments. Research shows that none of these interventions improves low-back pain in the short or long term. But these "passive modalities" remain popular for several reasons: "the patient's expectations of traditional physical therapy, the laying of hands as therapists gives satisfaction . . . and the patients' satisfaction at not having to exert themselves" (Nordin and Campello 1999, 80).

The demands of living daily with chronic conditions eventually prompt many people to take over managing their own care. The vast majority of persons with walking difficulties are not hospitalized for their underlying chronic conditions or are hospitalized only in later stages (e.g., for joint replacement surgery). Therapy must fit into their daily lives, so that it "encourages functional independence, emphasizes patient/client-related instruction, and promotes proactive, wellness-oriented lifestyles" (*Guides to Physical Therapist Practice* 2001, S97). Therapeutic exercise is the leading physical therapy intervention. Obviously, individual people have different needs and physical capabilities. "I have a gentleman who has dementia, Parkinson's disease, and a stroke," said Dr. Samuel Newton, a general internist. "He just sat in a wheelchair all day, not moving. He needs physical therapy because he's only going to deteriorate. He's never going to improve, but we need PT to keep him at a stable functional status, to move his legs, get him out of the wheelchair. And he's been OK. He spends a little bit of the day out of the wheelchair, which he never would have if he hadn't gotten physical therapy." The man participated minimally while the physical therapist exercised his limbs.

Other exercise programs involve people independently following physical therapists' instructions. Specific exercise regimens vary, such as to improve aerobic capacity or endurance or to enhance balance, coordination, flexibility, and range of motion. Depending on people's needs, an explicit goal of exercise training is preventing falls or minimizing fall-related injuries. Pool-based exercise programs use the buoyancy of water to ease people's movements and support weight. "You lose weight in the water," observed one woman. "Nothing hurts in the water. Even if you don't walk any better, when you get out, you feel great."

Physical therapists also intervene with assistive technologies. Although physicians typically must write prescriptions for these devices to be reimbursed, physical therapists often decide which equipment is appropriate, determine its exact specifications, and train people to use equipment properly. Physical therapists consider mobility aids (e.g., canes, crutches, walkers, wheelchairs), orthotic devices primarily for the lower extremities (e.g., braces, splints, shoe inserts), protective devices (e.g., braces, protective taping), and prostheses.

Motivating change in people's daily lives loomed large in the physical therapy focus group. Therapists, however, recognize their limitations in changing people's lifestyles and physical environments. "The first step is conscious acceptance that change needs to take place," said Gary McNamara, whose home-care agency serves south Boston.

"Your point is valid," concurred Tina Elliott. "I've been primarily treating patients with Parkinson's disease. A lot of them fall; it's a long-term problem. From the beginning, I spend a lot of time telling them, 'I'm going to try to help you figure out why you're falling, but then it's up to you. Are you ready to participate and make these changes? This is what I think needs to be done; however, the ball's in your court.' They have to buy into changing to fix it."

"The definition of 'fix' is negotiable for long-term conditions," said Edith Leder. "Parkinson's is chronic and ultimately progressive. So you may fix it today, but it's going to get all out of kilter again. Patients need to understand that. If they do make this change, they're probably going to have to change again. You can show them that they're safer using a piece of equipment, for example, but they don't see the benefit of it long-term. I think that's often why people don't do as we ask them. They don't see the benefit of it. It's an extra piece of equipment that's going to sit in the corner."

"We're trying to sell exercise programs," Gary said. " 'If you do this now, this is what you'll get.' Try selling it when patients have a progressive condition! All you do is delay a decline. You're telling someone they're going to get worse slower. And patients say, why bother? You can understand where they're coming from."

"Another thing with elderly patients is that many of them have never exercised," said Joan. "I've worked with women in their eighties who've never worn pants. We had a group exercise program and tried to convince this wonderful woman who's in her late eighties that she could do more if she bought a pair of pants. It was really hard for her. She'd come in her dress. The concept of sweating and getting down on the floor and stretching is difficult for some older people. Now we have a whole new group getting older that is going to be very different. We're going to have to tell them to slow down!"

"If you observe patients doing something functionally in their house, in their own setup, you adapt the exercise program to something that they're already doing," Lois suggested. "It should be something they're invested in rather than some meaningless exercise, like lying on their side lifting their leg. They could be standing at their sink and washing their dishes and doing some exercise."

"The only caveat with that is that, for somebody to really improve, unfortunately they need to practice and practice," said Edith. "If you want to improve your ambulation, you really have to work at it a lot, even if it's just repeating, repeating, repeating. I don't think you can soft-soap it: this *is* exercise. You need to do it as *exercise*. We can make it as pleasant as you want, but it's still exercise. You have to look at it that way to get better."

OCCUPATIONAL THERAPY

On its Internet web site, the American Occupational Therapy Association (2001) describes its profession,

> Occupational therapy is a health and rehabilitation profession that helps people regain, develop, and build skills that are important for independent functioning, health, well-being, security, and happiness. Occupational therapy practitioners work with people of all ages who, because of illness, injury, or developmental or psychological impairment, need specialized assistance in learning skills to enable them to lead independent, productive, and satisfying lives.
>
> Occupational therapy can prevent injury or the worsening of existing conditions or disabilities and it promotes independent functioning in individuals who may otherwise require institutionalization or other long-term care. Because of this, occupational therapy keeps health care costs down and maximizes the quality of life for the individual, their family, and other caregivers.

Over 50,000 occupational therapist and occupational therapy assistants practice nationwide. OTs must complete master's or doctoral degrees while OT assistants must have two-year associate's degrees from one of over 300 accredited educational programs. With shortening hospital stays, occupational therapists practice increasingly in home care as independent practitioners, either self-employed or affiliated with agencies (Ellenberg 1996).

Occupational therapy's underlying philosophy holds that through their actions, energized by mind and will, people can influence the state of their own health (Trombly 1995b, 20). The word "occupation" connotes purposeful activity, which can prevent or ameliorate dysfunction and help people adapt as well as possible to their daily lives within their environments. Therefore, the first step of an occupational therapy evaluation is to determine people's daily tasks and the activities they must and want to do within their own environments, their homes and communities. Occupational therapists' ultimate goal is to engage people in "occupations" or purposeful activities, not only by addressing their individual physical, emotional, and cognitive performance but also by improving their environments. Although various different ways of thinking have guided occupational therapists (Trombly 1995a), many today follow the model introduced in chapter 1, promulgated by the World Health Organization (2001) for its *International Classification of Functioning, Disability and Health.* Under this approach, disorders and disease interact with the environmental and social contexts to affect a person's impairments, activities, and participation in life situations.

Occupational therapy evaluations consider four factors: tasks causing people difficulties, including specific actions making up each task; exact reasons for the difficulty (ranging from physical or sensory impairments to emotional concerns to inadequate assistive technology to architectural barriers); whether patients themselves might modify these causes; and which occupational therapy interventions could improve the difficulties (Rogers and Holm 1998, 186). Occupational therapists gather information by asking questions, observing, and testing. All three approaches proceed from the general to very specific, breaking down tasks and barriers into their smallest components. Especially in the evaluation of environmental barriers, detailed questionnaires and on-site observation based on universal design principles help develop a comprehensive picture (Cooper, Rigby, and Letts 1995).

The six occupational therapists in the focus group—five actively practicing home care, the sixth teaching home care to OT students—appeared practical, grounded in reality. Unlike physical therapists, they evaluate walking not as an end but as a means for conducting daily life. When asked what they do on the first visit, they immediately emphasized safety: "Our first visit would be for home safety and accessibility. Can they get to the bathroom? Can they get their meals? Transportation? Look at everything."

"I try to distinguish myself as an OT," said Sherrie Little, who practices in a working-class neighborhood. "OTs look at the basics. What do you do day-to-day? Do you get up in the morning? Do you brush your teeth? Do you wash your hair? Do you make yourself a meal? From the start, I give patients a good understanding of what I address versus a PT, versus the nurse, versus the home-health aide, versus whoever else is coming in and out of the house. If someone has a home-health aide, I say, 'You're getting assistance with these things right now. The goal is for you to work toward independence.' "

"That's important," observed Heather Davis. "A lot of referrals are because the home-health aid needs to be decreased, and they want the OT to go in and do it. So you're going into someone's home trying to be all cheery: 'I'm going to help you be more independent.' And they look at you like, 'You're taking away my help.' Sometimes the home-health aide is the only person they see all day. That's difficult."

"How do you make them independent?"

"I make sure they're safe in the kitchen," Heather replied. "Can get to the refrigerator, the cabinets. They can get into the bathroom, that there's a clear path, there's no obstacles, no cords, no scatter rugs, especially if they use a mobility device. Make sure the environment is safe for them."

"I always looked at mobility aids," said Myra Markham, who now teaches OT. "People come home with a walker or the three-prong cane, but you wouldn't see it around their house. You'd realize they weren't using it or were using it wrong. They didn't want to bother with the walker; they'd leap from chair to chair; they'd carry the cane rather than using it for support. I'd talk to them about falls."

"I always think about setting goals," said Joanne Evans, who has practiced for many years. "I usually ask: 'Is there anything that you used to do that you can't do that you want to do?' It's like a story. The OT's story and the patient's story have to have the same ending. I can want someone to be able to get up, get dressed, go downstairs, make three meals, do everything because I think they're physically capable of it. But if that person does not have that same goal, it's never going to happen."

According to the American Occupational Therapy Association (2001):

> A registered occupational therapist develops and documents an intervention plan that is based on the results of the occupational therapy evaluation and the desires and expectations of the client and appropriate others about the outcome of service. . . . [Intervention plans include] client-centered goals that are clear, measurable, behavioral, functional, contextually relevant, and appropriate to the client's needs, desires, and expected outcomes.

Occupational therapy interventions vary widely depending on the nature of the person's impairments and potential for improvement, the specific task involved, and the social and environmental contexts (Holm,

Rogers, and Stone 1998a). Safe, efficient, and independent performance of activities requires a successful balance of three interacting factors: person, task, and environment. Treatments fall into three broad categories: remediating or restoring function (improving the ability to perform specific skills or actions comprising specific tasks, for example, through strengthening exercises); compensation (altering the method for performing the task, adapting objects used to perform the task or using assistive technologies, or adapting the environment); and educating people and, possibly, their family members or other helpers (Holm, Rogers, and James 1998b).

Although physical and occupational therapy share some therapeutic approaches, such as specific exercises and use of assistive technologies, occupational therapy explicitly aims to improve activities and participation within the patient's own environment, particularly the home. Joanne Evans had a patient with MS who "was sleeping on the floor because she could not get up, and when she went to do something, she fell. She felt it was just easier to spend her life crawling around her floor, and she did it for a long time." Joanne needed to think of everything, from grab bars, to wheelchairs, to repositioning furniture, to finding ways for the woman to perform routine activities. All the while the woman, who wanted to "be that independent ambulator," found it "really tough to accept" her physical limitations and the likelihood of progression. Joanne therefore needed to consider psychological factors and the emotional consequences of her interventions. All of this takes time.

"The trend in occupational therapy is client-centered goals," Myra observed. "Patients are part of the process from the first interaction."

"Things have changed a lot," observed Gina Lytton. "Years ago, we had the time to take people out in the community. We would have the bus schedule ready and take people shopping on the bus, show them what to do when they got to the store."

"There was that social component," Myra commented. "You really felt the relationship with the patient and with the family. I had patients who would bake cookies or have tea ready. They would look forward to your visit. You spent some time socially before getting down to work with them."

"Now we're all stressed." Everybody nodded. "Things take more time than you have scheduled."

Jennifer Kingsley agreed, especially when patients need extensive education. "Sometimes you have to teach people they need to conserve their energy but they also need to exercise. I have a MS patient right now who doesn't understand why she just can't do things the way she's always done them. I'm doing a lot of teaching on why she needs to conserve her energy.

She shouldn't make all these trips back and forth across her apartment. She should get everything at once and bring it over, but I know PT is telling her that she needs to walk certain distances. I'm trying to teach her to prioritize and to schedule exercise sessions and rest periods."

"We encourage people to be as independent as possible," stated Heather. "If they don't start doing something, they'll never be able to do it. I worked with a patient today. She must have said a hundred times in that half hour, 'I don't want to live like this. I don't want to live like this.' So I say, 'The reason I'm here is to help you to do more for yourself. You need to work with me so we can do that.' "

EXPERIENCES WITH PHYSICAL
AND OCCUPATIONAL THERAPISTS

Most people like their physical and occupational therapy experiences, although it was sometimes hard to distinguish between the two: did an occupational or physical therapist give Esther Halpern her much-used reacher? People generally like their therapists personally, feel that therapists explain situations well and understand their problems, and believe that therapists instill motivation and positive thinking. Some people do report negative experiences. Several themes summarize feelings about physical and occupational therapy and their general therapeutic approach.

People like the notion that exercises target specific muscles—it makes sense. They feel they are working on something they can understand and measure its progress. "I go to a wonderful physical therapist," said Margaret Freemont, who had MS for decades. "Her name is Anne. She explains to you why you do things, what you're trying to do with certain exercises."

"Does knowing that motivate you to exercise?"

"I'm very motivated," laughed Dr. Freemont. "I'm a very compliant patient. We're working on posture, really standing erect, recruiting muscles that will make me walk better. I will be more alert. I will stand up straighter."

"Will standing up straight improve your walking?"

"Yes, I'm sure of it."

Some people believe that physical and occupational therapy extends beyond addressing specific impairments to enhancing overall health and wellness, connecting the mind and body. "I was given a gift of this physical therapist named Alice," said Myrtle Johnson, who had a recent knee replacement. "She heals your leg with the mind and massage. She knows what I'm thinking and how I feel. After two months with her, I was walking great. I'm doing better all the time." Mrs. Johnson had tried various healers, including herbalists and a local celebrity nicknamed "The Russian," a hypnotist. "But only Alice's doing it. She's the one that got me walking."

"What are her goals for you?"

"She says, 'I want you to lead as full a life as you can for your age. But you do more than I do, so it's hard to know which way to go with you!' She wants to keep me on my feet. But she worries about me. She's about the only one who knows how tired I can get and not show it. She's afraid I'll get a stroke or I'll overdo it. But that's life. Why sit home and wait for it? I might as well do what I want to do."

Walter Masterson, who had ALS, had two separate therapists; one he equated with his body and the other with his mind. They worked as a tag team. "One is real physical therapy, and she does the torture stuff, the bending and the twisting," said Mr. Masterson. "The other is massage, who puts me to sleep after the first one has done her thing. I find that a very useful combination. It works some kinks out. It also coaches me and my wife in exercises that we do daily or almost daily, just to keep me loose, keep circulation flowing."

People are afraid of falling—legitimately so. Dr. Jody Farr spent two weeks in a rehabilitation facility after falling at work. That's where she met "a great physical therapist and a great occupational therapist. It worked out really well. They were full of energy and really good people. They were thinking of ways to make my house safe. We came out to my house and had a site visit." Dr. Farr had grab bars and railings installed, but she especially appreciated their ideas about making it easier to stand up from chairs: her muscular dystrophy impedes efforts to rise from low heights. "We got a six-inch cushion and a four-inch cushion, and put them on two chairs. That makes a huge difference. Now I only sit in those chairs because I can get up from them with ease."

Others share Dr. Farr's enthusiasm. "I just started with an OT," reported a woman in her early forties with ALS. "She's shown me a lot of little tricks around the house, and she gave me neat little gadgets that are pretty helpful. If I drop something on the floor, like my granddaughter's toy, I can pick it up with a reacher. It's a long stick; you squeeze it, and it grabs things. Or if my shoes are far away from me, I can pull my shoes to me with another little device. Also the shower chair and the sponge on the end of a stick. That's very helpful. The care that I'm getting makes me less scared and frightened."

Dr. Stanley Nathan feels that home interventions are one place where occupational therapy is clearly not only good for patients but also saves money.

I had this ninety-year-old patient living in Coolidge Corner. She was tripping because she had all this stuff in her house, all these little carpets. She fell at some point. An occupational therapist did a home safety assessment to help keep her from falling again. With managed care, it's one of those things that people actually feel is cost-effective—looking for things we could do at home to prevent falls that might lead to hip fractures.

Sally Ann Jones was not happy with the physical therapist who visited her. Her neurologist had perhaps contributed to the problem. "I asked the neurologist for a physical therapy prescription a couple of times. He finally wrote it. I called the PT department at the hospital near me, and a PT comes to my house and looks at the prescription. The prescription says 'strengthening exercises, range of motion, and gait training.' OK? I can't stand and pivot. So gait training is moot at this point." Her neurologist's prescription should have emphasized Mrs. Jones's functional deficit, standing up, balancing, turning to use the toilet. A good physical therapist would have evaluated the situation and customized treatment, but this therapist did not. She left Mrs. Jones instructions describing exercises impossible for her to do.

Mrs. Jones's experiences raise questions about the quality of care of therapists making home visits. "Home-care PT is a crapshoot," worries Dr. Lawrence Jen. "You never know exactly what you're getting. Home-care therapists are frequently really fine people, but they're isolated from any feedback. They don't have continuing education that's meaningful. In home care, they can't really get good oversight, and anyway doctors don't know how to give a PT order. A good therapist actually makes diagnoses and individualizes the treatment."

Other people also voiced concerns that therapists do not fully evaluate their situations or design interventions appropriate to people with chronic conditions. One woman in her mid forties who has had rheumatoid arthritis for over two decades observed,

> Over the years I have learned how hard it is to find physical therapists and exercise trainers who really understand how to put together a realistic, comprehensive fitness program for people with disabilities or limitations. Most professionals and programs are oriented toward people who are recovering from injuries that improve over time, not chronic problems that require a different approach or activity almost on a daily basis to prevent harm. Very few exercise programs are designed to address the problems that many people with disabilities have. Swimming and water aerobics programs are often taught in cold pools. Many pools have ladders that are very

painful to use if you have trouble gripping things and problems with painful feet. The pounding and repetitive motion of aerobics and typical exercise programs are completely out of the realm of possibility. Exercise bicycles have been helpful for limited periods of time, but the need to switch activities to avoid over-stressing the same joints makes it difficult to develop a realistic, affordable program.

Many people come up with exercise regimens that suit their daily lives. Sally Ann Jones says she exercises "every morning before I get out of bed. Then I go stand up in the bathroom half-a-dozen times a day and move this stupid foot as many times as it will move. I dress myself; I do my own housework; I do everything I can do because that's exercise." Jimmy Howard feels his "exercise bike is just as good as physical therapy. It does wonders. As soon as I get on the bike in the morning, hey, all the stiffness is gone. Why bother with physical therapy when I can do it on my own?"

ALTERNATIVE THERAPIES

Over the last decade, people have increasingly admitted using alternative or complementary therapies—remedies that are often as old as the hills, embedded within cultural and social traditions. Certainly, chiropractic has long received professional recognition, but other alternative therapies still remain outside the Western medical mainstream, including herbal therapies, acupuncture, homeopathy, megavitamins, energy healing, prayer, massage, and faith healing. Roughly 40 percent of Americans say they use some type of alternative therapy, with numbers of visits exceeding encounters with primary care physicians (Eisenberg et al. 1993, 1998). People with physical disabilities are much more likely than others to report using alternative therapies, especially to treat pain, depression, anxiety, insomnia, and headache (Krauss et al. 1998).[5] Massage, relaxation techniques, and self-help groups are especially popular; people with back problems also frequently seek chiropractic care.

I asked every person whether they use or have used alternative or complementary therapies, such as acupuncture, chiropractic, herbal medicine, or massage. Many people had not. "I don't want to try a chiropractor," said Marianne Bickford, reflecting views held by others. "I'm afraid for my back. I've often wondered about acupuncture, but when I think of needles, I freeze up, and I don't know many people who've used it." According to Stella Richards, "The chiropractor can make you worse off than when you started. You've only got one back, and I don't want them to make it worse. I think I could stand acupuncture better," but Mrs. Richards hasn't tried it.

She worries about what her surgeon might think. Walter Masterson has tried various alternative therapies:

> I'm getting massage now. In the early days, I got acupuncture. It was an exotic experience. A couple of years ago, the thought of seeing an acupuncturist would have been ludicrous to me. But at the end of the session, there was a sense of internal cleanness in my legs which impressed me. Now, there's no evidence that these sessions actually had any impact. But when there's no cure, it's really impossible to say that something has no impact. There's nothing to compare it with. It might have delayed the next step for months. It might have made zero impact. I stopped going when it became apparent to me that it wasn't going to make this go away. Then I went to a different guy. He did herbal medicines. They tasted terrible, but I stuck with it for a couple of months just to see what impact it would have. Then a length of monkey arm became part of my prescription. Monkey arm, quite literally—probably about an inch and a half of monkey arm chopped up into five or six pieces. That's when I dropped out.

Lillian Lowell, in her late seventies, has a thick thatch of white hair and alert, inquisitive eyes. Her tiny house is neat as a pin, the living room filled with glass animals—cats, dogs, penguins. She recently had her second hip replacement for osteoarthritis. "The first thing is the hurting. I started acupuncture shortly after I started hurting, and that worked beautifully for a year."

"What made you do acupuncture?"

"I was talking to somebody whose opinion I respect, and she said it was helping her. So I felt what do I have to lose? For a year I went four days a week. I *loved* the woman who did it, Dr. Siu. It was very relaxing, very fun, and that kept me going for at least a year before I really thought of an operation." That was Mrs. Lowell's first hip replacement, five years previously.

"When the acupuncture stopped working, what did you do?"

"I was going to an orthopedist at the same time. He told me it was osteoarthritis and the cartilage was degenerating, the bones rubbing against each other—he described it fairly callously. He gave me big doses of pain pills."

"Did you tell the orthopedist about the acupuncture?"

"I'm sure I mentioned it to him. I don't think he thought much of it. My internist said, 'Anything that's good therapy for you is good therapy.' I thought that was a very smart approach." Four years later, when her second hip had become painful, Mrs. Lowell tried acupuncture again but did not return to Dr. Siu, whose office was on a busy turnpike. She tried several practitioners, but "I wasn't getting the same results from the acupuncture—the nice relaxed feeling."

One woman had tried chiropractic and found it useful—so useful that the local television news station wanted to feature her story in a piece about chiropractic. "I refused because I didn't want my neurologist to know that I was seeing a chiropractor. At that point, I realized I was starting to take over my own medical care. I was feeling guilty about going to see a chiropractor because it was an alternative medicine. So I didn't even tell my primary care doctor"—the physician who had referred me to this woman.

Some people try techniques, such as massage or prayer, they do not necessarily see as formal interventions. Myrtle Johnson and her husband intoned Buddhist chants over her knee. Lester Goodall is "still exploring the school where it's mind over matter. I really try to find that inner spot. My wife thinks I'm crazy. I do things just for the theatrics, to force feeling. I put my hands like this here," Lester held both hands out straight in front of him, "and I try to communicate with my immune system. They now say the immune system," which might affect MS, "is controlled by the brain. And I say two things: 'heal and protect.' Sometimes I think it works; other times I'm not sure. But that keeps me doing it at times where I'm feeling real bad. That's when I revert back to it: heal and protect."

PAYING FOR SERVICES

In the end, how health insurance—private policies or public programs (Medicare or Medicaid)—covers therapy determines whether people get these services. Wealthier people can afford to pay out-of-pocket for care, but costs accumulate over time. About 20 percent of people say they do not get physical or occupational therapy because they cannot afford it. Thus, people with fewer resources must rely on insurance coverage. Physical and occupational therapy were built into Medicare and Medicaid almost forty years ago, but with explicit limitations. Private coverage varies widely by plan, with insurers typically circumscribing the number and types of visits, setting strict limits. Insurers have only recently started paying for certain alternative therapies, primarily chiropractic.

Esther Halpern feels that pool-based therapy is best for her painful back. "I had physical and water therapy."

"It was warm water," nodded Harry Halpern.

"It was wonderful. The pool was nice and warm, and it's much easier to do exercises in the pool."

"At first it was free."

"I got it free as long as they felt I needed the physical therapy. When they felt that I no longer needed it, I had to pay for it if I wanted water therapy."

Esther looked agitated and Harry muttered under his breath. "You could not afford it?" I asked.

"That's right," exclaimed Harry. He saw benefits to Esther, beyond improved physical function. "It was really good for her. She got out among people. She was able to get herself dressed and undressed and—"

"I was able to get dressed and undressed by myself before that," Esther interrupted.

"Yes, but it was better."

"It wasn't quite as easy after I stopped," Esther conceded. "All the therapy helped me. It really did."

"I don't know whether her doctor will give her a prescription, but she really needs it."

"They did arrange for me to have home therapy," said Esther, making clear this was second best. "I've been getting it now. I don't know how much longer they'll give it to me. But I'll take it as long as they'll give it to me."

"Sounds like money is the real problem," I stated the obvious.

"Oh, it still is," replied Esther. "Absolutely."

11 Ambulation Aids

I had no choice about using a cane. One day during my surgical rotation in medical school, my right leg suddenly collapsed, and the fall broke a small bone in my foot—the fifth metatarsal. The fracture was minor, the pain abating within a week. The cane aided bone healing by off-loading weight from the foot. Afterward the cane steadied my veering, unbalanced gait.

Despite its utility, the cane embarrassed me—I'm not sure exactly why. It precipitated a barrage of eerily identical questions: "Did you have a skiing accident?" I had never skied in my life, unless you count the hour or so in high school. Taking the rope tow up the beginner slope, unsteady on rented skis, I felt an unpleasant choking sensation. The twisting rope tow had somehow latched onto the fringe of the scarf peeking out below my parka. After they stopped the tow and unwound me, I sat out the rest of the day.

So how do you respond to such questions? "No, I didn't have a skiing accident," sounds inadequate. Somehow social convention demands a more complete explanation, but my MS was private. If I, a medical student, mentioned my MS, I reasoned, patients may lose faith in me or think I'm seeking sympathy. After all, they're the sick people, lying in hospital beds. Burdening them with my disease, even by explaining my cane, seemed presumptuous. Plus, the cane was clunky. When propped in a corner, it invariably fell, with a clatter, to the tile floor. If placed on the floor in cramped hospital rooms, someone, including me, could trip over it. Girded by these rationalizations, I began stashing—hiding—the cane at the nurse's station or utility room before entering patients' rooms, carefully clutching the doorjamb. That way, maybe patients wouldn't notice I had trouble walking.

Mobility aids are always visible, and they are explicitly utilitarian. Unlike Fred Astaire's glossy, svelte walking stick, real mobility aids clearly aim to support or transport persons. These aids generally do their jobs well, easing pain, enhancing balance, maximizing safety, helping people get around. Mobility aids can restore independence and conserve energy drained by enervating struggles to walk.

Users of mobility aids openly admit—both to themselves and the external world—their lost physical function and consequent need. After injuries, walking short-term with canes or crutches evokes sympathetic inquiries about that presumed skiing or other accident. When I fractured my foot and adopted the cane, surgeons regaled me with stories of their own broken bones (but never asked about my injury). Long-term, however, mobility aids carry not only weight, quite literally, but also a hefty symbolism. As Tom Norton said, "Company presidents don't use canes."

Not surprisingly, many people with progressive chronic conditions express tremendous ambivalence about using mobility aids. One study found that about half of people with great difficulty walking one-quarter mile do not use any assistance; they probably simply avoid walking that far (Verbrugge, Rennert, and Madans 1997, 386). Using equipment to aid mobility, however, enhances people's sense of autonomy and self-sufficiency. With increasing technological sophistication, mobility aids can offer efficient alternatives to costly personal assistance and institutionalization, even for people with significant physical limitations.

Chapters 11 and 12 explore the contradictions surrounding mobility aids, juxtaposing their important advantages with persisting individual and societal unease. Chapter 11 considers ambulation aids (canes, crutches, walkers) but not potentially useful items fabricated for particular needs (special shoes, splints, braces, orthotics, or limb prostheses). Chapter 12 examines wheelchairs and scooters.

As a bottom line, decisions about mobility aids and all assistive technologies (AT) must reflect the user's needs, circumstances, and preferences. "Assistive technologies should be adapted to persons with disabilities, not the other way around. AT choice should include the right to choose or to reject AT" (Olkin 1999, 291). Almost inevitably, others weigh in—family members, physicians, physical and occupational therapists, AT vendors, and health insurers. Decisions about mobility aids can become complicated and emotionally charged.

THE HIERARCHY OF MOBILITY AIDS

According to the NHIS-D, 3 percent (estimated 6.1 million) of adults living outside institutions use some mobility aid: over 2 percent (estimated 4.5

TABLE 15. Use of Mobility Aids by People with Major
Mobility Difficulties

	Mobility Aid (%)		
Difficulty	*Cane*	*Walker*	*Wheelchair*
Arthritis	44	26	16
Back problems and sciatica	34	10	5
Heart conditions	30	15	14
Lung conditions	16	11	12
Stroke	48	28	44
Missing lower limb	57	30	23
Diabetes	37	40	35
Multiple sclerosis	36	29	66

million) use canes; 0.3 percent (510,000) use crutches; almost 1 percent (1.7 million) use walkers; 0.8 percent (1.5 million) use wheelchairs or scooters; and 0.7 percent (1.4 million) use more than one mobility aid.[1] The majority of these people anticipate using mobility aids for one year or longer.[2] Among people with major mobility difficulties, almost everybody with arthritis, stroke, amputation, diabetes, or MS uses at least one type of mobility aid, while those with heart or lung disease use mobility aids less often (Table 15).[3] Many live alone: 37 percent of cane and crutch users; 35 percent of walker users; and 26 percent of wheelchair users. After accounting for various personal factors,[4] we find that cane users live alone 50 percent more frequently than other people, and walker users 30 percent more often. The survey has no information on whether mobility aids allow people to live alone more independently and safely than without the equipment.

Mobility aids have their own hierarchy, from low-tech wooden canes with crook handles, to multifooted canes, to crutches, to walkers, to manual wheelchairs and scooters, to sophisticated power wheelchairs. People generally start with the lowest practical option, then, if impairments progress, they move up the hierarchy, as did Walter Masterson (chapter 3).

Over the last two decades the sophistication, design, and diversity of mobility aids have grown dramatically, offering consumers wide-ranging options for most tastes and requirements. Yet little systematic evidence is available about the technical pros and cons of different mobility aids and their safety and biomechanics in routine use. Most studies involve few participants, often "normal" volunteers. Research including persons with actual mobility problems is generally conducted in laboratories, with few studies examining how people use mobility aids in daily life or whether these aids save societal costs (e.g., by allowing people to work and pay taxes, by reducing personal assistance expenses).

Choice of mobility aids must consider many factors beyond lower-extremity functioning, including people's cognitive status and judgment, vision, vestibular function (which affects balance), upper-body strength, and global physical endurance, as well as home and community environments. Ambulation aids fall at the low-tech, higher-functioning end of the mobility device continuum. Dr. Stuart Hartman, an orthopedic surgeon, encourages patients to use ambulation aids by emphasizing that they will still walk independently, albeit now with mechanical assistance:

> People don't normally want these things—they just don't want to be seen that way. They feel like everybody is looking at them, like they're getting old and that's the final chapter. But I say to people, "Look, you would walk much better, much farther, more comfortably, and you'd walk more places because you'd feel supported and steadier on your feet." People still say, "Doc, I just won't use it. You can give me the prescription, but I'm not going to use it." A lot of people later discover, hey, it was a good idea and they like it. They go farther because they're not as exhausted, they're not huffing and puffing. It's an aid for ambulation. It's not like a wheelchair.

Canes are simple but remarkably useful. They help off-load weight, such as from painful arthritic joints. Canes augment muscle action and provide stability, especially for people with neurologic conditions. For balance, a single finger lightly touching fixed objects, like walls, actually improves stability better than canes (Maeda et al. 1998). People often "furniture surf" at home, placing objects strategically to balance themselves, but in open spaces have nothing fixed to grab. Canes can convey tactile information and enhance balance, as fingers touching walls do (Jeka 1997; Maeda et al. 1998). Canes also improve stability by increasing a person's base of support.

Unfortunately, most people get little instruction in proper use of canes (Kuan, Tsou, and Su 1999), although, as Dr. Hartman notes, "somebody with a balance disturbance should use a cane differently from someone with a bad hip or knee who uses it for weight-bearing." People often buy canes from drugstores or receive them from family or friends, without getting professional advice or training. Up to 70 percent of canes are the wrong length, faulty, or damaged (Joyce and Kirby 1991; Kumar, Roe, and Scremin 1995; Alexander 1996). Many people, therefore, do not get the maximum benefit from their canes.

Although canes are the least sophisticated ambulation aid, several variants are available, differing at their handles and bases. Canes come with crook tops, spade tops, and straight tops; they can have a single rubber-capped tip or three or four short legs attached to little platforms at their base. Functional differences among these variants are unclear, and studies are limited and contradictory.[5] Cane selection largely reflects personal tastes.

Crutches primarily off-load weight rather than improve balance. Depending on users' upper-body strength, underarm crutches can bear up to 100 percent of their weight, while forearm crutches (i.e., with a cuff and piece fitting under the forearm ending in a handle) can bear 40 to 50 percent (Joyce and Kirby 1991, 538–39). Cuffs free the hands of forearm crutch users for actions like opening doors. Various styles of crutches offer different benefits for people with weakness in specific arm muscles (Ragnarsson 1998). Again, choosing the most suitable crutch depends on individual circumstances. As with canes, training and proper fitting maximize their usefulness.

Walkers provide additional stability for people with poor balance and lower-extremity weakness and come in many styles, from standard rigid models without wheels to collapsible wheeled walkers, with handbrakes, seats, and baskets. As with canes, walkers must be the proper height, and training is essential. Wheeled walkers are dangerous if they roll forward unexpectedly, but they are easy to propel on smooth surfaces (Joyce and Kirby 1991), demand less energy (Foley et al. 1996), and require less mental concentration to operate (Wright and Kemp 1992) than standard walkers. Rigid walkers appear institutional, symbolizing serious debility—anathema to many people. Colorful rolling walkers with baskets and seats, in contrast, are practical (e.g., for navigating shopping malls) and seem friendlier. People who refuse standard walkers often welcome the rolling version.

A USEFUL TRADE-OFF

After initial reluctance, Dr. Hartman's patients generally appreciate their ambulation aids—after all, they still walk. But the decision to try one is often complicated and reflects a conscious trade-off, balancing recognition of practical realities against the symbolism of debility. Interviewees' pragmatic reasons to use ambulation aids fall into five categories:

- to assist postoperative recovery after joint, back, or other lower-extremity surgery
- to minimize pain by giving mechanical support

- to compensate for neurologic problems, such as weakness or imbalance

- to assuage personal fears, such as fear of falling

- to convey something to the outside world, such as alerting strangers to stay clear

But almost no one welcomes ambulation aids with open arms.

Stella Richards had back surgery to alleviate intractable excruciating pain: "You have to be able to walk, and they outfit you with a walker after that operation because you can't walk without it." After her first back surgery, "I went home with my walker. But after two or three days, I was off it." Unfortunately, her pain returned, and she had a second operation that also failed. "I have never been able to get off this walker since the second operation," she stated grimly.

Immediately after surgery, people readily agree to use ambulation aids. They really have little choice, given the compelling mechanical rationale—to avoid putting weight and pressure on healing bones and joints. Some people first use walkers for more substantial weight-bearing, then graduate to crutches or canes as they mend. Many people also do physical therapy or other exercises to strengthen muscles and speed restoration of function. Most expect to jettison these postoperative ambulation aids soon afterward, as did Mrs. Richards following her first surgery, although sometimes it doesn't work out.

"It Took the Pressure Off"

Mike Campbell resisted using a cane for years, despite deepening arthritis pain in his knees. When he finally gave in, "at least it took the pressure off." Canes off-load weight from painful joints and thus reduce the mechanical causes of pain, but people balk. Why?

Despite his physician's plea and pain like a "hammer and chisel," Jimmy Howard also resisted. "I was trying to be cool. I don't need no cane. I'm walking around trying to find something to grab onto," Mr. Howard laughed. "Then I decided he's right. I think I better get a cane. So I got a cane. It was a big help. I call this my assistant," he said pointing to an aluminum cane with a crook handle. "I tell my wife, 'Be careful with my assistant—it's very temperamental!' And she cracks up."

"Do you use your assistant around your house?"

"Oh, yeah. I use it everywhere I go. As soon as I get out of bed, I reach and grab it, right next to me."

Dr. Josh Landau, a rheumatologist, was Mr. Campbell's physician. He believes that canes significantly lessen pain for some patients.

I've often recommended canes and had patients turn me down. I barely have the words out of my mouth that the patient might consider a cane, and they are shaking their head "no"—before I'm even done suggesting it, or telling them how to use it, or why I would recommend it. I think it's the stigma issue. Patients feel they're giving in or broadcasting that they've got this problem, even though they're limping so their problem's evident anyway. A lot of patients would rather have the pain or the balance difficulty or go slower than they might otherwise rather than get a cane.

Mike Campbell claimed that he didn't care what other people thought about him, while Jimmy Howard originally was intent on "being cool." Both eventually recognized the cane's value, Mr. Campbell temporarily (until after his knee replacements healed) and Mr. Howard for the foreseeable future.

"For Balance"

"Why did you start using a cane?" I asked Margaret Freemont, who had MS.

"Balance. For a while, I just would use it outside, and when I got into the house, I could sort of cruise—there were always things I could use for balance if I needed it. But outside, I needed the cane for balance because there weren't things I could grab. Then I started using the cane inside the house, too." When I met her, she used a rolling walker at home, somehow threading through rooms crowded with low furniture, plants, and scatter rugs. Outdoors, she traveled by scooter.

Concerns about balance motivate other people with neurologic conditions to use ambulation aids, despite some misgivings. "I needed to use a cane for balance, for security, for safety," stated Louisa Delarte, who also has MS. "I thought the cane with three prongs helped more, gives more stability. But I didn't go for that because I was too vain." She felt the three-point cane looked "more disabled" than the simple, single-point version. "To tell you the truth, I didn't want people staring at me." At home, Mrs. Delarte now uses a bright blue rolling walker, with a seat and handbrakes, while outside she rides a scooter.

Reflecting the fears of many people, Gerald Bernadine was quite explicit about his concerns: "A fractured hip. That's actually my biggest fear—if I fell out here on the pavement and I fractured a hip. That's all I need. That was one of the reasons I started using the cane. It was really as a safety thing because I was afraid. If I fall, I'm going to be a hell of a lot worse off than losing a little vanity. Vanity had prevented me from using the cane."

Regardless of the cause, many people who have trouble walking are afraid of falling. Ambulation aids can give a greater sense of security and help prevent falls (Tinetti and Speechley 1989; Tinetti et al. 1993). Mildred Stanberg went to her corner drugstore and bought a cane. "Why?" I asked.

"I don't know, I think I was afraid of falling. The sidewalks are a little uneven. . . . The cane helps a lot. I have a little security and that makes a difference. I don't use it in the house to do things, but the minute I go out, I use it, and I feel very secure with it."

"It Identifies Me"

Finally, some people use ambulation aids for specific physical reasons but find one additional benefit—the aids caution strangers to stand clear, to get out of their way. At risk of being shoved or tripped in a crowd, people welcome the explicit symbolism of the ambulation aid.

Lester Goodall cited several reasons for using his cane. "I have times when I lose my balance. That's why I walk with a cane when I'm on the street, when I travel on the public transportation. It just gives me something to brace myself." Lester likes to sit when he's on speeding, swaying subways, but the cars are often crowded. Each car has seats marked with the wheelchair logo for disabled passengers, and Lester believes that carrying a cane validates his claim to the designated seats. "It identifies me to the average person out there. It's a general statement."

ENCOURAGING CHOICE

Dr. Ron Einstein, a primary care physician, has trouble getting his patients to use a cane.

> Even my mother! I think she should use a cane, but I cannot convince her. She has this wide-based gait. I know she's going to fall, but she will not use a cane. She says, "I will not be seen dead with a cane, and I will not leave my house. Forget it!" She's probably embarrassed. It's not so strange. You don't want to be too tall, short, heavy, fat, or thin. You don't want to be different. I remember when I first got glasses. I didn't want to admit that I needed glasses. I went for half a year where I would squint and say I didn't need them. I was very embarrassed. You'd think older people would be more comfortable with themselves, but they're still embarrassed.

If ambulation aids can help, using them seems logical, but people aren't always logical. Dr. Einstein is genuinely concerned about his mother's safety and comfort but feels powerless. He risks sounding paternalistic, condescending, or disrespectful by constantly urging his mother to use something she fervently wishes to avoid—even if it could spare her a nasty fall, ease her pain, or speed her way. Everybody grows frustrated.

Unless people themselves choose to use an ambulation aid—or at least give it a solid try—they often won't use it properly and get little benefit, confirming their original objections. Some people agree to carry the ambulation aid but won't let it touch the floor, defeating the purpose. The physical therapist Gary McNamara finds,

> Until they've taken a first step and realize that it's going to take change to create change, you can't do anything. You go to someone's home and they say, "Yeah, I've fallen and my doctor told you to come." They're sitting there and the cane has four inches of dust on it. "I'm not using the cane." . . . It's someone who's not ready. They're convinced that they're stuck in this rut and there's nothing they can do. There's a lot of preconceived notions in their head about assistive devices and what they mean. Some people are just anti, no matter what. Other people think it's the best thing since sliced bread. "Hey, I got a cane. Look what I can do now." It varies. The first step is conscious acceptance that change needs to take place.

The psychologist Rhonda Olkin (1999, 285) argues that acceptance of assistive technologies, such as mobility aids, requires that they "be perceived as enablers of activities and functions that would otherwise be difficult or impossible. This half-full perspective comes more readily to some than to others." But the person needs to make the choices: "loss of function does not equal loss of control—decision making and self-determination as they relate to function should be retained" (285). Even the informed opinions of clinicians ultimately must defer. "It is the people who have the problem (in this case persons with disabilities) who are the experts; the experts aren't the experts" (291).

Since mobility aids are visible, family members often hold strong opinions, and long-established familial dynamics come into play. Sometimes "a family might resist the implications of an AT and insist that the family member rely on his or her own limited facilities, despite the drain on personal energy and emotional resources" (Olkin 1999, 291). I heard this from younger women whose husbands became deeply disturbed when their wives used mobility aids. The husbands do not outright forbid it, recognizing their wives' needs. Nevertheless, the husbands are terrified by the implications—presumed permanent debility and inevitable downward spiral. Other times, family members are persistent advocates, and physicians enlist their help to persuade patients. Dr. Einstein finds, "The spouses are much more receptive than the patients. The spouses know there's a problem. They try to get patients to use the device, but they don't always succeed."

Dr. Johnny Baker navigates delicate terrain between his patients and their family members. Although family members want his professional opinion to validate their positions, Dr. Baker simply doesn't know exactly what is right: after all, little scientific evidence exists to guide decisions about ambulation aids.

> Frequently there's a family member who says, "Mom does fine here in your examining room, but she totters around at home and I'm concerned about her. Don't you think she should use a walker?" The family member comes to the visit, and I hear an earful from them. Then I try to redirect things to the patient: "How do you respond to what your daughter's saying?" . . . The family member usually wants more assistance than the patient has accepted—like moving from a cane to a walker—and wants to go home and quote the doctor: "The doctor said you have to do this."
>
> It's a delicate discussion, a social interaction as opposed to medical. But whether this person who's using a cane would be better off with a walker, I don't know. If I can get the patient and family member to agree with each other, I'll assume that's what's right. I need to maintain my therapeutic alliance with the patient. I'm not the family member's doctor—I'm the patient's doctor.

As Dr. Baker and other clinicians noted, the symbolism of specific ambulation aids is off-putting. Clinician interviewees suggest that carved or painted canes and colorful walkers are more palatable, ornamental as well as practical. "The stigma is heavy duty for some people," observed Myra, an occupational therapist. "They're not going out if they must use a walker or cane, especially young people. People look at you, especially if you're young. It's not considered cool, hip, sporty. Thank god now the equipment is less nursing home–looking. Like the canes. They're a little bit sporty, and they have all these carved canes. So the equipment looks more young and healthy." Myra thinks therapists must be creative, redefining symbols of disability, ways that "feel more comfortable or interesting. Each person needs to find a way to make equipment less of a barrier with other people. They have to go through a process where they feel OK, that it's OK."

Harry Halpern knows when he will finally use a cane. The Halperns' house was an obstacle course, jumbled boxes and stacked papers strewn among sheet-draped furniture. A standard rigid-frame walker leaned, folded, in one corner. Esther Halpern doesn't like that walker, rejecting it immediately after the physical therapist delivered it. Instead, Mrs. Halpern loves her "carriage"—an aluminum walker with four wide gray rubber wheels, brakes on each handlebar, and a stretched cloth seat. Mrs. Halpern demonstrated walking, moving confidently up the short hall. A four-pronged cane, once Mrs. Halpern's, stood in the middle of the cramped living room. She wants Harry to use it, but he objects.

This was clearly a bone of contention between this couple who were about to celebrate their fiftieth wedding anniversary. Emotions escalated, as Mrs. Halpern recounted recent instances of her husband falling out of bed or falling while pulling in the trash barrels. Several times, Mr. Halpern rose from his recliner and lurched around the room, snaring photographs to show me, while his wife pantomimed her distress at his not using a cane: "He's supposed to use the four-prong cane."

"Why won't you use it?" I asked.

"It's not a question of not wanting to use it. When I have to get out, I'm sure it will be different. Until that point arises, which can be any time, I've been hoping . . . ," Harry's voice trailed off.

"How will you know when you reach that point?" I asked.

"I think I'll know."

"What will tell you?"

"When the Lord thunders out, 'Harry, start using that thing.' "

GETTING AND USING AMBULATION AIDS

Tina DiNatale gets around her house by grabbing everything in sight and running her hands along the walls at shoulder height. As do many people with MS, Tina has trouble with balance. Despite conventional wisdom that crutches offer less help with balance than other mobility aids, Tina often uses crutches when she goes out—the standard underarm crutch in pale wood, with gray rubber tips. Barefoot, she demonstrated walking, the crutches splaying widely on either side. "That's interesting," I observed, privately appalled. "Having the crutches out that far gives you a broad base of support." Tina walked awkwardly, with her crutches needlessly heavy and long. Her technique looked exhausting.

"No," she replied. "I'm usually wearing heels so I'm much taller, so the crutches don't go out so far."

Wearing heels? "How long have you walked this way?"

"Sixteen years. They only had wooden crutches when I started, so I'm quite accustomed to the weight of the wooden crutches. They just drop; you don't have to place them anywhere. They fall into place. That helps me. I don't use the pad under my arms because it's just for balance." Unlike for weight-bearing, Tina did not keep the upper part of her crutches tucked into her armpits. Holding the canes away from her body extended their length even further to each side and undoubtedly required more energy. Tina DiNatale's ambulation technique seems a case study in what not to do: wrong ambulation aid, wrong length, needlessly exhausting, potentially dangerous to herself and people straying near her. But she seems satisfied. It's worked for her for sixteen years.

Unlike wheelchairs, most ambulation aids are readily available at neighborhood drugstores. Some products, such as certain rolling walkers, are sold only by medical supply vendors or must be ordered through professionals. But Esther Halpern saw her rolling walker in her local pharmacy's window—it was even on sale. Ready availability of ambulation aids makes them easy to obtain; yet often people receive little instruction about their equipment or its proper use. Mildred Stanberg bought a cane but only discussed it with her primary care physician when he noticed it at her checkup. "I didn't discover until I had it almost a year that you can adjust it," said Mrs. Stanberg, describing her aluminum cane with its crook top. "He told me it was a little high, and if I had it a little lower, it would work better."

Physicians Are "Worse Than Clueless"

Mrs. Stanberg is lucky that her primary care physician recognized that adjusting the cane's height could make it more useful. Some other primary care doctors have little training or skill in prescribing or evaluating ambulation aids. "I haven't a clue how to think through what someone needs," admitted Dr. Alan Magaziner. "I have no idea how to decide whether someone needs a one-pointed cane, a three-pointed cane, a walker, a walker with wheels—worse than clueless. I never had a single talk from anyone on assistive devices—ever!"

Some clinical specialists (e.g., specially trained rheumatologists, geriatricians, neurologists, and orthopedists) know about when to prescribe ambulation aids, and this is obviously a core interest of physiatrists. Dr. Melinda Whittier, a physiatrist, chooses her timing carefully before suggesting ambulation aids.

> You begin that discussion only after you've done a history and a physical examination. We really need all the facts about what is going on medically. I make sure that I have done all my homework and have a good rapport with the patient. Depending on where the person is, you might recommend an assistive device as potentially a temporary measure: "What's important right now is to keep you moving." Don't even broach the long-term issue: "This may be forever." Depending on the disease process, it may do enough to turn

things around. You may reverse the deconditioning and the inactivity, so patients could get back to a level that satisfies them. Where patients have advancing illness and gait isn't really feasible anymore, I talk about potential options: "I don't know which ones are right for you." If they're ready to hear or can deal with it, they will. If not, they'll drop the subject, and they won't come back. It may take six months or a year to decide. But it's your role as a physiatrist when your patient's in distress and facing difficult issues to be friendly and educate them, thoughtfully, sensitively, about the potential options.

Dr. Whittier admits that there is no conclusive evidence about what is best over time for individuals with progressive chronic conditions. Her patients make the decisions, guided by her suggestions.

Determining options, writing proper prescriptions, and training people to use ambulation aids generally involve referrals to other professionals (American Medical Association 1996; DeLisa, Currie, and Martin 1998). And most of the physician interviewees refer people needing ambulation and other mobility aids to physical and, sometimes, occupational therapists. Dr. Lawrence Jen, a rheumatologist, finds that many patients use a cane incorrectly: "They carry it in the wrong hand, and they use it as a gentle support, not really pushing down." He works closely with physical therapists. "I send them to PT to have cane evaluation and training. If people have fallen, I have to talk them into using canes or a walker. I almost always try to do that with a therapist." Dr. Jen worries that most physicians do not use rehabilitation professionals. "They'll say, 'Mrs. Jones, get a cane,' and Mrs. Jones will go out and get some cane. It may not fit, she may not have the upper arm strength to use it, and she may not even know how to use it."

For Therapists, "The Focus Is All on Safety"

With many physicians "worse than clueless," recommendations about specific ambulation aids often fall to physical or occupational therapists. Generally, physical therapists play four roles: evaluating people's physical capacity; delineating appropriate equipment options; training people how to use their equipment for maximum advantage; and following up, to see how people actually use ambulation aids in their homes. In this latter activity, they sometimes overlap with occupational therapists, who typically focus on how people can best use equipment to perform daily tasks. On the day of our focus group, Donna Hitchcock, a physical therapist, had seen a man who falls repeatedly. In this first encounter, she began his workup.

The focus is all on safety. This man said that yesterday he mowed four lawns, yet he falls. He uses the lawn mower for support. So I joked, "Next time you come in, make sure you bring the lawn mower!" In the appointment today, I couldn't do all the functional testing, like the balance test and the six-minute walk. Obviously, I don't think I'll need the six-minute walk test with him if he can mow all those lawns, but some of the more primary measurements—addressing his strength and tone and just standing, balance, and other things to get an idea of what's going on. The man has a really bad memory. He couldn't remember who referred him.

Ms. Hitchcock must consider factors beyond the patient's physical capabilities, including cognitive functioning, to address fully his safety.

People's performance with their ambulation aids in the clinic may not equal how they will do at home. Visiting homes to see how people use their mobility aids is therefore essential; after all, the greatest risk for falls is at home (Tinetti and Speechley 1989; Tinetti et al. 1993). After many home visits, Gary McNamara is realistic but believes ambulation aids can improve people's lives.

I've got patients who will use their cane all around their house, but there's no way they'll go outside with it. A lot of them have lived in their neighborhoods their whole lives. Everybody on the block knows them, and they know everybody. You know the Irish neighborhoods in Southie. I saw a woman today; she's having a difficult time getting around. She's very unsteady. At times she could run across her house as if it's nothing. Other times she sways. It's frightening.

So we got her a walker, a rolling walker with nice glide caps so that it won't catch and make the horrible sound on her floors. We took her for a spin around her place and she's like, "This is great. It moves wonderful." So I'm excited. "Do you think it helps?" She says, "Yes, it does help." I say, "Do you think you'll use it?" She says, "No." The home-health aide's watching me, and she just burst out laughing. This happens all the time.

So then you sit down and see how you can adapt it to their situation. Sometimes, if I stand up and put on my big voice, they think I'm authoritative, and they'll listen. Other times, it's pleading and begging. And sometimes it's demonstrating with facts and numbers that statistically your fall chance is 20 percent without it. You've got to be flexible. The image of being seen with it makes them think they're old. So I try to sell: "Look at what you can do with it. Look how much more you can do."

Despite Gary's safety arguments, ultimately his patients make their own choices.

LIVING WITH AMBULATION AIDS

Jimmy Howard calls his cane his "assistant" and uses it everywhere, keeping it at his bedside at night. Sometimes his wife humorously rebukes the cane, but Jimmy would rather use his assistant than rely on her arm: "I'm very independent. That's what she hates about me! Why should I depend on her, when she's not with me all the time?" He does things independently, after carefully studying how best to move with his cane. "I know I can't move this way; I know I can't move that way without hurting myself. You sit there and figure it out."

Irritations with ambulation aids inevitably arise. Despite their rubber tips, canes slip on shiny floors or in tiny puddles, making people fall. Cynthia Walker always leaves her crutches upstairs when she needs them downstairs. One woman repeatedly misplaces her cane, but since her husband continually loses his glasses, they go back and forth, searching for both. People with arthritis in their wrists or hands cannot grasp ambulation aids or use them maximally to off-load weight and alleviate pain. Ambulation aids with multiple moving parts, like sophisticated walkers, malfunction more often than lower-tech devices.

Even so, people still walk, not only at home but also outside. Virtually by definition, ambulation aids are themselves easily mobile. Canes can go anywhere. Folding canes fit into purses; walkers load easily into cars. With his bilateral amputations, Arnis Balodis occasionally needed his cane to rapidly restore his balance. His cane, a standard single-footed wooden model, was beautiful, the crook head carved with a basket-weave pattern and parallel spiraling lines encircling the shaft.

"I carved that for self-preservation," explained Arnis. "It slips and slides when it gets wet. I just picked up a knife and carved it so it has a grip if it gets wet."

"Did your doctor give you a prescription for the cane?"

"No, I just went out and bought it—one to fit me. I have another cane that's identical. If it's slippery or I go shopping, I take two of them along."

"Have you ever used a walker?"

"Yeah, when they took the legs off. I was bouncing with one artificial leg and no leg at all, and I had a walker to get around. But I wouldn't use a wheelchair except right after surgery. I wasn't interested *how* I walked, but I was *going* to walk." The canes helped him do that.

The year after medical school, Reed and I went briefly to London in early November. I still walked with one cane and thought I could use taxis and rest frequently on benches. Most importantly, I had Reed's willing arm. The first day it rained, so we headed to the National Gallery, entering through a little foyer up several stairs. The guard in his navy blue uniform immediately accosted us: "Do you want a wheelchair?"

"No, thank you," I answered, somewhat taken aback. Did I look like I needed a wheelchair?

"You might as well take it. You're going to need it sooner or later."

"No, thank you," I said, trying to be firm. How could he know I'd need a wheelchair sooner or later? The guard shrugged his shoulders.

This conversation unnerved me. Despite my bravado, was the guard right? I spent that morning searching for benches: I had no choice. My legs held me upright only briefly before threatening collapse. Fortunately, wide sturdy benches are strategically placed throughout the gallery so I saw the major treasures, albeit from bench-distance. Nevertheless, my confidence was rattled.

So passed our trip. I lurched from bench to bench, with some good stretches in between. The unexpected "silver lining" was our encounters with people. Instead of moving at breakneck speed as do many American tourists, we took our time; because we were slow, often stationary, people talked to us. The down side was obvious. Every vertical moment, I had to concentrate on remaining erect. I could not look around, only at my feet below, and Reed inched along, bearing and feeling responsible for a heavy load. Overall, the trip was wonderful—of course, it would be. But the guard had been right.

12 Wheeled Mobility

Several years elapsed before I acceded to the guard's prediction—that I would need a wheelchair sooner or later—and purchased my scooter-wheelchair. I raised all the usual objections: using a scooter conceded failure; I would never walk again; my remaining muscle strength would wither; riding was embarrassing; and I didn't want to be seen that way. Having left an awkward girlhood, I relished being tall. And in a wheelchair, I would constantly gaze up at the world rather than look it straight in the eye. But the countervailing arguments won. My legs carried me shorter and shorter distances, more and more slowly; even brief walks sapped strength; I occasionally fell; and I could not travel alone, as my job increasingly demanded. I wanted independence and control over getting around. I desperately wished to walk, but since I couldn't go far, I decided to roll. Now I do, and it's terrific! In a real sense, this book is a paean to my wheelchair.

In some situations, such as paralyzing strokes or advanced ALS, people have no choice about using a wheelchair. With progressive debility, however, the decision to use a wheelchair often emerges slowly, borne of practical necessity counterbalanced by visions of the future and sense of self. John Hockenberry had no choice about using a wheelchair after his spinal cord injury:

> It took years of being in a wheelchair before I could be truly amazed by what it could do, and what I could do with it. On a winter night in Chicago, after a light snow, I rolled across a clean stretch of pavement and felt the smooth frictionless glide of the icy surface. I made a tight turn and . . . I saw two beautiful lines etched in the snow. They began as parallel and curved, then they crossed in an effortless knot. . . . My chair had made those lines. The knot was the signature

of every turn I had ever made. . . . It was the first time I dared to believe that a wheelchair could make something, or even be associated
with something, so beautiful. (1995, 207)

This chapter examines wheeled mobility, starting with three brief stories emphasizing the diverse roles of wheelchairs in people's lives.

Walter Masterson's ALS was progressing, and he had climbed the mobility
aid hierarchy, from cane through power wheelchair. "Did the decision to
use a wheelchair seem bigger than your decision to use a cane?" I asked.

"You'd think the answer would have to be yes. But I'm not really sure.
They were both rather traumatic because each was an admission that I'd
gotten to a point of no return, and I did not want to admit to points of no
return." Mr. Masterson's voice was failing because of the ALS, and he anticipated the day he could no longer breathe. Mobility problems felt
smaller than these other impairments. "The wheelchair was in many ways
a release, because as I got worse with the cane and then with the walker, I
was only transporting myself between places where I could sit down. And
those places had to get closer and closer together, which meant that my
range was really decreasing. Christmas shopping takes on lots of new
meanings in this circumstance. The wheelchair was an immense aid in
Christmas shopping."

Gerald Bernadine and I first met at the local college where he taught
night courses pending resolution of his disability discrimination lawsuit
(chapter 7). Despite the chilly day, I rode my scooter to his office. Gerald
walked slowly and tentatively, leaning constantly against the wall, his free
hand extending a wobbling cane for counterbalance. He collapsed into a
chair, collecting himself, before talking: "I'm so exhausted by the end of the
day. My legs feel like they weigh a thousand pounds. I feel like an old
man." After the interview, he eyed my scooter. "How did you get over
here?"

"I rode over."

"Really? Can you really do that?" Gerald had never thought about a
scooter and his physician hadn't suggested it. Several months later, Gerald
won his lawsuit, and shortly thereafter, he bought a scooter. I found him
zipping around his office in a bright red scooter. "I don't have limits now
about where I can go. Fortunately, we live in the United States, so there are
lots of elevators and lots of handicapped ramps and accessibility. I can do
lots of things that I used to dread, like going to the Registry of Motor Ve-
hicles recently to get my driver's license. You know what that's like—an
absolute horror show. No sweat! I just rode up on my little cart, I waited in

line with everybody. As they went, I went. I got my license and, zoom, I was out of there."

"Do you feel less tired on days you teach?"

"The other day I taught a three-hour class. No problem. I zipped around in my cart, got everything I needed, and I drove it right into the classroom. I saved all that physical energy, and afterward, instead of being ex-hausted—even after a three-hour class—I still had energy." Gerald said that his colleagues laughingly warned him to control his speed. "I need a cow catcher on the front of it so I can knock people out of the way! The biggest thing is being careful not to drive too fast, especially in the build-ing. There's a wicked temptation on these long straightaways to go fast." For Gerald, his scooter restored not only his energy and mobility but also his control over major aspects of daily life.

Cynthia Walker flatly rejects a cane, openly blaming vanity and desire to keep pushing forward, but she has temporarily used a scooter and loved it:

> I was in Tennessee this past summer. We went to Dollywood. To see the entire park comfortably, I rented a scooter. It was $5.00. Some people have a problem with that because you're giving into your physical condition. I didn't see it that way at all. I saw it as assisting with my physical condition, so I could enjoy the park thoroughly with the rest of my family. So the people who are renting out the wheelchairs saw a woman walking toward them with a slight limp: why would she need this? Because, if I didn't use it, by a quarter into the trip, I wouldn't be limping anymore. I'd be dragging, and I wouldn't see a thing. So, it's wonderful for people who can't go the distance, quite literally."

For Cynthia, *selective* scooter use preserves her sense of personal perse-verance but permits great vacations.

"WILL I END UP IN A WHEELCHAIR?"

In our society, perhaps nothing symbolizes frailty, dependence, and loss more completely, definitively, and succinctly than a wheelchair: "The as-cription of passivity can be seen in language used to describe the relation-ship between disabled people and their wheelchairs. The phrases *wheel-chair bound* or *confined to a wheelchair* . . . imply that a wheelchair restricts the individual, holds a person prisoner" (Linton 1998, 27). The threat of needing a wheelchair terrifies persons newly confronting chronic disease. S. Kay Toombs remembers her fear on being diagnosed with MS.

Just two days earlier, by a strange coincidence, I had read a magazine article about the plight of a young woman with M.S. The photos accompanying the story are still imprinted on my mind. In one, the woman posed coquettishly in a bathing suit with a "Miss Michigan" sash emblazoned across her chest. In the other, she sat dejectedly in a wheelchair, appearing broken and helpless. The author explained that she was paralyzed, unable to care for herself . . .

Not surprisingly, on hearing my diagnosis, my first question to the physician was, "Will I end up in a wheelchair?" (1995, 4)

One barrier to outright rejection of wheelchairs as symbols of debility is obvious: they *are* used only when people cannot walk. So we must look beyond specific physical limitations to the whole person. How ironic it is that wheelchairs symbolize dependence and lost control since they build on that most enabling of early technologies, the wheel. In fact, wheels and chairs probably developed contemporaneously, albeit separately, somewhere in the eastern Mediterranean region around 4000 B.C. (Kamenetz 1969, 5). Chairs certainly improved personal comfort, but wheels literally transformed human beings' sense of space in the world.

Although canes, crutches, and walkers also symbolize dependence, they carry less stigma than wheelchairs, perhaps because their users remain upright. The distinction is not based on practical functionality: wheelchairs can be fast, safe, and flexible. As Nancy Mairs said of her power wheelchair, "Certainly I am not mobility impaired; in fact, in my Quickie P100 with two twelve-volt batteries, I can shop till you drop at any mall you designate, I promise" (1996, 39). James Charlton, who uses a lightweight manual wheelchair, wonders why people struggle to remain erect:

> When I see old people using "walkers" I am always struck by the generation and development gaps in how people with disabilities live. Someday people will be liberated enough to discard such ridiculously antiquated aids. The idea that slowly hobbling around is better than briskly moving about in an electric wheelchair would be shocking if I did not see it practiced every day. (1998, 162)

Very slowly, the symbolism of wheelchairs is changing as more wheelchair users participate in public life and appear on the street (chapter 4). Instead of using metaphors of confinement, they "are more likely to say that someone *uses a wheelchair.* The latter phrase not only indicates the active nature of the user and the positive way that wheelchairs increase mobility and activity but recognizes that people get in and out of wheelchairs for different activities" (Linton 1998, 27). Today's wheelchair users go many places, independently and with confidence, because they control equipment designed specifically for their needs. New technologies allow people to do for themselves rather than rely on others.

WHEELCHAIR OPTIONS

Since early times, many people who could not walk rarely left their homes or even their rooms. Occasionally, generally for the convenience of others, they needed to be moved. As Herman Kamenetz, a physiatrist, recounted in his history of wheelchairs, in ancient times people with limited mobility rode on litters or palanquins, carried by slaves, servants, or family members. By the 1700s some chairs had devices for self-propulsion, including pulleys, cranks, springs, and large wheels. The most common wheeled chair was the Bath chair, named after the English spa. Bath chairs typically had two large wheels in the rear and a smaller wheel in front. While an attendant pushed the chair from behind, its occupant steered using a handle connected to the front wheel, offering everything "which the safety of invalids requires" (Kamenetz 1969, 20).

Wheelchairs first appeared in America to transport wounded soldiers during the Civil War. Made of wood and cane, these heavy chairs had large wooden wheels up front, and designs changed relatively little over ensuing decades. At the time of Franklin Delano Roosevelt,

> Rather than struggle with such a contraption, Roosevelt had a chair built to his own specifications and design. To the seat and back of a common, straightback kitchen chair he had a sturdy base attached, with two large wheels in front, two small ones in back. . . . Roosevelt seldom sat for long in his wheelchair. Rather, he used it to scoot from his desk chair to a couch, from the couch to the car. He used his chair as a means of movement, not as a place to stay. (Gallagher 1994, 91–92)

Throughout the centuries individual consumers, like Roosevelt, had devised wheelchairs for their own needs. In 1918 Herbert A. Everest, a mining engineer, became paraplegic following an industrial injury. He enlisted the mechanical engineer Harry C. Jennings to design a sturdy transportable model. They founded a company in Los Angeles that, in 1933, manufactured the first folding metal wheelchairs, weighing 50 compared to the usual 90 pounds (Shapiro 1994, 215). A consumer had finally assumed control of wheelchair design and production. Their company, Everest and Jennings (E&J), dominated the market for the next fifty years.

With size and success came complacency as E&J catered increasingly to institutional clients, such as hospitals and nursing homes, rather than consumers.[1] One dissatisfied consumer was Marilyn Hamilton, who in 1978 crashed her hang glider into a California mountainside and became paraplegic. Unhappy with existing wheelchairs, she challenged her friends and fellow glider pilots Don Helman and Jim Okamoto to build an ultralight wheelchair from aluminum tubing, as used in their gliders (Shapiro 1994, 211). The resulting wheelchair weighed 26 pounds instead of the standard 50 and sold under the name "Quickie."

> Hamilton's wheelchairs put people—users and those around them— at ease. Instead of chrome, Hamilton's chairs came in a rainbow of hot colors. The customer could personalize a chair in candy apple red, canary yellow, or electric green. . . . A Quickie chair was fun, refuting the idea that the user was an invalid. (Quickie's biggest competitor today is Invacare, a name that is an abbreviation for "invalid care.") Quickie chair riders were neither sick nor objects of pity. They just got around in a different way. "If you can't stand up," Hamilton likes to say, "stand out." (Shapiro 1994, 212)

Some give partial credit to Quickie designs for furthering the disability rights movement of the 1980s, by expanding the independence of wheelchair users and separating their image from "the institutional feel of the older design. The world saw more of the person, less of the chair" (Karp 1998, 6).[2]

The market success of Quickie and continuing demands for new technologies, such as lightweight power wheelchairs, attracted many competitors to the wheelchair market. Companies now sell directly to consumers, through magazines, the Internet, and other venues. Compared to twenty years ago, today's wheelchair market is vibrant with new ideas and diverse options for people who no longer walk, helping them to ride where and how they wish.

Wheelchair technologies span the gamut. The old standard chrome model with leatherette sling back and sling seat remains ubiquitous in institutions, to ferry patients around. Now comparatively inexpensive, these relatively heavy and uncomfortable wheelchairs are sometimes all people can afford, even for home and community use. But for people with money or generous insurance coverage, countless options exist, ranging from ultralightweight three-wheeled chairs for marathoners to plastic chairs with bulbous wheels for rolling along sandy beaches to all-terrain four-wheeled power wheelchairs for traversing rugged surfaces to technologically sophisticated power wheelchairs controlled by pneumatic switches. The majority of people have manual wheelchairs (90 percent), with 8 percent using power equipment and 10 percent scooters—about 8 percent have more than one type of chair.[3]

Given this diversity, this brief description covers only wheelchair basics. The list of selected resources at the back of the book offers suggestions for obtaining information about wheelchairs and other assistive technologies. Extensive additional information is available elsewhere (Scherer 2000; Currie, Hardwick, and Marburger 1998; Karp 1998, 1999) and through such sources as the Rehabilitation Engineering and Assistive Technology Society of North America (RESNA), magazines, the Internet, and advocacy groups. But in most instances health insurers ultimately determine which wheelchair people get (chapter 14).

Independence and Safety

The most basic decisions about which wheelchair to try revolve around independence and safety. Sophisticated technologies now allow even persons with severe physical debilities to operate power wheelchairs and move independently.[4] Depending on individual circumstances, however, including cognitive functioning and judgment, the safest option may require someone to be accompanied and pushed in a wheelchair. Trading off independence for safety becomes complicated.

If people choose independence, deciding between manual and power wheelchairs depends primarily on having the physical strength and stamina to self-propel a manual chair. Most manual wheelchairs have push handles, so that other people can help tired users. But being pushed defeats the goal of being independent and in control. Addressing users, Karp suggests: "be honest with yourself about your strength and energy—you'll need plenty of both to operate a manual chair" (1998, 49). Nevertheless, compared to power wheelchairs, major benefits of manual chairs include:

- lighter weight
- range not constrained by the charge capacity of a battery
- lower purchase and maintenance price
- more discreet appearance, less bulk, and little noise
- easier to transport in cars, airplanes, trains, and buses
- greater ability to surmount environmental barriers (persons who master the "wheelie" can "jump" a curb or step; some even use escalators) (1998, 49; 1999, 226–27)

For people without adequate strength or endurance, "introducing powered mobility equipment . . . can truly be liberating" (Warren 1990, 74). Power wheelchairs offer the following advantages over manual chairs (Karp 1998, 50; Karp 1999, 227):

- conserves energy and minimizes exhaustion
- reduces the likelihood of needing assistance when traveling long distances
- climbs slopes that are not unduly steep
- leaves one arm free to do other things, such as carry packages
- offers technologies, such as powered tilt or reclining, which can lessen risk of pressure sores and improve comfort

After the choice of manual or power wheelchairs, many decisions remain, such as solid rubber versus pneumatic tires, fixed or swingaway footrests, seat depth and width, flat back versus lumbar back support, and type of cushions (e.g., foam, gel, air flotation, or urethane honeycomb). Given this diversity and the complex technical decisions, the advice of knowledgeable professionals (e.g., in a "seating clinic") can prove essential. "Do your best to remember that you are not buying a ball and chain," advises Karp (1998, 32). "You will not be confined to a wheelchair; you will be liberated by it."

Manual Wheelchairs

Manual wheelchairs are either rigid-frame or folding-frame. With fewer moving parts, rigid-frame wheelchairs are very lightweight, strong, and energy-efficient. Streamlined and unobtrusive, they are the "de facto standard for those who want to reduce the visual emphasis on their disability" (Karp 1999, 229). Rigid frames are extremely responsive—even minor movements of riders' bodies can cause changes in direction. Athletes, especially, find this sensitivity essential to their quick maneuverability, while others are unnerved by it. On uneven surfaces, rigid-frame wheelchairs give a bumpy ride, becoming dangerous when one or more wheels lift off the ground. Rigid-frame wheelchairs do not fold neatly for easy storage (although their wheels pop off) and are too bulky for some cars.

The major success of E&J was designing a sturdy and reliable folding chair. Although flexible-frame chairs are heavier, they offer some advantages over rigid-frame models. They are safer on rough terrain, fold easily for storage, and fit into most cars. They routinely have push handles just in case the user cannot self-propel (many rigid-frame chairs do not). But their weight undeniably demands more energy to propel, and they appear more like the prototypical wheelchair.

The choice of rigid- or flexible-frame wheelchairs involves more decisions: about wheel size; placement and angle (camber) of wheels; width of hand rims for pushing wheels; and wheel locks or hand brakes. These decisions must consider not only the users' physical attributes (e.g., height, strength) but also their lifestyle and ways they will use the wheelchair. The optimal design for a marathoner or rugby player differs significantly from that for a person who still walks but uses a wheelchair for traveling to and from work.

Power Wheelchairs and Scooters

Power wheelchairs and scooters both rely on batteries to transport users. However, their different designs have important consequences. Power wheelchairs roll on four wheels, with the battery power pack below the seat, flip-up footplates, and swingaway footrest hangers. Users typically maneuver them using a short, vertical joystick positioned on the armrest. People unable to move their hands operate power wheelchairs using sophisticated technologies, which respond to chin movements or puffs and sips of air blown through a strawlike device (Warren 1990).

In contrast, scooters—undeniably wheelchairs, given their function and purpose—place their users behind the controls. Scooters are built on a platform, with a rotating "captain's chair" rising from the back, battery underneath the seat, and a steering column on the front, sometimes bearing a basket, horn, and headlight. Because of their configuration, scooters can carry packages and suitcases (e.g., when traveling, I tuck luggage under my legs). Users drive scooters by pulling or pressing levers on the handlebars. Most scooters are three-wheeled, but because of their potential instability, four-wheeled versions are also available. Scooters are safe and appropriate only for people with good hand and arm strength and upper-body balance. Many users still stand and walk short distances, riding the scooter only for longer trips.

Power wheelchairs and scooters are either front- or rear-wheel drive (i.e., the drive wheels are positioned either in the front or back; mid-wheel drives are now available for some power wheelchairs). Front-wheel drives have a small turning radius, so people can rotate fully in tight spaces. Surmounting low obstacles is easier, although the weight of power equipment generally precludes curb jumping. Rear-wheel models give a greater sense of control but need wider spaces for turning. Rear-wheel-drive power wheelchairs can tip over, when the front casters lift off the ground as heavy rear wheels accelerate.

Power chairs and scooters operate off either gel-cell or wet-cell (lead acid) batteries. Gel-cell batteries are slightly less powerful and shorter-lasting than wet-cell, but they need less maintenance and do not spill; wet-cell batteries require users to maintain specified water levels, and they can spill or leak dangerous acid.[5] My scooter salesman asserts that my gel-cell batteries go 25 miles, but I never tempt fate. Meticulous recharging of batteries is essential to avoid power failures. Automatic battery chargers typically plug directly into standard electrical outlets.

ADVANTAGES OF WHEELS

Most interviewees who used wheelchairs were matter-of-fact: they use a wheelchair because it helps them get around. Some people, like Mr. Masterson, had little choice. Other wheelchair users who still walk emphasize two primary reasons for sometimes riding—fatigue and frequent falls.

"Sometimes I'm so tired I could drop," said one woman with MS. "It's just not worth it to get exhausted. You have to take precautions, to husband your energy. Using the scooter, that's husbanding my energy." People carefully calculate how far they can walk, using their wheelchair for distances beyond their limits. "I have a handicapped apartment, and the apartment's OK," said Bobby, whose serious heart disease reduces his endurance. "Once I get out of the apartment, that's where I have problems. I need the wheelchair for distances."

Louisa Delarte likes to grocery shop, but long supermarket aisles daunted her.

> I said, gee whiz, it's going to take me a long time to walk through that supermarket, even holding onto a shopping cart. I liked going to the supermarket, because you can hold onto the cart and walk around. You felt like a normal person. But then I noticed the store had these electric carts, scooters. "This is great," I said. "This is marvelous." I knew about them from the MS magazine. I never tried one in the store, but I just knew I wanted one. So almost ten years ago, I decided to buy one. I bought a new car, too, at the same time— I gave up my convertible! I traded it in for that old bus [a minivan] and got a little crane to lift the cart. It is really great.

Edith Leder, a physical therapist, echoes Louisa's comments, saying "walking isn't really the most important thing most people do. You might conserve energy so you can tend to your child, for example. You can do that by using a wheelchair or scooter." She still urges her patients to walk as much as possible, but acknowledges, "ultimately, a lot of people decide that maybe walking isn't the number one thing in their lives."

For about a dozen years Jamie Johnson, in his mid fifties, has had cerebellar ataxia, a degenerative condition of the cerebellum (the part of the brain that controls balance), marked by progressive unsteadiness in walking and standing. "I've been using the wheelchair now for a couple of months," said Mr. Johnson, who had used a walker. "I'd done quite a bit of falling, and I would fall as much as I would walk around. This disease that I have is getting worse. I'm adjusting to the fact that I have the wheelchair. It's really an asset to me, because I suffer with my balance and my walking, my gait, they call it. I've been falling more than I really want to talk about."

For safety, Mr. Johnson had little choice about using a wheelchair. The only question was when. Sometimes a fall dictates the answer. Dr. Jody Farr had danced around using a wheelchair for years: "It's definitely a decision you have to come to yourself. It's not one that anyone else can make for you." Occasionally, people urged her to consider a wheelchair. She refused and continued walking until a bad fall hospitalized her for a week, followed by two weeks on the rehabilitation unit.

"I finally got out, but I needed some way to get around."

"Who came to that decision?"

"I can't even think of who said I needed something. It was kind of a group decision. The physical therapist whom I worked with was partially responsible. Warren, who was my senior colleague and treated me like gold, really wanted me to stop walking. I would not do that just for him, though, as good as he was to me, a father figure. Initially, I was going to get a wheelchair. Just the image—I couldn't accept it at that time."

"The image of a wheelchair is different from that of a scooter?"

"Yes, very much so. A wheelchair is an invalid thing, and I couldn't manage pushing it myself. I would not be independent. The guy from the medical supply store wanted to just drop off this wheelchair one afternoon, and I said, 'Wait, I'm not sure that I want this.' So I went into the city and looked around at what was available. I wasn't even conscious of something called a scooter. When I saw it, I said, 'This is neat. I really like this.' I thought it would be fun." Dr. Farr has used a scooter ever since, although she has a manual wheelchair for airplane travel.

ADMITTING FEARS, FINDING FREEDOM

Tom Norton wouldn't use a cane until he retired ("Company presidents don't use canes"). Not surprisingly, he avoids wheelchairs. Nelda Norton's mother had used a wheelchair before she died, so they had one at home. "I went with him to his doctor," said Mrs. Norton, "and I was very cross. I said, 'I'm not going to travel with him anymore. He uses all his energy in the airport just trying to get to the plane.' And the doctor said, 'What's the matter with you that you won't take a chair to the plane?' The doctor didn't realize Tom wasn't getting help like that."

"I haven't felt a need to use the wheelchair where I can confine the distance I must walk," argued Tom. "Going to a wheelchair, I would fear the dependence. I'm trying to hold off as long as I can." Tom took his mother-in-law's wheelchair on vacation but spent much of the time in his room.

Many share Tom Norton's fear of physical dependence on a wheelchair. These fears are ironic given that today's wheelchair technologies increase independence and control. Perhaps the contradiction arises from differing frames of reference: a focus on specific physical losses or on the *whole person*. People who fear dependence often emphasize their psychic determination to endure and push on.

The interviews suggest that this frame of reference flips at some point, prompted by increasing physical debility or frustration with existing limitations. People decide that the prospect of independence trumps fears of dependence, and they start using wheeled mobility. At that point, many become less afraid—of falling, of getting stuck when their walking fails. People who can still walk do walk when they can, using their wheelchair selectively (Hoenig et al. 2002). They do not see wheelchair use as an "either/or decision"—they make choices throughout each day, often reversing long-held images and substituting empowerment for loss. Other people, including physicians, can impose their own perspectives on these decisions.

"I'll Never Walk Again"

Esther Halpern walks happily with her rolling walker, her "carriage," saying, "I feel safer now that I have this, than I felt before." She does fall sometimes. "One of the first times I used the carriage was on the East Point beach. We had walked, and we were going to sit down on a bench. There's a little hill to get there. I had the brakes on, and I had let go of them because I was turning around. And the thing started to go, and I went with it. I had to let go of it completely. I fell down and rolled over and over. Fortunately, I didn't hurt myself."

"What about using a wheelchair?" I asked.

"I'd rather not use a wheelchair. I figure that once I go into a wheelchair, I'll never walk again. As long as I can walk, I'd rather walk, and it's not hard for me to walk. As a matter of fact, when we go on level ground, when we go into a mall, I can keep up with Harry."

"All I have to do is worry," interjected Harry Halpern.

Other people share Esther Halpern's all-or-nothing view of using a wheelchair—that they will never walk again. Some needed wheelchairs at certain points, as Myrtle Johnson did after her knee surgery, but worked hard to resume walking. They refuse to return to the wheelchair. "That's not for me. That's not my direction," Mrs. Johnson asserted. "I would get into the wheelchair and relax, let other people push me around. I would never get out."

Louanne Mawby, now in her early sixties, was only forty years old when she had a stroke: "They said I'd never walk again, but I did." Now Mrs. Mawby walks slowly with a four-point cane, but her physician told me he's worried. Her gait is unsteady, and she rarely gets out. Her physician wants her to consider a scooter. "I think it's OK," said Mrs. Mawby, "but I'm just not ready for that, yet. I figure if I get one of those scooters, my walking will just go away, that I would never walk again. I'd start depending on that scooter too much."

Joanne Evans, an experienced occupational therapist, observed that people with chronic conditions often say that they are not yet ready for a wheelchair, even when debilities progress significantly.

> That's the hardest population. It's so hard to accept the wheelchair. I had a guy with MS. He was huge—a big guy. He had been fine for years and years and then got worse. Another OT and I were trying to move him around his apartment, and we were holding him up with all our weight. We were praying to God; you could see us both looking to the sky. If this guy went down, the police were getting called because there was no way we were lifting this guy off the floor. We finally got him to get an electric wheelchair.

"Use It or Lose It!"

Louanne Mawby fears that if she starts using a scooter her "walking will just go away." Her fear resonates with the "use it or lose it!" philosophy—a strongly held disincentive to wheeled mobility. I first heard the phrase "use it or lose it" from Dr. Josh Landau, a rheumatologist, who could not remember ever having prescribed a wheelchair. "Maybe I should have," Dr. Landau confessed. "I've probably had shut-ins who could do a lot more if they were in a wheelchair. But there's a tendency on the patient's part, as well as on my part, to see wheelchairs as a last resort. I want to keep them ambulating independently rather than utilize a wheelchair, despite its benefits."

The "use it or lose it" dictum certainly carries mechanistic truth. Even elite athletes lose peak conditioning after several days without exercise. For many people with progressive chronic conditions, however, this belief isolates the legs from the whole person. It assumes that the primary objective is to maximize failing muscle function rather than consider the totality of a person's daily life. Those who look beyond physical functioning "believe it is ultimately more important and cost-effective to enhance a person's quality of life, not merely to restore capability; to meet an individual's need for independence" (Scherer 1996, 440). Wheelchairs can do that.

Max Cleland, former U.S. senator from Georgia, whose right hand and both legs were amputated following a grenade explosion in Vietnam, was exhorted to "use it or lose it" during rehabilitation. With arduous effort, he learned to walk upright using heavy wooden bilateral leg prostheses. Years later, after a grueling day of political campaigning,

> I fell on my bed completely exhausted. Mom gave a cry when she saw the ends of my stumps. They were bleeding. By now I knew I could not take the hellish torture of the pain I was putting myself through anymore. The next day, Saturday, my doctor confirmed it.
> "Get off your legs, Max," he ordered, "until your stumps heal."
> Somehow my machismo had been involved in walking on those legs. To hear him order me off them was a welcome relief. At least he had *told* me to do it. That provided some balm to my bruised masculinity.
> On the following day, Sunday, I attended a coffee. It was the first time I had ever gone out campaigning without my artificial limbs. As I sat in the living room in my wheelchair, I felt completely relaxed and comfortable. I was able to answer questions better. Before, while struggling on my limbs, I began to get uptight after a half hour. Now, I felt affable and relaxed. (1989, 134–35)

Soon afterward, Senator Cleland abandoned his prostheses forever.[6]

Joe Warren had experiences similar to Cleland's after he partially injured his spinal cord: "I went to the hospital every day for therapy with the leg braces that came up to the very top of my leg. It got to a point where it wasn't going anywhere. I was able to walk maybe 50 feet, and I'd be wiped out." Joe felt let down, but he also admitted that "trying to walk was more of a hassle than anything. I got the wheelchair." One of the things he likes best now is being with his children. "If I was to try to walk, I wouldn't be able to hold their hands. Basically, I'd need to concentrate on trying to walk instead of enjoying them. With the wheelchair, my kids sit on my lap, and I can enjoy them a lot more. In a chair, getting around's a lot faster. So walking'd be good for circulation. That's about it."

For Cleland, his physician's order to get off his legs validated his move to a wheelchair. Physicians, however, sometimes exhort patients, especially younger persons, to "use it or lose it," without fully considering the daily implications. Eleanor Peters, now in her mid forties, contracted polio as a toddler. She had walked for about thirty years before needing a wheelchair. "I've been using the chair for somewhere between eight or nine years. I had started to fall a lot, especially in the winter. I would slip and fall and bust my face, bust my mouth. I went to my doctor and told him it would be good if I had a wheelchair or else I'm going to have a head injury soon. At first he recommended that I try crutches, which was impossible because I can't use my left arm at all and my right arm is too weak to hold a crutch. So I told him I needed to have an electric wheelchair, and after a little bit of fighting, I got it."

"Fighting with whom?"

"The doctors. They didn't think that I should use a wheelchair. They felt that if I started using the chair I was going to lose more muscle in my legs. That wasn't the case because I don't just sit in a wheelchair all day. When I go to work, I usually get out of my wheelchair, and I sit in my chair at the desk and walk around the office for different things. I don't really use the chair in my house. I usually park it, and I walk around the house when I can. When I used to travel and I wore a long leg brace, it was really difficult getting on and off buses or trains and hard to get a seat sometimes. And I would fall because I couldn't hold on. So when I'm in my chair, I can just get on the buses. I don't have to worry about a seat, and I don't have to worry about falling anymore. So the wheelchair's a real asset."

Eleanor Peters believes that people must advocate for themselves. "Whatever assistance you can get, don't feel bad about taking it. There's some people that say, 'Oh, I'm never going to use a wheelchair. I don't want it.' I'm not saying that people should jump into a wheelchair if they don't need it. But I'll tell you one thing, I thank God that I can get out of my chair when I can, but I wouldn't trade my wheelchair in to anybody. This is my transportation. These are my feet."

CHOOSING AN IMAGE

Wheeled mobility technologies offer not only mechanistic variety but also diverse public images. Everybody carries pictures, in their minds, of their corporeal selves. Nancy Mairs (1996) caught an unanticipated glimpse of herself in a mirror.

> "Eck," I squealed, "a cripple!" . . . I love my wheelchair, a compact electric model called a Quickie P100, and I've spent so much time in it, and become so adept at maneuvering it, that I have literally incorporated it—made it part of my body—and its least ailment sends me into a greater tizzy than my own headaches. But the wheelchair I experience is not "out there" for me to observe, any more than the rest of my body is, and I'm invariably shocked at the sight of myself hunched in its black framework of aluminum and plastic. (46)

Some people have little choice about their equipment (e.g., persons with high-level quadriplegia need sophisticated heavy-duty power wheelchairs). But others have options. Various types of wheeled mobility carry different public connotations—what's cool versus what's not. On the cool end, "Jocks get a lot of attention in their sporty wheelchair basketball chairs or their tennis outfits. There are the crip skiers, and most impressive of all are the runners in their three-wheel track chairs" (Hockenberry 1995, 120). At the not-so-cool or frankly fuddy-duddy end are scooters. Even Rhonda Olkin (1999, 277), who uses a scooter, describes them as "wheeled cousins of the golf-cart."

Nevertheless, only a few people can be wheelchair jocks—then there are the rest of us. As with other products, the media can shape images. Scooter manufacturers market directly to the public. Typical television advertisements depict well-groomed, contented elders rolling around at leisure in lush tropical settings. To generate sales, these ads must send inherently contradictory messages, distancing scooter-wheelchairs from dysfunction, making them "fun" and unthreatening but reliable conveyors of potential purchasers. Even the word "scooter" has a sporty, carefree connotation divorced from its serious purpose. Many large stores now offer scooters for their shoppers, which customers gratefully borrow. Nonetheless, this association reinforces views of scooters as optional aids for pleasurable pursuits. Unscrupulous vendors sometimes cajole vulnerable people into purchases, offering unrealistic promises that scooters will restore something missing from their lives. Persons considering wheeled mobility must choose not only practical mechanics but also external images of equipment.

Manual or Power?

As noted above, the first technological choice is manual versus power. Karp (1998) cautions that people must be realistic about whether they can propel themselves. Sally Ann Jones first got a manual wheelchair but confronted an unanticipated problem. "I am the mother of sons. I lived in a household with three impatient males who always said, 'Oh mother, we can do this. We're only going up a fourteen-inch curb.' They figured the way to do it is to start in the middle of the street and then run over the curb. Oh, they were just awful! Regular wheelchairs make me enormously uncomfortable because there's somebody back there pushing." After investigating various options, Chet, Sally Ann's husband, discovered scooters, which were uncommon back then. "I've got the strength in my arms to work scooter controls myself. This is mine. I do this myself. I'm in control."

One manual wheelchair user refuses to consider power equipment. "I have good upper-body strength. With an electric chair, I wouldn't be using the muscles to push the chair. I'd rather stay in shape as long as I can. It's more of a necessity for me to stay in shape than an image thing." Nowadays, however, long-term manual wheelchair users are developing shoulder problems and injuries associated with repetitive stress. Hugh Gregory Gallagher was concerned about his image but confronted the physical realities of postpolio, losing muscle power and endurance. He increasingly needed friends to push him.

> Incrementally, yet absolutely, I have become less independent, more invalid.
>> Clearly, time to think of an electric wheelchair.
>> I resisted the thought. Electric wheelchairs are for *crippled* people, not for folks like me. In my mind's eye, I am one of those lean, mean athletic wheelies who compete in the marathon and get their pictures on the back of Wheaties boxes. And besides, electric wheelchairs are *so big*, like Sherman tanks, nothing at all like my lightweight chair, which goes so fast and turns on a dime. (1998, 217)

Gallagher spent a year looking for the right power wheelchair and found one the same size as his manual chair. He feels that people react slightly differently to him in his manual versus four-wheeled power wheelchair.

> I think the manual is perceived as personal equipment—like crutches, or perhaps a blindman's cane. The electric, on the other hand is seen as a thing—a vehicle something like a golf cart. . . . In motion, the electric chair moves from A to B so effectively, so efficiently, that it imparts to its occupant a dignity that is somehow missing in a hand-propelled chair. It is a *very sensible* way to go about your business. . . . I have had my Invacare 9000 for six months. It has changed my life. (219)

Scooter Images

Some interviewees eschewed regular wheelchairs and got scooters because they are "fun." Scooter users employ euphemistic words to describe their equipment—using the brand name or "cart," "go-cart," "motorized cart," "buggy"—never "wheelchair." Mattie Harris is considering a scooter: "I don't want to ride around in a wheelchair. People stare at you."

"How does that make you feel?"

"Like I'm an invalid. I don't think I'm an invalid. I have problems, but I don't think I'm an invalid. I don't want anybody coming up to me, asking, 'What's wrong? Why are you in a wheelchair?' You know how people are—they talk."

"Do scooters seem different from regular wheelchairs?"

"Yeah, 'cause that don't look so like an invalid. The wheelchair makes you seem like your legs're broke or you just can't walk. But I know with those the people can walk—they just need help. That's why I feel different about them."

At one focus group, all participants reported seeing scooters at stores. Eva said she would never use it: "As much pain as I'd be in, I'd be embarrassed because it's me. I know a lot of people. So I just go ahead and walk pushing that grocery cart."

"The only problem I have with it is the up and the down to get the articles off the shelf," observed Martha. "But I wouldn't be embarrassed to use it, no. A few people will stop and ask, 'Are you looking for something? Or can I help you get it?' There's a very few people out there that do it."

"I'm trying to get one now, as we speak," repeated Nan. "I'd rather have a scooter than a wheelchair. It would make it easier to go to the store and to the laundromat. I could do those little things for myself. That way I don't have to depend on my daughter to leave work and come over and do it for me. I'd feel more independent."

"My girlfriend, they all went to Las Vegas," reported Dora, "and she took hers. It's electric. They couldn't keep up with the woman. She was all over the place!"

"It's God sent," said Jackie, who had just moved to a scooter. "If you feel embarrassed, you have to get over it. It's there for *you.*"

PRACTICAL CONSIDERATIONS

During a focus group of wheelchair users, I asked their advice: "What would you say to people who have trouble walking and stay at home because they're too embarrassed to use a wheelchair?"

"Have fun," responded one man. "Treat it like a fun thing, like it's a ride. When I first had to be in this, in the beginning, we had a great time. We'd go real fast. I wasn't embarrassed. I just felt very elderly all of a sudden, but then we started having fun with it."

"I would say that they need to try it for a week," said Eleanor Peters. "See how much more freedom they have. Usually I have both of my grandsons with me. The three-year-old stands on the front; the five-year-old gets in the back. Everybody gets out of my way, because I usually speed wherever I go. Police officers say, 'Hey, you better slow down. I'm going to give you a ticket.' I tell them, 'If you can't catch me, you can't give me a ticket.' That's my motto. Other than problems with transportation and the curb cuts—things that have to do with the system and the city—I love my chair. I wouldn't trade my life for anything. I would not trade having my disability. I really wouldn't. That's just me."

Others echoed Eleanor's sentiments—that their wheelchairs have opened the world. But the urban environment still presents barriers, both physical and interpersonal. Although wheelchairs restore day-to-day mobility, constraints remain. Wheeled mobility also carries physical realities (e.g., risk of injury). Sometimes people find their equipment doesn't work for them, and they abandon it—the wheelchair just gathers dust.

Views on the Street

Much of society remains uneasy with persons who roll rather than walk. The anthropologist Robert Murphy, who had a spinal tumor, found that something changed when he started using a wheelchair:

> Not long after I took up life in the wheelchair, I began to notice other curious shifts and nuances in my social world. After a dentist patted me on the head in 1980, I never returned to his office. . . .
>
> I used to be invisible to black campus policemen. . . . They now know who I am and say hello. I am now a white man who is worse off than they are, and my subtle loss of public standing brings me closer to their own status. We share a common position on the periphery of society—we are fellow Outsiders.
>
> During my first couple of years in the wheelchair, I noticed that men and women responded to me differently. My peer group of middle-aged, middle-class males seemed most menaced by my disability, probably because they identify most closely with me. On the other hand, I found that my relations with most women of all ages have become more relaxed and open. (1990, 126–27)

Murphy's experiences are familiar. A department of medicine chairman once patted me on the head—affectionately, I think. When I roll around the hospital, the cleaning staff often greet me, while many physicians gaze fixedly above my head. These behaviors symbolize societal attitudes and have practical consequences too. If people don't look down, they can't see you. Traveling by wheelchair on busy Manhattan streets is particularly unnerving. Stereotypical New Yorkers look straight ahead, rushing forward at full throttle, intent on their destination. They pirouette away in near misses that are heart-stopping (my heart, that is), surging onward, not glancing down. Yet other New Yorkers are at my eye level: I face the beseeching pleas of homeless people huddled on the pavement. Once at National Airport in Washington, D.C., a woman running to catch her plane collided with me. Hair flying, arms cradling her briefcase, she sprinted, eyes fixed on the television monitor overhead. I didn't veer out of her way quickly enough, and she went sprawling. Luckily, she wasn't hurt, and she made her plane. I felt terrible and now stop dead in my tracks whenever I see anyone running toward me. After the collision, a man lambasted me for recklessness. To him, I was a driver who had hit a pedestrian.

Because wheelchair users are the height of children, Mairs suggests, society will "demand little of her beyond obedience and enough self-restraint so that she doesn't filch candy bars at the checkout counter" (1996, 62). Perhaps this is sometimes true. Sally Ann Jones was ticketed for speeding in her car:

> The town's courtroom is upstairs from the police department, and there's no elevator. So I go to the police department in my Amigo [brand of scooter]. They don't know what to do with me exactly, and they're very deferential: Do I want a cup of coffee? The bailiff came down after about half an hour, and he said, "The judge apologizes, Mrs. Jones, that the building isn't accessible and that you have to stay down here. But he'll come down and hear your case in about a half an hour if you can wait." Then people scurry around to get me another cup of coffee, and somebody wants to run out and get me a donut.
>   In about another half an hour, the bailiff came down and said, "We're just so busy the judge is not going to get down here. The judge *really* apologizes. He sent me down to ask you where you got this ticket and why." He went upstairs and told the judge. And then the bailiff came downstairs, and he said, "The judge is sure you probably won't do that again, that you'll be more sensitive. He said we're going to waive the ticket because you've been sitting here for so long. We apologize." So I didn't have to pay any fines because I'm handicapped. I laughed. I actually thought to myself, well, finally there's some benefit to being handicapped—NOT! I would gladly pay the tickets.

Faulty Equipment

With increasingly complicated mechanisms and electronic circuitry, equipment can falter or fail. Sometimes this is not the wheelchair's fault. Once an airline bent the heavy metal steering shaft of my scooter so badly that it no longer worked. In Phoenix, far from home and my scooter salesman, I fought mounting waves of panic while being passed up the hierarchy of baggage claim representatives. The airline sent my damaged scooter to a local repair shop and rented equipment for my business trip. At least the Phoenix outfit unbent the steering shaft, and the scooter limped back to Boston where it received a thorough overhaul.

Sometimes people neglect routine care of their equipment. A few weeks after Gerald Bernadine got his scooter,

It went dead on me. I was zipping all over this place. One day, I got back on it, and it wouldn't go. I turned on the key, and I checked all the connections. It wouldn't go. So my colleague helped me push it down to the car. I read the instruction book, and it talked about when the battery is dead. I learned that instead of going a month between recharges, it wouldn't hurt to charge it every week.

Charging scooter batteries is easy: after you attach the batteries to the charger unit, plug the charger into a standard electrical outlet.

Mr. Bernadine's power failure fortunately occurred near help. The experience can be terrifying, as for Toombs:

> I was crossing the plaza outside the university library when my scooter stopped dead in its tracks. I was surrounded by a sea of concrete embedded with decorative pebbles, marooned in the middle of a flat, completely open area with no trees, no lampposts, no benches anywhere within reach. I did not have my crutches. There was no one in sight. The nearest "object" was the building, but it was impossible to reach on my own two feet with nothing to support me. Nor could I easily crawl the distance, given the hard uneven surface of pebbled cement. . . . The space of the plaza, which a moment before had been bright, sunny, inviting, now suddenly appeared ominous. (1995, 15)

This happened before people routinely carried cellular telephones, although Toombs did have a car phone in her van. Nowadays, in case of emergency, people should always carry cell phones whenever rolling out on the streets—yet who will provide this service to people who can't afford it?

Getting repairs often poses problems. Dr. Boris Petrov uses a black, four-wheeled, power wheelchair operated by a little joy stick; it swivels and turns within a tight radius. The wheelchair looks well traveled. When Dr. Petrov's wheelchair failed, he couldn't get to the bathroom: since both of his legs were amputated almost to his groin, he cannot crawl. He called his wheelchair vendor, Devi-Deals (a pseudonym). "When they came, I told them about my problems," Dr. Petrov reported. "They wrote it down and forgot about it. I called them a few times, and they said they hadn't received parts." His batteries were finally replaced, but the speed control mechanism malfunctioned, unintentionally and precipitously changing the speed. "I offered them all the time to come to your shop, and you fix it there. I don't want to fix one part and then another part and then another part." Devi-Deals didn't respond. Dr. Petrov made his own repairs, although his screws didn't quite fit the holes. "I wouldn't move at all if I would wait for them."

Choosing Wisely

Myrtle Johnson laughed, looking out her living room window into her quiet urban side street jammed with parked cars.

> This lady walks up and down here all the time pushing her wheel-chair. She's fantastic. She's a big black woman. She has many things wrong with her, and she hates that wheelchair. She'll go to the su-permarket pushing the chair, and she's got her bundles in the chair. I laugh every time I see her. I say, "Molly, when are *you* going to get in the chair?" "The latest I can," she says. "I'm using it for a grocery cart." She doesn't want to get into it.

People sometimes seek equipment they later find they don't like; others receive wheelchairs they never really wanted in the first place. One expert emphasizes, "The value of offering trial periods before finalizing a technol-ogy selection cannot be overstated. The consumer must try the device in the actual situations of use (home, work, school)" (Scherer 2000, 124). But unfortunately, most equipment is not available for rental or test drives be-fore purchase, so people have little sense of how the technology will work in their daily lives.

People abandon mobility aids more than any other assistive devices (Scherer 1996, 2000; Olkin 1999), with canes, walkers, and braces rejected most often. Marcia Scherer, an expert in rehabilitation psychology, argues that "there is a dynamic interactive relationship among assistive device use, quality of life, and the user's functional capabilities and temperament" (2000, 117). Most assistive devices are abandoned within the first year, es-pecially in the first three months.

> Technology abandonment can have a series of repercussions. For in-dividuals, non-use of a device may lead to decreases in functional abilities, loss of freedom and independence, increases in expenses, and risk of injury or disease. Device abandonment also represents ineffective use of limited funds by federal, state, and local govern-ment agencies, insurers, and other providers. . . . The single most significant factor associated with technology abandonment is a fail-ure to consider the user's opinions and preferences in device selec-tion—in other words, *the device is abandoned because it does not meet the person's needs or expectations.* (118)

Scherer offers detailed advice on maximizing use of assistive technologies (120–43), emphasizing the match between people and technology and the mi-lieu or setting in which the device will be used. Molly, Mrs. Johnson's neighbor, will not use her wheelchair, no matter what—perhaps this refusal reflects her personality or maybe just her preferences. Environment is crucial. One stroke survivor wants to use a wheelchair but finds "the problem is getting it into and around inside our house, which is very small, has stairs at the outside doors, and very small doorways inside. How do you cope with that?"

Lonnie Carter walked slowly while pushing her wheelchair, its seat loaded with parcels. Asked if she preferred being pushed, she shook her head firmly, declining. She leaned heavily on the manual chair, a cheap model with black vinyl sling back and seat on sale for $279 at J. C. Penney. Lonnie paid it off $17 a month. She also had a scooter. "Who paid for the scooter?" I asked.

"Medicaid. I work. If you work, they'll do anything to keep you on a job. At first, Medicaid deferred me because they wanted more information. The doctors gave more information. I said I'm going to the grievance board for this if I have to. The next thing I knew, I got it. I got it six months ago, but I haven't used it."

"Why not?"

"I have to break it in. It's being used by something else, but it ain't being used by me.

"Who's using the scooter?"

"My bags of Avon! They're on it, but not me!" Lonnie laughed. So Lonnie, a part-time Avon saleslady, stored her cosmetics merchandise on her scooter.

"The scooter's being used as a piece of furniture?"

"Yes, and it's beautiful. It's that color of yours, blue. It's a beautiful thing; it has the keys with it. See, I was gonna move it because the building manager was coming to clean my rugs, but I hadn't charged it yet." Uninterested in using the scooter, Lonnie hadn't maintained its batteries during the six months she'd had it. "Well, I charged it, and it didn't work. I called the company and they said, 'When was the last time you used it? When did you charge it last?' They said the batteries are busted because I ain't used it or charged the battery. So I got a slip from my doctor and mailed it last week to Medicaid to get a new battery. Medicaid might give me a hard time, because they'll wanna know why this battery is defective this early. That's what I'm worried about. Medicaid is very fussy."

Lonnie never explained exactly why she hadn't used her scooter. Perhaps she legitimately feared that her near blindness from diabetes made scooter riding dangerous. Whoever ordered the scooter for her—and perhaps Lonnie herself—should have better understood Lonnie's needs and expectations.

Consequences of Sitting

"Sitting continuously is not a neutral event," Walter Masterson observed. "It becomes an extremely painful process." Because they are seated, wheelchair users are assumed to be comfortable, safe, and at ease. Their experience tells them otherwise. Mr. Masterson saw any exercise he did as "strengthening to endure sitting." Without adequate back supports, padding for vulnerable sites (e.g., ischial tuberosities), and appropriate seating angles, wheelchairs, especially those with sling backs and sling seats, are incredibly uncomfortable to sit in.

"I buy pillows," said Mr. Masterson. "This funny looking thing that I'm sitting on here is a very expensive pillow. The idea is that you sink into this and these cells make a personal impression of you. I don't fully understand it myself. Of course, that makes it a rather intricate thing to put together. They charge a price that reflects that—this is around $400. I've seen other pillows at significantly higher cost. But no matter how comfortable it is, my butt can only take it for maybe a couple of hours, and I've got to move."

People who must sit for long periods need to adjust their positions periodically, so their body's weight will not cause the skin to break down at prominent pressure points. Compression between bone and a hard surface cuts off blood flow to soft tissues, which can die in as short as one to two hours (Lewis 1996, 263). Pressure ulcers result, sometimes taking months and surgery to heal, and contributing to feelings of hopelessness and depression.

The most common wheelchair injury, however, involves falls, either from tipping over or from falling out of the wheelchair (Currie, Hardwick, and Marburger 1998; Gaal et al. 1997). Using standard wheelchairs, most people tip or fall forward, but scooters (especially three-wheeled models) can tip to the side. People can also tip backward, especially during acceleration of rear-wheel drive power wheelchairs. Falls are obviously dangerous and terrifying. Jenny Morris had taken her daughter to the park: "I was on a three-wheel scooter, with Rosa on my knee, when suddenly the scooter overbalanced on the steep gradient and we were in a heap on the grass. . . . I had felt such panic at this sudden reminder of my physical vulnerability" (1996b, 168). Fortunately, neither was hurt.

OBTAINING WHEELCHAIRS AND SCOOTERS

New wheelchair technologies give people options and a challenge—finding the right equipment. The federal Technology-Related Assistance for Individuals with Disabilities Act of 1988 (P.L. 100–407, the "Tech Act"), reauthorized in 1998, aims to heighten access to products for improving function and independence. Through the National Institute on Disability and Rehabilitation Research (NIDRR) in the Department of Education, the Tech Act allocates over $39 million annually to state programs to help people identify and understand assistive technologies (Brandt and Pope 1997, 151). Although Tech Act projects generally do not provide assistive devices directly, some do give practical guidance and legal advice on navigating insurance hurdles (Appendix 2 lists these sites). Nevertheless, Tech Act programs have not yet reached many people.

People obtain their wheelchairs through different routes. Lonnie Carter bought a wheelchair from J. C. Penney on sale, while her Medicaid-funded scooter sat unused in her apartment. Gerald Bernadine searched the Internet, finding his scooter and a lift device for his car. A scooter salesman visited Louisa Delarte at home. One man bought his scooter secondhand, through newspaper want advertisements; another inherited several wheelchairs from dead friends. Tina DiNatale seeks an ultralightweight manual wheelchair but cannot find one at local medical supply stores.

Wheelchairs are serious equipment with important physical, mechanical, practical, and emotional ramifications. Although diverse technologies exist, "there are no menus of assistive devices, and consumers simply are not aware of their options" (Olkin 1999, 277). The Internet offers dozens of sites about wheelchair technologies, although questions remain about the completeness and veracity of information. While primary care physicians sometimes discuss ambulation aids with their patients, few physicians I interviewed discuss wheelchairs or know much about them.

The best way to select a wheelchair is to work with experienced professionals, potentially including a physiatrist, occupational and physical therapists, social worker, equipment manufacturer, vocational rehabilitation counselor, and even health insurer (Warren 1990; Currie, Hardwick, and Marburger 1998; Karp 1998, 1999). Proper wheelchair evaluations can take time. After people receive equipment, they must be trained to use it, especially on how to avoid falls and other injuries.

Gary McNamara, a physical therapist, considers wide-ranging practical implications when suggesting wheelchair technologies. "People call in for a wheelchair versus a scooter evaluation. So I ask, can they get in and out of their house? If they have a manual chair now, are they dependent on another person propelling because, for whatever reason, they can't propel themselves? With this power chair, they'd be able to drive themselves. But someone's got to dismantle it, to carry it downstairs, and to put it back together. Unfortunately, a lot of the homes and housing projects in Boston are not accessible. The main thing in my mind is whether they need it in the home. Usually a wheelchair gives them a little more maneuverability through narrower places, but the scooter lets you go longer distances."

"If you have a power chair, you still need a manual chair," added Edith Leder, another physical therapist. "You can't take your power chair everywhere. Then you have that whole problem of having two pieces of equipment and insurance will only pay for one. Of course, it's usually the manual that comes first. It's cheaper. People need to find a rich uncle!"

13 Who Will Pay?

When I bought my first scooter over a dozen years ago, I had a gold-plated indemnity insurance policy, now virtually extinct, from Blue Cross–Blue Shield. The benefits package clearly included wheelchairs, but Blue Cross rejected my claim, arguing that a scooter-type electric wheelchair is a "recreational vehicle" analogous to a "golf cart"—a convenience item. Two neurologist friends intervened with letters and telephone calls, but Blue Cross stood firm. The insurer did offer to pay for a four-wheeled power wheelchair (then about $4,500), but not a scooter-type wheelchair (roughly $2,300), never mind that the scooter better suited my mobility needs. We bought the scooter ourselves.

"I can't keep up with this walker," said Erna Dodd, moving along slowly and laboriously, breathing oxygen from a canister dangling from the walker's handlebars. "I had a wheelchair, but I didn't like it because people has to push me around. I don't want people pushing me in a wheelchair. . . . So Max [her nurse] put in to get me a scooter. He had my doctor fill out some paper for it. This was a letter they send, telling me they wouldn't give it to me." Reaching into her bag, Erna retrieved a legal-size envelope containing a single sheet of paper.

"Medicare sent this to you?" I asked, looking at the letterhead, then read aloud, " 'We have received a prior authorization request for the above named beneficiary for a power operated vehicle. This request has been denied because the information did not support the medical necessity of the equipment. If you do not agree with this decision, you may request a review in writing within six months of the date indicated in this letter.' Did Max appeal this for you?"

"I don't know. I was going to call my doctor and talk to him about it. It would help me a lot."

"Would you use a scooter to do errands, go to church?"

"Yes, I'll be able to go," she sighed, "but who knows?" Erna's rented house had stairs at both front and rear entrances. How would she get the scooter in and out? Dr. Baker, her primary care physician, contested Medicare's denial, but Erna Dodd died during the appeals process (Iezzoni 1999).

We could afford to buy my scooter; others, like Erna Dodd, cannot. Innumerable services and strategies can enhance mobility or compensate for its loss, ranging from medical and surgical treatments to therapies for physical functioning to assistive technologies to home modifications to improved public transportation to enhanced accessibility of public spaces. Various interventions target different levels of this multidimensional problem, from an individual's specific pathological processes to communities, but each costs money up front. Each may also offer downstream savings, for example by reducing the risk of costly secondary conditions, such as hip fractures and depression, and bolstering people's ability to live independently and contribute productively to their communities. Each doubtless enhances quality of life. Services denied or delayed represent lost opportunities to improve mobility, reduce struggle and pain, and restore active life.

But who will pay, and what will they pay for? This book concentrates on health-care interventions. But their boundaries are blurry—what falls within the reimbursable health-care purview? Services provided at hospitals and by physicians typically do, as do those of physical and occupational therapists, if they're short-term and supervised by physicians. But what about long-term PT, to maintain physical functioning or prevent its decline? What about OT-recommended grab bars, shower seats, widened doorways, and ramps? What about when Erna Dodd, who had a manual wheelchair, requested a scooter to permit *independent* mobility? Given nineteen million adults with some mobility difficulties, mightn't improving physical access, broadly speaking, be an important *public* health goal, in this instance, to prevent epidemics of injuries and needlessly constrained lives?

This chapter reviews payment policies, focusing on public and private health insurance. Insurance is central to current health policy debates, with rising costs of the major public programs—Medicare and Medicaid—and concerns about whether and how employers will continue to provide private health insurance to their employees. Public and private plans are actively experimenting with different reimbursement strategies, endeavoring to control costs and to care for populations increasingly burdened by chronic disease. No strategy has yet achieved both goals, widely and over time.

With the human genome deciphered and significant medical advances hovering nearby, funding health care into the future is a pressing concern. Important causes of mobility problems, such as diabetes, Parkinson's disease, and ALS, may succumb to genetic insights. Major progressive chronic causes of mobility difficulties—degenerative arthritis, back problems, heart and lung disease, stroke—might escape gene-derived "silver bullets." Many factors underlying these conditions are hard to crack, such as obesity, smoking, inadequate exercise, poorly controlled blood pressure, and occupational hazards. Nevertheless, even without fundamental cures, treatments will improve, including targeted pain medications, longer-lasting artificial hips and knees, and new approaches to restoring cartilage eroded from joints. Funding the fruits of medical discoveries, even if expensive, will likely prove politically popular. Such new treatments epitomize the physician-hospital-science enterprise long accepted as meriting reimbursement. But will function-related therapies, assistive technologies, home modifications, and related services remain on that reimbursement boundary line?

This chapter describes basic policy issues raised in decisions to fund function-related items and services, while chapter 14 looks at how these policies specifically affect provision of physical and occupational therapy, mobility aids, and home modifications. For both chapters, I draw heavily on Medicare policies, publicly available in statute and regulation. I also touch on policies of state Medicaid and private insurers, which vary widely.

HEALTH INSURANCE MATTERS

Americans without health insurance, estimated at 15 percent of the population—forty-two million people—in 1999 (Institute of Medicine 2001b, 23), provide a critical backdrop to this discussion. A 1999 poll found that 57 percent of Americans believed that uninsured persons are "able to get the care they need from doctors and hospitals" (Institute of Medicine 2001b, 21). But this notion ignores the facts: among uninsured people, chronic diseases and disabling conditions are often neglected or poorly managed medically (22). Over the past twelve months, 10 percent of working-age people with major mobility problems did not get care they say they needed, and 28 percent say they delayed care because of cost concerns (Table 16).[1] Uninsured people with major mobility difficulties are 40 percent less likely

TABLE 16. Working-Age People Who Did
Not Get or Delayed Care in the Last Year

Mobility Difficulty	Did Not Get Care (%)[a]	Delayed Care (%)[b]
None	3	10
Minor	10	22
Moderate	13	28
Major	10	28

[a]Any time during the past 12 months, when a person "needed medical care or surgery, but did not get it."

[b]Any time during the past 12 months, when a person "delayed seeking medical care because of worry about cost."

to have wheelchairs or walkers than insured persons.[2] So health insurance matters.

Being uninsured is primarily a problem of younger persons. Almost 98 percent of elderly people have Medicare (Medicare Payment Advisory Commission 1999, 5). Voluntary employer-based private health insurance covers roughly two-thirds of the population, although it accounts for less than one-third of national health expenditures (Reinhardt 1999, 124). This statistic is not surprising. Medicare and Medicaid cover people who on average have greater health-care needs than workers and their families. Nonetheless, working-age persons who do not qualify for Medicare or Medicaid are often out of luck, even if they are employed.

Over half of uninsured people who have any disability work (Meyer and Zeller 1999, 11). Some employers avoid hiring disabled workers, fearing higher health insurance premiums (Batavia 2000). The ADA does not address employment-based health insurance explicitly, although it does prohibit employers from discriminating in "terms or conditions of employment" against an employee. Such terms presumably encompass benefits, like health insurance. The ADA's legislative history suggests that employers and health insurers can continue offering health plans with restricted coverage "as long as exclusions or limitations in the plan are based on sound actuarial principles" (Feldblum 1991, 102).[3]

Among persons eighteen to sixty-four years old, 6 percent report some mobility difficulty. But only 76 percent of those with minor and moderate mobility problems have health insurance, while 83 percent of younger

TABLE 17. Health Insurance Coverage among
Working-Age People

Mobility Difficulty	Health Insurance (%)			
	Any	*Medicare*	*Medicaid*	*Medicare and Medicaid*
None	80	1	4	< 1
Minor	76	9	20	3
Moderate	77	16	27	5
Major	83	28	35	10

persons with major mobility difficulties are insured, primarily through Medicare and Medicaid (Table 17). More unemployed than employed working-age people with major mobility problems have insurance (86 versus 79 percent), because of these public programs.[4] Younger people with mobility difficulties are denied health insurance more frequently than others, especially because of preexisting conditions or poor health risks, such as smoking or obesity.[5]

Health insurance doesn't cover everything. Even persons with health care insurance "are rarely covered for (and have access to) adequate preventive care and long-term medical care, rehabilitation, and assistive technologies. These factors demonstrably contribute to the incidence, prevalence, and severity of primary and secondary disabling conditions and, tragically, avoidable disability" (Pope and Tarlov 1991, 280). Health insurers typically decide what to reimburse in two stages: organizationwide decisions about what services are "covered" by a particular plan; and case-by-case decisions about the "medical necessity" of covered services for individual persons (Singer and Bergthold 2001). A third-order decision, potentially critical for persons with mobility problems, is the setting of care: can patients receive services at home? For mobility-related services, two major concerns generally underlie coverage decisions for private and public health insurers:

- How long will the person need the service? Chronic needs raise more questions than short-term demands.

- Will the service result in measurable improvement of physical deficits caused by medical illness or injury?

Neither issue is especially propitious for persons with progressive chronic conditions, who, by definition, generally need services long-term and are unlikely to improve.

COVERAGE DECISIONS

All health insurance plans specify the types of services or items they cover or will reimburse—their benefits packages. Plans covering more services typically cost more. Coverage policies reflect their historical roots. Private health insurance appeared about seventy years ago, partly to help acute-care hospitals make their increasingly costly services affordable to "the patient of moderate means" (Law 1974, 6). To ensure their financial survival during the Great Depression, hospitals organized prepaid health insurance or Blue Cross plans, writing contracts with employers to insure their workers. Over ensuing decades, as new hospital-based technologies offered "medical miracles" to combat acute threats to life and limb, costly but time-limited hospital interventions became the cornerstone of most health insurance plans.

Therefore, early and subsequent commercial plans primarily covered short-term, acute hospitalizations and physician services. Given today's competitive pressures, private health insurers offer numerous plans to meet diverse demands. Private health plans typically cover acute medical and surgical hospitalizations and primary and specialty physician visits but differ widely in coverage for other services. "Indemnity, preferred provider, and HMO [health maintenance organization] insurance products combine variations in cost sharing in myriad ways with variation in coverage, including or excluding physical therapy, rehabilitation, mental health, . . . and durable medical [equipment]" (Robinson 1999, 54).

Medicare and Medicaid, enacted in 1965, reflect decades of political maneuvering and compromises (Marmor 2000; Fox 1989, 1993). As with private health insurance, Medicare's roots reach back to the Great Depression. Although President Roosevelt wanted to add health insurance to his 1935 Social Security bill, he did not, concerned that opponents (such as organized medicine) could derail his entire Social Security plan. Decades later, Johnson administration officials underscored Medicare's focus on acute care in short-stay hospitals to gain congressional support. Policymakers feared that adding chronic care would exacerbate concerns about uncontrollable costs and derail political approval (Fox 1993, 75). Thus, Medicare explicitly did not cover long-term chronic care.

> The structure of Medicare as enacted—Social Security financing and eligibility for hospital care (Part A), and premiums plus general revenues for physician expenses (Part B)—had a clear political explanation, not a clearly understood social insurance rationale. . . . The structure of the benefits themselves, providing acute hospital care and intermittent physician treatment, was not tightly linked to the special circumstances of the elderly as a group. Left out were provisions that addressed the particular problems of the chronically sick elderly: medical conditions that would not dramatically improve and the need to maintain independent function rather than triumph over discrete illness and injury. (Marmor 2000, 153)

In 1972 Congress extended Medicare coverage to SSDI recipients who have received cash benefits for two years, but it did not broaden the general benefit package.[6]

As stipulated in the Code of Federal Regulations (C.F.R.), Medicare explicitly covers only services that are "reasonable and necessary for the diagnosis or treatment of illness or injury or to improve the functioning of a malformed body member" (42 C.F.R. Sec. 402.3).[7] Statutory exclusions—such as routine physical checkups, routine foot or dental care, hearing aids, and "personal comfort" items, such as grab bars (42 C.F.R. Sec. 411.15)—have important implications for specific mobility-related services (chapter 14).[8] Expanding coverage to include more function-related services proved politically unpalatable: "the cost implications of disability-related services . . . frighten policymakers away from contemplating all but the narrowest of expansions. What looks like a half-empty glass when benefits are being designed may be a bottomless pit once the payments begin to flow" (Vladeck et al. 1997, 88).

Medicare beneficiaries themselves pay for uncovered services or items, filling in two broad gaps: covered services for which Medicare pays only a portion of the expense; and services not covered at all (such as outpatient prescription drugs in traditional Medicare, sometimes covered by Medicare managed-care organizations).[9] In 1995, community-based (noninstitutionalized) Medicare beneficiaries with the highest 10 percent of expenses averaged $895 out-of-pocket for medical equipment and supplies, although Medicare Part B typically covers 80 percent of these costs (Medicare Payment Advisory Commission 1999, 8).

People fear the financial risks of relying solely on standard Medicare. "I have Medicare," said Fred Daigle.

"Part A and B," nodded Martha Daigle.

"They don't pay nothing," Mr. Daigle scoffed.

"It only pays 80 percent of hospital costs. So if you're in the hospital for, say, two days, can you imagine what 80 percent of that bill would be?" Mrs. Daigle kept working solely for private health insurance to supplement Fred's Medicare. About three quarters of Medicare beneficiaries purchase these private "Medigap" policies, roughly one-third through employers (Rice 1999, 112). Enriched standardized Medigap packages cover home health and long-term care services, although because of high premiums they are less popular than cheaper options (McClellan and Kalba 1999, 144). "I have Blue Cross and Blue Shield Gold," said one elderly woman, describing her Medigap plan as comprehensive. "That costs a fortune. It's $800 for each quarter, four times a year. That's a lot of money."

Because it explicitly covers poor people, Medicaid (a joint federal and state program) presents a different picture. Recognizing the inability of low income people to purchase care, Congress adopted broader benefits for Medicaid than Medicare, including medications, preventive services, eyeglasses, and long-term care in nursing homes.[10] Fox (1989, 1993) argues that Medicaid grew from a public welfare tradition, where eligibility and benefits generally reflect moral imperatives (such as long-standing interests in protecting vulnerable populations) rather than the medical considerations that drive Medicare. All states must cover core services (e.g., acute-care hospitalizations, home-health care, skilled nursing facility stays); individual states may offer any or all of thirty-two optional services, including physical and occupational therapy and durable medical equipment. Some states even fund modest home modifications like grab bars. Disabled enrollees do cost more than poor mothers and their young children. In 1995, 17 percent of Medicaid enrollees were blind or disabled, but they generated almost 34 percent of expenditures, costing $8,784 per year compared to $3,789 for the average recipient (Regenstein and Schroer 1998, 14).

Few insurers pay for "wellness" care—services aimed at promoting general health rather than treating or preventing disease. Medicare explicitly does not cover "services related to activities for the general physical welfare of beneficiaries (for example, exercises to promote overall fitness)" (42 C.F.R. Sec. 409.44[c][1]). Private insurers also rarely reimburse exercise services (Manning and Barondess 1996, 61). Some Medicare managed care organizations (MCOs) have offered free memberships at fitness clubs, although these benefits may erode with tightening costs.[11] Otherwise, despite its clear benefits, routine exercise generally falls outside health insurance coverage.

Although private and public health insurance plans document their covered benefits, enrollees often remain unaware of the details. Frustration erupts when plans deny uncovered services. "I don't think that patients really understand the distinction between the people who design their benefits and the people who pay the claims," observed the medical director of an eastern Blue Cross–Blue Shield plan. "Insurers pay the claims for services, but it's the employers who choose the benefit packages." Extensive benefit packages cost more than some employers or governments will pay; packages must meet budgets and, presumably, the enrollees' major needs. But, as the medical director said, "It's the insurance company that gets the blame when there's a discordance in expectations."

The health insurance system's complexity overwhelms some people. Esther and Harry Halpern can't agree on who pays for the home-health aide who helps them with grocery shopping and routine tasks around the house—their supplemental Medicare insurance or themselves, personally. After they disputed back and forth, Harry threw up his hands. "It's beyond belief," he sighed. "I just don't know how the system works. We're told all about it, but it takes special information to know how to work the system so it can help you." Myrtle Johnson, who has both Medicare and Medicaid, believes that people must educate themselves about their covered benefits. She was especially interested in orthopedic shoes for arthritis.

> I go to my doctor with a whole plan. I get all the numbers and names of everything I want. I went to school, and I studied Medicaid. I know exactly what I'm entitled to—and I get what I'm entitled to. I've worked hard all my life so I can do that. I don't want nothing less. I want what's mine. I needed shoes that are $125 a pair. I said, "Hold it. Medicare covers those shoes." I went to the State House, and I looked it up in the computers. I found it. Medicare covers two pair of shoes for anybody with arthritis or diabetes. They just need a prescription from the doctor. So I told that to everybody. I put it in our neighborhood newsletter. I put a sign in the lobby of the neighborhood health center.[12]

Mrs. Johnson wants *everyone* to know what they're entitled to.

MEDICAL NECESSITY

Before reimbursing covered services, insurers often require case-by-case determinations that specific items or services are "medically necessary" for individual persons. Debates about "medical necessity" wend throughout all health-care settings, from disease-oriented acute services to chronic care, and often pit patients' personal physicians against health plans. For persons with progressive chronic impairments, the issues are especially vexing. Insurers often reduce the arguments to a simple distinction: is the item or service medically necessary or is it primarily desired for convenience? Was it *medically necessary* that people like Erna Dodd leave their homes, enhance their safety, independently conduct their daily activities, possibly improve their quality of life? Medicare didn't think so.

Medicare's medical necessity language ties directly to the statutory definition of covered services quoted earlier—"diagnosis or treatment of illness or injury" or *improvement* of functioning. In the pamphlet *Medicare & You 2001*, the Health Care Financing Administration (HCFA, renamed the Centers for Medicare and Medicaid Services, or CMS, in June 2001), which runs Medicare, informs beneficiaries that Part B covers physical and occupational therapists and supplies that are "medically necessary" or that

- are proper and needed for the diagnosis or treatment of your medical condition

- are provided for the diagnosis, direct care, and treatment of your medical condition

- meet the standards of good medical practice in the medical community of your local area

- are not mainly for the convenience of you or your doctor (HCFA 2000a, 70)

The prohibition against "convenience" items, in particular, compromises efforts to obtain assistive technologies and other devices. Medicare probably turned down Erna Dodd because it viewed her requested scooter as a convenience item; it was clearly not "medically necessary" to diagnose or treat her many medical conditions.

While some Medicaid programs closely follow Medicare's definition of medical necessity, others set their own standards. "The Medicaid policy of finding 'medical necessity' in the functional aftermath of medical acuity makes its disability coverage more complete than that provided under Medicare" (Tanenbaum 1989, 295). For Medicaid managed-care contracts with health plans, most states have put together definitions of medical necessity, if not details of decision criteria (Rosenbaum et al. 1998). Medical necessity definitions from three states underscore the diversity of language.[13] California's language is terse and strongly medical; Pennsylvania emphasizes achieving or maintaining "maximum functional capacity in performing daily activities"; and South Carolina takes an even broader view, aiming to prevent, correct, alleviate, or cure conditions causing "malfunction," "handicap," or "infirmity."

Private health plans are numerous and have differing benefit packages. Their language about medical necessity is often vague or open to interpretation. The standards of medical necessity vary widely, and private plans' decisions on medical necessity ultimately come from physicians, typically the insurers' medical directors (Singer and Bergthold 2001). In making decisions, medical directors depend to varying degrees on contractual language, expert opinions, scientific evidence, professional experiences, local practices, and the enrollee's characteristics and preferences.

For mobility-related services, questions about scientific evidence showing the effectiveness of interventions loom large. Although the activities of physical and occupational therapists make theoretical, clinical, and practical sense, few clinical trials or large observational studies have analyzed the outcomes and effectiveness of these services. Research on OT outcomes is especially rare, particularly for home-based services. PT has a larger evidence base, focused primarily on inpatient rehabilitation or short-term outcomes. Mobility aids attract little research; studies generally involve small numbers of nondisabled volunteers in laboratory settings. The scarcity of research evidence about the effectiveness and clinical outcomes of therapy and assistive technology compromises efforts to make objective medical necessity decisions about the merit of mobility-related items and services.

Medical necessity decisions frequently appear idiosyncratic and subjective. As one disability rights activist said, "Health plans are pretty much free to manipulate the definition of medical necessity. It's whatever the doctor says it is. It's so open-ended it can be used as an excuse. 'Medical necessity' can be used to deny services to people who need them." Deficient communication compounds the problem. "Denial letters rarely explain who made the decision, the reason for the decision, what sources of evidence were considered, what coverage policies were applied, or anything else about the process of making the decision" (Singer and Bergthold 2001, 204). Conflicting motivations heighten concerns:

> The need to control costs and generate profits also brings into question the reliability and soundness of decision making by insurers. The sine qua non of scientific research is the production of objective results, and objectivity is ensured through a process of open and vigorous debate among persons who have no financial stake in the outcome. Yet much of the decision making about insurance coverage is based on unpublished, proprietary, and unreviewed data. Furthermore, methods are undisclosed and unexamined unless litigation ensues. (Rosenbaum et al. 1999, 231)

Growing numbers of lawsuits are questioning health plans' medical necessity decisions.

Thus, decisions about medical necessity often encounter that uncomfortable nexus, balancing personal needs against plan costs. "There is a tendency to vilify insurance companies—rightfully so in some cases—but keep in mind that, in order to keep your premiums low and stay in business, insurers must control the costs of what they provide to you and other policy holders," wrote the wheelchair user and expert Gary Karp (1998, 24). "You will be looking to get what you need so that you can live a full and comfortable life; your insurance company will be looking to place limits on what you get." Unfortunately, decision-making approaches do not engender tremendous confidence. "It's pretty loose," replied the medical director of a large western Blue Cross plan when asked to define medical necessity. "It means what a reasonable physician thinks is needed for his patient. It has to be a skilled service." Wheelchairs fit this definition but not "something that's just being done for convenience. That isn't a benefit."

CARE IN THE HOME

For mobility-related items and services, the home-care question cuts two ways. On the one hand, persons may have such severe mobility limitations that traveling to an office or clinic for physical or occupational therapy would be a hardship. Receiving care at home maximizes convenience and perhaps the benefit of therapy, by eliminating travel fatigue and thus enhancing the ability to exercise. OT in homes is essential for therapists to identify safety hazards and help modify people's daily routines. On the other hand, an explicit purpose of therapy and of mobility aids is to allow people to leave their homes comfortably and safely. But this goal directly conflicts with policies such as Medicare's coverage rules for power wheelchairs (described in chapter 14). In addition, Medicare and most private insurers view such equipment as grab bars and shower seats as "convenience items," and therefore not covered benefits.

Since the 1970s, Medicare regulations have stipulated that to qualify for home-based services, people must be "homebound," having "a condition that results in a normal inability to leave home except with considerable and taxing effort, and absences from home are infrequent or of relatively short duration or are attributable to receiving medical treatment" (U.S. General Accounting Office 2000, 6). A law enacted 21 December 2000 loosened this requirement somewhat: attending religious services was deemed permissible.[14] New guidelines announced 26 July 2002 broadened allowances for leaving home (see chapter 14), although people must still demonstrate that "considerable and taxing effort" is required. Persons must require skilled care, under a physician's explicit treatment plan. In contrast, Medicaid home health care beneficiaries "need not be homebound nor require skilled care" (Tanenbaum 1989, 296). Medicare beneficiaries who also have Medicaid therefore frequently get their home care financed by Medicaid (Foote and Hogan 2001, 248).

Scooter-user Louisa Delarte can't understand why Medicare stopped her home PT. Going back and forth from her rural residence to office-based PT services requires some effort. Mrs. Delarte does have a household handyman who drives her to shop and visits with her son. "The home-care people dropped me because they said I went out. I can't believe this! They drop you just because you're not home all the time! What am I to do? Stay home and vegetate? If someone drives you, naturally you're going to go out." Despite decades with MS, Mrs. Delarte's shopping and social engagements suggest she is too robust to merit Medicare home PT. Her trips do not demand considerable and taxing effort. Medicare sees Mrs. Delarte's home PT as a matter of convenience.

Medicare home-based care epitomizes that "bottomless pit" anticipated by Vladeck and colleagues (1997, 88). From 1989 to 1996, Part A home health care spending grew from $2.8 to $11.3 billion (U.S. General Accounting Office 1997b, 5). Many factors explain this increase, including changes in Medicare coverage policies (e.g., eliminating requirements that home-health services be tied to hospitalization), various court rulings that liberalized coverage criteria, and perhaps people like Mrs. Delarte. Policy changes between 1980 and 1989 "essentially transformed the home health benefit from one focused on patients needing short-term posthospital care to one that serves chronic, long-term care patients as well. . . . [From 1989 to 1996] the average number of visits to home health beneficiaries also more than doubled, from 27 to 72" (U.S. General Accounting Office 1997b, 6). Funding for "program safeguard" activities—a euphemism for preventing fraud and abuse among care providers—fell.

To control costs, the Balanced Budget Act of 1997 significantly changed Medicare home health-care payment policies. Between 1996 and 1999, the average number of home health visits per user fell by 21 percent for physical therapy and by 13 percent for occupational therapy (U.S. General Accounting Office 2000, 14). Some worry that these cuts have gone too far, especially for home-care recipients who are frail and medically vulnerable. Exactly how home-based care will fit into Medicare and private health insurance plans in the future is unclear.

WHO DECIDES THE DETAILS

At the global level, benefit and coverage policies are set politically or by the marketplace. Yet when it comes to day-to-day detailed decision-making about whether individual persons will get specific items or services, physicians rule. Medical directors of health plans determine medical necessity. On the front lines, physicians must write prescriptions and devise and oversee treatment plans for their patients to receive therapy and assistive technologies. Public and private plans will not pay without explicit physicians' authorization. For example, for Medicare PT and OT, physicians must review and sign plans of care at least every 62 days for home-health services (42 C.F.R. Sec. 409.43[e]) and at least every 30 days for outpatient services (42 C.F.R. Sec. 410.61[e]). How ironic: as described in prior chapters, most physicians have little knowledge of physical or occupational therapy or of assistive technologies. Yet physicians are in charge.

Cynthia Walker has commercial HMO insurance through her husband's employer, which required her to change her rheumatologist: "My insurance is set up that I am forced to work with this man, and I want to make the best of it." She feels the physician doesn't know about mobility aids and other devices that could improve her daily functioning. "To find specific things that would be helpful to me, I have to do my own homework." Mrs. Walker searches the Internet, scanning arthritis-related sites. "Then I go to my doctor. . . . The HMO requires prescriptions. The insurance doesn't want to cover everything if they don't have to. That's a shame, isn't it? It all comes down to a price tag."

Walter Masterson worries that requiring all decisions to channel through his primary care physician, Dr. Burton, wastes time and doesn't recognize the varying expertise of different clinicians. "Burton is a really nice doctor. I like him a lot," said Mr. Masterson, "but look at his position as a primary physician. It's an impediment to the natural flow of medical care. It's very centralized. The ball always seems to have to come pinging back to the middle, to Burton, before it can go anyplace else. Everything has to await a chain of approval."

Mr. Masterson acknowledges that his neurologist's clinical role is limited, given that no effective treatments yet exist for ALS. "Now, what I'm discovering in the last year is that, as the disease progresses, there are peripheral impacts of ALS that do have treatment. There are roles for other specialists to play where there didn't appear to be any in the beginning. Physical therapy. What they call occupational therapy. People for sleep disorders. People for depression." Mr. Masterson must wait for Dr. Burton to approve these services, which he does, but it can take time to get through the "chain of approval."

Dr. Patrick O'Reilley, a primary care doctor at a neighborhood health center, generally ignores what he sees as byzantine rules about prescriptions and approvals set by health insurers. "I'm pretty much blind to what they'll do or what they won't do. If they kick out something I prescribe, then I'll find out about it, but I just go ahead and do it. I'm not really sensitive to what I'm allowed to do." But Dr. O'Reilley does worry about his patients, who are poor, being sent large bills by providers because their insurer denies coverage and he didn't follow rules. "I would feel bad if somebody ended up having to pay a big bill."

A nationwide survey of persons age sixteen and older performed in 2000 found worrisome disparities, even among those with health insurance. Of the insured people with various disabilities, including mobility problems, 28 percent report they have special needs that are not covered—for particular therapies, equipment, medications—compared to 7 percent of those without disabilities. Among those with very severe disabilities, 40 percent note uncovered special needs (Harris Interactive 2000, 56, 57). Overall, 19 percent of disabled persons report that they needed medical care within the last year but didn't get it, compared to 6 percent of nondisabled persons (Harris Interactive 2000, 60). Disabled people attribute these failures to lack of insurance coverage (35 percent), high cost (31 percent), difficulties or disagreements with physicians (8 percent), problems getting to physicians' offices or clinics (7 percent), and inadequate transportation (4 percent).

In its Healthy People 2010 initiative, the U.S. Department of Health and Human Services (2000, 6-5) recognizes that, "As a potentially underserved group, people with disabilities would be expected to experience disadvantages in health and well-being compared with the general population." These types of findings concern the public policy analyst and disability rights activist Laura Remson Mitchell (personal communication, 5 August 1998):

> People with disabilities are the "canaries in the mine" of the health care system. You know how canaries used to be the warning system for miners? When the canaries keeled over, the miners knew the air wasn't good—they'd better get out. People with disabilities tend to be the most vulnerable persons in the health care system. Unless there's a lot of advocacy, their needs tend to be put on the back burner and dealt with as an afterthought. Problems in the health care system hit people with disabilities first, but ultimately almost everyone is affected. That's why I find it really ironic and sad that

people fail to realize that they have a stake in making sure the
health care system works for us.

No solutions are yet in sight. Basic restructuring of our health-care system is essential, but intractable societal forces and cost concerns have, thus
far, blocked fundamental reforms. While often maligned, public and private
health insurance has protected much of the public from the full brunt of
acute health-care costs, although uninsured and chronically ill people
might tell different tales. As a country, we have not yet explicitly confronted what the health-care system should pay for and why.

Even Christopher Reeve had trouble getting his private insurance company to extend his stay in a rehabilitation facility and to purchase equipment. "I talk to some of the executives of insurance companies," wrote
Reeve (1998, 290). "And I say, Why is this? Why don't you take care of
people? People who have paid their premiums, people who are in need. And
they say, Well, we're in the risk management business. And I say, You
should be in the people business."

Reeve argues, "One of the reasons that insurance companies deny essential equipment and care is because only 30 percent of patients and their
families fight back" (129). Could many of the interviewees fight this one
alone?[15] Should the government and private insurance companies take all
the blame?

14 What Will Be Paid For?

A colleague who lives in a small mountain town described his neighbor. "Mary Jo is her name. She lives three blocks from us. She's thirty-nine or forty, and she has diabetes. She's had one leg amputated, and the other leg is constantly in danger. She lives in a low-income apartment, one of those little places like a motel room. Some friends raised the money and gave her an electric wheelchair—a real cheap one, but it allowed her to get out the door and up to a small park. On a nice spring day, she can go out and sit under a tree and come back in. That's all she ever did with it."

Mary Jo has a home-health nurse to treat her ulcerated leg, among other things. "One day, the home-health nurse saw the electric wheelchair sitting in the apartment, and she said, 'You know what? I can't come anymore.' Mary Jo is disabled under Medicare, and Medicare won't pay for home health unless the person is homebound. So the wheelchair has now been folded up and is gathering dust in the corner. It's been retired from use, and every time a home-health aide comes, she tries not to see it."

"Mary Jo doesn't go out anymore?"

"No, except on Sundays. What happens—and nobody from home health sees this—is that this team at her church comes and gets her on Sunday and packs her up and takes her over and then brings her home afterward. She's overweight. She's very difficult to get around. The people are scared to death they'll drop her, but they take her. The home-health person doesn't know this."

"Could she go to church herself in her electric wheelchair?"

"That's right. It'd be a lot easier. And she could go into town. She could actually buy a loaf of bread. In our town, you can still buy a loaf of bread a couple blocks away."

Mary Jo is entrapped by paradoxical payment policies. Her friends rightly assumed that Medicare would refuse to purchase her power wheelchair since she does not need it within her tiny apartment—as for Erna Dodd, it would not have been deemed "medically necessary." They bought it themselves. The independence and ease conveyed by the power wheelchair, however, could put at risk her eligibility for home-based nursing care for her remaining leg ulcerated by diabetes: if Mary Jo leaves her apartment without considerable and taxing effort to sit under a tree in her power wheelchair, she might lose home-health care. Going to church is permitted, but neither Mary Jo nor her friends wish to risk a strict interpretation of Medicare's rules, and so her power wheelchair sits unused. Remaining homebound when she could venture out diminishes Mary Jo's quality of life and could compromise her overall health.

To commemorate the twelfth anniversary of the ADA on 26 July 2002, President George W. Bush addressed one concern raised by Medicare's homebound definition: that home-care coverage ceases if people go out for reasons other than health care or church services.[1] Urging people to meet friends, join family reunions, and even attend baseball games, President Bush announced that "we're clarifying Medicare policy, so people who are considered homebound can occasionally take part in their communities, without fear of losing their benefits."[2] Because these trips still must require considerable and taxing effort, Mary Jo may be stuck. It's too soon to tell how Medicare will interpret President Bush's pronouncement.

Insurance covers health-care costs at premiums that governments, employers, and individuals are willing to pay. Therefore, controlling costs is completely reasonable and even essential to keeping premiums affordable, presumably allowing more people to remain insured. Chapter 13 described how insurers typically invoke several strategies to limit function-related expenditures: delineating covered items and services; requiring proof of "medical necessity"; limiting the setting of services; and demanding physician authorization. Chapter 14 examines the consequences of these strategies for provision of physical and occupational therapy, acquisition of mobility aids, and home modifications.

THERAPIES TO MAINTAIN PHYSICAL FUNCTIONING
OR PREVENT ITS LOSS

People with chronic conditions know the jargon of today's health-care marketplace. Tina DiNatale, who has had MS for many years, has "Master Medical" private health insurance through her husband's job. "With good physical therapy, my walking can be improved greatly," said Tina, remembering her prior treatments. "The endurance was much much better. The posture would be better if I continued the physical therapy." Tina stopped PT for various reasons, including the arduous drive from her suburban home to the inner-city hospital where she received services, but she worries what will happen if she again wants long-term therapy. "Doctors have to write a prescription, but doctors writing a prescription *ad infinitum* is almost unheard of today. Also, the way the insurance companies are, it's limited. They think you only need physical therapy if it's to get better, not for maintenance. Insurance companies put time limits on physical therapy."

Physical and occupational therapy aim to restore, enhance, and preserve function. But restoring function is generally not realistic for people with progressive chronic conditions. The goal shifts to maintaining function or preventing more loss. This process lasts a lifetime, although the intensity of necessary services would wax and wane. Not surprisingly, health insurers balk at writing what they see as blank checks—covering services with no end in sight. Therefore, they set endpoints: when people meet some target functional goal or cease making progress, therapy stops. As the medical director of a western Blue Cross plan said, "When people plateau in terms of their functioning, then health insurers get reluctant to pay for something that's not going to have a significant benefit over time. So people's insurance contracts often limit benefits for rehabilitation or physical or occupational therapy." Anecdote and limited reports suggest that private plans impose annual or lifetime caps on rehabilitation expenditures (Brandt and Pope 1997, 185).

Medicare's regulations are explicit: "There must be an expectation that the beneficiary's condition will improve materially in a reasonable (and generally predictable) period of time based on the physician's assessment of the beneficiary's restoration potential and unique medical condition" (42 C.F.R. Sec. 409.44[c][2][iii]).[3] Medicare does reimburse therapists' services to set up a "maintenance program," specifically to train the beneficiary or family in what to do, paying only for "necessary infrequent reevaluations of the beneficiary" by the therapist. Thus, an Institute of Medicine committee concluded,

> Common to Medicare, Medicaid, and private policies . . . is the stipulation that reimbursement will continue only for as long as the person receiving rehabilitation services continues to show improvement in functional capacity. Yet for many people—for example, those with head injuries or chronic heart conditions—improvement in functional capacity may not be apparent until long after the start of

therapy. This restriction also ignores the rehabilitation goal of maintaining capacity and of halting or slowing declines in function in people with degenerative conditions. (Pope and Tarlov 1991, 255)

Judgments about the value of staying on that functional "plateau" obviously differ from person to person. To persons with progressive conditions "maintenance of function . . . may be as important or more important to the patient than modification of the disease activity per se" (Manning and Barondess 1996, 5). Alan M. Jette, Ph.D., dean of the Sargent College of Health and Rehabilitation Sciences at Boston University and a physical therapy professor, views such distinctions as spurious. "Separating restorative from maintenance physical therapy is not a substantive distinction," said Professor Jette (personal communication, 19 January 1999). "It comes purely out of the Medicare legislation. If the services you are providing are restorative, then they would be reimbursed. If they are for maintenance, they are not reimbursed. I never see this distinction discussed within the profession of physical therapy." Professor Jette considers prevention of functional loses as essential for persons with progressive chronic diseases. Nevertheless, "most rehab professionals work in an environment where restoration is the ticket for reimbursement, and so you write and speak in a way that allows you to get paid for your services."

Insurers use different strategies to limit physical and occupational therapy expenditures. Some plans approve limited numbers of therapy sessions, reevaluating patients' progress before authorizing more visits. Stella Richards's private health insurer counted visits. "Did you have physical therapy after your back operations?" I asked her.

"Definitely. After both."

"Are you still doing physical therapy?"

"No. My insurance company is cheap. They thought I'd had enough. I could use more physical therapy, but I can't afford to pay for that. When I had to retire because of my back, I lost half of my pension."

"What did your insurer say about the physical therapy?"

"They give you eleven visits. And then they gave me eleven more, and I don't remember if they extended it another time. I was just getting ready to do more. A new program opened up out at the rehab hospital. They were gonna have water aerobics, which I really needed." Many people find they move more easily buoyed by water. "I bought a new bathing suit. I'm all set to go. Then the insurance company said it wasn't medically necessary so I couldn't go." After Mrs. Richards stopped therapy, "I just felt myself sinking, sinking, sinking. Then I reached the magic age of sixty-five! I was able to get back in therapy because of Medicare."[4]

Another strategy for limiting expenditures is setting functional targets. The medical director of a midwestern health insurer does not specify fixed numbers of physical therapy visits for his company's private plans. Instead, the company monitors functional progress. "We primarily evaluate what's medically necessary for restoring function—as long as patients are making progress and if they continue to make progress. For restorative therapy, we're usually talking five sessions a week, once or twice a day. Once they've reached the level at which patients are fairly functional—in other words, they walk 100 feet with or without an assistive device but without assistance from any person—that's the cutoff."

"So when the person walks 100 feet, you say that physical therapy is no longer medically necessary?"

"Right—not for walking. As far as whether or not they need continuing maintenance therapy, almost all of the benefit plans exclude maintenance therapy."

I asked Jim Allerton, a senior physical therapist, about this 100-foot threshold. "For me, a functional goal has to do with real-life behavior," said Mr. Allerton. "Say I'm working with an older woman client who's fractured her hip. I can't imagine her saying her goal is to walk 100 feet. She wants to be able to live on her own, to get up and out of bed in the morning, to get dressed, to cook, to see her friends, to get out to social activities or church. She wants to be able to climb stairs so she can get into her house. Those are functional goals." The question then becomes what is needed to achieve these goals, both to improve her physical functioning and to adapt her living environment. "Being able to walk 100 feet is only a proxy for these other activities. It loses sight of what the real goals are."

In assessing coverage for occupational therapy, the policies of private plans and Medicare alike are highly variable and less systematic than for physical therapy. Because of its emphasis on acute-care hospitalization, Medicare covers home-based occupational therapists "only if they are part of a plan that also includes intermittent skilled nursing care, physical therapy, or speech-language pathology services" (42 C.F.R. Sec. 409.44[c]). These restrictions make little sense: OT more than PT deals directly with conducting daily activities at home, yet Medicare beneficiaries cannot get home OT without concomitant PT or other services. During their focus group, occupational therapists described home visits and constraints imposed by public and private insurers.

"Our time is more limited now than it used to be," stated Joanne, who has practiced OT for over fifteen years. "We're doing tons more things in one visit than we used to. I'm fighting with the case manager to get one more visit with a woman who's ninety-two. She has all the equipment to do her ADLs [activities of daily living], but I don't feel comfortable that she's able to do them safely. I'm probably going to lose the battle, and there's nothing we can do about it."

"When do you start feeling pressures from insurance?"

"The first visit. We're getting told we have one visit—one eval [evaluation]. You call the case managers, and it's a huge negotiation. Some case managers are fabulous. They respect our clinical judgment. Our agency's policy is that we see people if you really feel that a visit needs to be made. But then, on the other hand, money at the agency is tight. We're getting patients who've had a stroke right out of hospital, and we're getting a couple weeks of visits. If they're not better, the insurer says sorry, no more services. I think it's getting worse. Before we could push a little more."

"What's the average number of times you're allowed to visit patients for private insurers?"

"Five, ten," said Joanne. Others concurred. Standards are different for Medicare. "You can have as many as you want within the period if patients are achieving active, measurable goals and the patient remains homebound," Joanne added. "I saw a patient the other week, but all three disciplines had to go in on the same day: PT, nursing, and myself. Patients are totally overwhelmed. They have no clue who we all are. We're all nurses as far as they're concerned. So how much teaching can you actually do in that first visit? Forget it!"

"It's a wasted visit."

"But you have to go because it's all the time you have. At least you have something on paper to tell the case manager so you can hopefully go back, but the patient hasn't benefited from that OT visit."

Finally, tight restrictions on physical and occupational therapy services, such as limiting the numbers of visits, may reflect years of soaring costs and insurers' frustrations. As Stan Jones, a health policy expert in chronic-disease care, saw it (personal communication, 6 February 1998),

> From the insurers' standpoint, services like rehab, physical therapy, and occupational therapy are suspect. Providers see them as money-makers. Payers, both public and private, are convinced that there's enormous overuse of services going on. I don't know if one could ever document this. But I'll bet much of this goes back to practices that have, in fact, gone on with rehab centers and hospitals and clinics who are trying to raise revenues anyway they can to pay for the cost of complicated patients whose insurance is inadequate.

Admittedly, providers learn to shade the literal truth, trying to protect patients from what they see as foolish regulations. "It's been that way for years," said Jim Allerton. "The best anecdote is from when I was a student in physical therapy. I had a rotation in home care. I was working with one of my patients on helping her with safety, going outside, being mobile, walking on level ground. I had written a nice note about the progress she was making. My mentor took me aside and said, 'You have to redo that note. To be reimbursed by Medicare for home care, patients have to be homebound, and therefore you cannot write that you're taking her outside.' "

"What did you do?"

"I rewrote the note. The note didn't reflect the reality because we didn't want her to lose her reimbursement. So you play the reimbursement game."

Patients sometimes witness this firsthand. "I get this 'Explanation of Benefits' from my insurer—for me, it's Blue Cross—that says this physical therapy claim has been rejected," recounted a man whose chronic progressive condition necessitates periodic physical therapy. "So I pick up the phone and call the physical therapist and say, 'Gee, I'm concerned. This claim has been rejected, and since that bill went to Blue Cross, I've had four more sessions. I face a fee of $700.' I've been told again and again, 'Don't worry about it. We just need to put a different code on it.' " In fact, insurers often reject claims containing one specific diagnosis code but accept another. "One time, I had a buildup of claims that was a couple thousand dollars. The physical therapist kept saying, 'Don't worry. You're not gonna have to pay it. It's just a matter of finding the right code.' That took five or six tries before Blue Cross finally paid them. I couldn't help but think, holy mackerel! No wonder there's distrust on both sides of that fence."

I asked Stan Jones whether payers think such practices constitute outright fraud. "I'm always nervous about that word," he replied. "There's so many diagnoses and so many ways you can describe a patient. Physical therapists can say that treatment is for pain. But if the insurer won't pay, no, it wasn't for pain. The therapy was for dysfunction. Oh, you don't pay for that? Well, how about if it were for something else? But it's all the same treatment or largely the same treatment."

Jim Allerton recognizes "medical necessity" stipulations, in particular, as a way that public and private insurers curb excess in physical therapy services:[5]

> Medical necessity has a gatekeeper function. In the absence of more meaningful criteria as to what therapy is appropriate and what's not, it's a gatekeeper to cut down on abuse of the system. I fully acknowledge that, in the past, there have been abuses. There's been a lot of over-provision of rehab services, and there's been a reaction against that. The professions have been unwilling to police themselves, and now they're paying the price for that.

In this context, the obvious question is who's looking out for the patient. It's harder to count patients' mobility difficulties than mounting dollars spent on their care. Little objective evidence supports the value of these services, as an Institute of Medicine committee reported,

> The investment in these expenditures is expected to be outweighed by the economic, social, and personal benefits accrued from getting people back to work or school and living independently. Unfortunately, very few studies have adequately examined the extent to which rehabilitation achieves these goals—and the relationship of achieving these goals to costs. In today's climate of rising health care expenditures and emphasis on cost-containment, it is incumbent on the rehabilitation community to demonstrate what works best and at what cost. (Brandt and Pope 1997, 174)

Professor Jette agrees (personal communication, 19 January 1999). He believes that scientific evidence about the benefits of rehabilitation is strong in selected areas, notably care following strokes. But for other conditions, such as low-back pain, "It's shakier. There's evidence in support of some approaches and not for others. The question is how tough a standard do you want. That's a judgment call. In most fields of health care, not just rehab, we have less evidence than we really need to make evidence-based decisions." He acknowledges that fields like physical and occupational therapy are slow to produce credible research supporting their interventions. "There's even a lack of theory behind a lot of what people are doing in some areas. We've come late to science."

The geriatrician Muriel Gillick fears the consequences for her patients, who tell her that when "therapists terminate their services, they begin to deteriorate. They often feel—and their therapists concur—that they are more likely to maintain their gains if they are in a long-term rehabilitation program. . . . Once a patient has reached a plateau, once he is not making further progress, he is no longer eligible for services" (1995, 198).

MOBILITY AIDS

Health insurance policies make no sense to several women wheelchair users. Marcia, in her mid thirties, has recently "been nursing a rotator cuff injury"—an injury in her shoulder joint caused by self-propelling her manual wheelchair. She wants an ultralightweight wheelchair, but it is more expensive than the standard heavier model, and her health insurer will not cover it. "How can this understanding of better equipment get into the heads of the medical community and the insurance companies? They should understand that if you've got a heavy wheelchair that was giving you a repetitive stress injury on a shoulder or a wrist or an elbow, the cost to them for putting you in rehab and getting you back to 100 percent health is ten, fifteen, twenty times greater than just paying the few extra bucks for the better wheelchair."

"The problem I've had is knowing what I need," said Penny. "For instance, if you could go to a store and look at what they have, that would be great, but you really can't because they don't have an inventory. You can look at pictures and stuff—they have that. But you don't know how it feels, so you end up buying something that may not work out for you."

"Right now we're going through Medicare to get my new wheelchair, but I'm supposing that the chair I want is going to have zero coverage," Maureen stated. "My insurance is written that I'm eligible for a $1,200 wheelchair, which I wouldn't go for because I can't get a good enough chair for that. The insurance company won't apply that $1,200 and let me pay cash for the extra. They're protecting the disabled person because the wheelchair manufacturer is going to talk you into a more expensive, light-weight chair. That's what the federal government said!" True. Presumably to stymie unscrupulous vendors, Medicare precludes people from paying cost difference themselves, at least for now: "You must accept the chair they are willing to buy, or they will not cover you" (Karp 1998, 27).[6]

"I once had an insurance company that wouldn't pay for a new chair, but they would pay for the continual rentals of anything," recalled Marcia. "So I never got a chair out of that company."

"I'm in the process of waiting for a new chair," Samantha reported. "My doctor wrote the prescription. Last April I went to the wheelchair clinic. I haven't seen the chair yet, and I've been waiting since April." It was then late September.

"Did they tell you why?" I asked.

"It's just jumping through hoops," Samantha sighed. "I've heard the same issues with other people. I've gotten approval. But the dealer won't give you the chair until they get paid by the insurance company. It takes so long for them to get paid now that it creates a backup of chairs. They could have your chair in their shop, but since it's not paid for, they won't give it to you. That should be a federal crime."

These women, all active persons in early middle age, needed wheelchairs, otherwise they could not get around. From their perspective, such payment policies are, at best, "penny wise and pound foolish"—for example, covering only heavier manual wheelchairs, which are more likely to cause upper-body injuries than lighter-weight models. At worst, the policies are simply mean-spirited—withholding someone's wheelchair while the insurance company, having certified approval, delays paying the bill. A business perspective might offer more nuanced interpretations. Insurers do need to contain costs. Dealers seem entirely justified for not delivering a wheelchair until paid; less defensible is the delayed insurance payment. Karp finds that, "Although you may have to assert yourself to get the right wheelchair, it's possible that approval from your insurance company will go smoothly" (1998, 25). Nevertheless, rifts frequently arise between payment policies and practices and the needs of the people who require mobility aids—a class of so-called durable medical equipment (DME).

Insurers often impede requests for wheelchairs and other mobility aids from persons with chronic progressive debilities, by outright denials or repeated demands for extensive justification or substitutions of less desirable equipment for preferred options. They might ultimately grant approval, but, as Samantha observed, people and their doctors must first "jump through hoops." Dr. Ron Einstein, a primary care physician, concurs: "It's very hard to get good wheelchairs from health insurers. They really fight you." Some faith-based and advocacy organizations, such as disease-specific associations, offer equipment or organize trade-ins and redistribution of used devices, but these opportunities address only a fraction of the need for mobility aids.[7] An Institute of Medicine committee summarized the situation:

> Applying commercially available technology to the needs of people with disabling conditions would seem to be a relatively straightforward exercise in technology transfer. Unfortunately, a major impediment exists in the form of the reimbursement criteria of public and private insurers. Tailored to the treatment of acute conditions, reimbursement criteria emphasize curative medicine and rarely recognize the importance of maintaining health and improving functioning. Thus most assistive technologies, which are tools of preventive care, do not qualify for reimbursement. . . . This shortsightedness is also reflected in the inadequate coverage that most insurers provide for long-term maintenance and replacement of the few assistive technologies they do fund. (Pope and Tarlov 1991, 227)

What Will Insurers Cover?

Medicare Part B covers only "medically necessary" DME, requiring 20 percent coinsurance from beneficiaries. Part A covers mobility aids furnished to qualifying homebound persons under an authorized treatment plan, with beneficiaries again paying 20 percent coinsurance. The 20 percent coinsurance adds up. A rolling walker, for example, can cost $400, while good-quality standard manual wheelchairs typically cost $2,000, scooters are roughly $2,000 to $5,000, four-wheeled power wheelchairs generally run $10,000, and technologically sophisticated power chairs can exceed $30,000.

Medicare sets strict dollar ceilings for specific types of DME, generally far below the actual costs of good-quality mobility aids. Maureen's Medicare carrier, for example, only allows $1,200 for manual wheelchairs, much lower than the price for a good-quality standard model, let alone an ultralightweight wheelchair. Medicare imposed these dollar limits following congressional investigations of fraud and abuse among DME vendors (Wickizer 1995, 384). These limits affect all types of mobility aids, including artificial limbs. Arnis Balodis was dissatisfied with his bilateral leg prostheses: they were different heights, heavy, and less functional than new technologies. "Medicare. Money," Arnis explained why he didn't upgrade his prostheses. His present legs had cost about $2,700, and higher-tech legs would cost more. "It's what Medicare will allow."

Medicaid coverage policies for DME vary by state. The underlying philosophy of Medicaid supports more expansive coverage of DME than Medicare allows. "Medicaid was created as a welfare program and as such, made it a program policy to (re)establish functional independence in individuals and families . . . [and] to blur distinctions between medical and social services, professional and practical care giving, so as to move a recipient toward disenrollment" (Tanenbaum 1989, 303). This policy might explain Lonnie Carter's rather cryptic response when asked who paid for her scooter: "Medicaid. I work. If you work, Medicaid'll do anything to keep you on a job."

Some states are less generous than Massachusetts: even people with spinal cord injuries occasionally cannot get Medicaid coverage for wheelchairs (Karp 1998, 27). Medicaid often denies mobility aids, describing them as "non-essential," or pays only for obsolete equipment (Perry and Robertson 1999). One Florida woman observed, "If you are going to die if you don't get [this piece of equipment], then you get it. But if you are going to have a poor quality of life because you don't get it, that doesn't qualify as essential" (32).

Private health insurers carefully circumscribe DME benefits, including mobility aids, if they cover them at all. A representative of a national health insurance trade association told me that such devices as wheelchairs fall outside the scope of legitimate "health-care" services: insurance covers acute services to restore function, he said, not equipment to compensate for its loss. Insurers also must guard against nefarious wheelchair vendors charging unnecessarily high prices since the "rich insurance company has deep pockets." Many private insurers use Medicare standards, including 20 percent copayments (Pope and Tarlov 1991). Anecdotal evidence suggests that commercial MCOs, in particular, restrict DME coverage, either refusing requests outright or placing such tight caps on allowable costs that only low-end equipment is provided (Karp 1998). Although MCOs generally allow appeals, reversing denials is time-consuming and requires tenacity.

Beyond compromising users, buying cheaper equipment sometimes costs insurers money in the long run, as Marcia suggested. Jody Greenhalgh, an occupational therapist at Stanford Rehabilitation Services, finds,

> We see patients who have severe skin ulcers. They've been on bed rest for months. A specialized wheelchair is medically recommended but denied by the insurer. The patient then requires a $50,000 surgery, after which he returns to the inadequate wheelchair. This causes the surgery to fail and the pressure sores recur. The patient has to go back on long-term bed rest and repeat hospitalization.
>
> The insurance companies seem to be short-sighted, preferring to spend money on surgical intervention rather than paying for the right cushion and specialized wheelchair—which would ultimately save dollars and help the patient return to a productive and independent life. (Karp 1999, 213)

When Are Mobility Aids Medically Necessary?

Unlike physical and occupational therapy, most mobility aids will not improve baseline physical function (although they certainly may enhance safety and ambulation techniques). Judgments of medical necessity therefore cannot rely on that traditional standard of restoring function. For Medicare, the focus shifts to whether the equipment allows someone to perform minimal activity—moving around *within* one's home. Medicare Part B "pays for the rental or purchase of durable medical equipment" only "if the equipment is used in the patient's home or in an institution that is used as a home" (42 C.F.R. Sec. 410.38[a]). Getting around *outside* the home is a "convenience," not medically necessary, as Erna Dodd found.

By this stringent standard, many people with progressive chronic conditions who still get around inside their homes (e.g., by furniture surfing) cannot qualify for mobility aids through Medicare. Requirements are even stricter for power wheelchairs. To obtain a "power operated vehicle" (POV)[8] for their patients, physicians must complete the "Certificate of Medical Necessity" (Form HCFA 850[4/96] and OMB No. 0938–0679).[9] Section B of the form asks six questions,[10] including:

Does the patient require a POV to move around in their residence?

Have all types of manual wheelchairs (including lightweights) been considered and ruled out?

Does the patient require a POV *only* for movement outside their residence?

Thus, Medicare's intent is clear: to pay for the more expensive POV only if cheaper options are "ruled out." Standards for ruling out manual chairs nevertheless remain unspecified, leaving considerable leeway for subjective judgment and denials. A social worker told me of a man paralyzed by a stroke whose POV request was refused. Medicare asserted that his elderly wife could push him in a manual wheelchair within their home—never mind that she is also frail and weak. This stringency seems unnecessary. Compared to certain other types of DME, POVs are relatively rarely requested, and no evidence suggests that they are overprescribed (Wickizer 1995). As one woman whose husband has severe MS said, "I don't believe there's a massive abuse of DME—that people are buying things that they don't need. There's a copay. My husband's wheelchair is $20,000. That's a $4,000 copay. Do you think I'm going to spend $4,000 just for the fun of it?"

No information is publicly available on the language covering mobility aids across the myriad of private health plans, but medical necessity figures prominently in decisions about their coverage (Karp 1998). The medical director of a midwestern health insurer (mentioned earlier) told me he does not argue with wheelchair prescriptions for people with stroke or spinal cord injury—the most common conditions generating these requests. If their arms are paralyzed or weak, he also does not question the medical necessity of powered equipment. But he wonders how one really decides what is medically necessary when there are so many technological options.

> People are disappointed when they don't get the exact chair they
> want. They want the Cadillac models when they don't really, in our
> view, need the full Cadillac model. We always go back to the clini-
> cian ordering the wheelchair and ask them to justify it. Tell us why
> it's necessary. The Cadillac wheelchair may be a little more comfort-
> able at times, but it doesn't seem like they truly need it.

Appealing medical necessity denials can be daunting, time-consuming, and ultimately unsuccessful. "I will write a lengthy justification if a wheelchair prescription is denied," said the occupational therapist Greenhalgh, who has helped contest many denials. She often argues that the equipment will save money by preventing expensive complications. "If I persevere it really does pay off, but the process can extend for months. It means I have to spend a lot of time on the phone and paperwork rather than treating patients" (Karp 1999, 214).

Should New Technologies Be Covered?

New medical treatments and technologies appear constantly, each requiring approval for insurance coverage.[11] New mobility aids also must undergo this vetting process. One particularly exciting invention is Ibot, a novel gyroscope-guided wheeled technology that climbs stairs and raises riders to standing height. Ibot must first get Food and Drug Administration approval (as a safe and effective medical device) before Medicare will consider coverage. Ibot's developers might argue that, despite the hefty $25,000 price tag, their technology makes major structural renovations of homes unnecessary since the device climbs stairs (Samuels 2001). Such technologies may allow people to function independently in communities, preventing costly institutionalization. While these arguments have merit from a broad societal viewpoint, Medicare does not pay for home renovations or long-term institutionalization. Manufacturers are therefore asking Medicare to pay to achieve downstream savings that the program will not realize.

Medicare makes coverage decisions consistent with the program goals articulated in its regulations (chapter 13), including cost considerations:

> From the beginning of the Medicare program, one of the goals has been to provide a health insurance system that would make "the best of modern medicine" available to Medicare beneficiaries. Over the last 35 years, there have been significant advances in medical science that have changed the Medicare program and improved the health of beneficiaries . . .
>
> While the Congress has demonstrated a strong interest in providing access to necessary medical care for Medicare beneficiaries, the Congress has been equally concerned with ensuring that the Medicare program operates on a sound financial basis. . . . [The Social Security] Act requires that "no payment" may be made under Part A (hospital insurance) or Part B (supplementary medical insurance) for any expenses incurred for items or services that "are not reasonable and necessary for the diagnosis or treatment of illness or injury or to improve the functioning of a malformed body member." (HCFA 2000b, 31125–26)

Thus, the language surrounding coverage decisions for new technologies reflects Medicare's general focus on acute care and on "body members" rather than the entire person and daily functioning.[12]

In most instances insurers, like Medicare, seek objective, clinical, scientific evidence to make coverage decisions. A study comparing a technology like Ibot with standard power wheelchairs would be time-consuming and prohibitively expensive, and it would present numerous logistical and scientific challenges. Although Medicare aims eventually to add quality of life to these evaluations, methods for doing so remain unresolved (HCFA 2000b, 31127). In the end, how will Medicare decide whether the special capabilities of an Ibot-type or other novel mobility technology represent sufficient "added value" *for the Medicare program?* For individual beneficiaries, Medicare purchases power wheelchairs only after eliminating manual options. Given that, global Medicare-wide decisions to cover new mobility technologies face significant hurdles.

Mary Harroun, a geriatric psychologist, worked as a nursing home administrator for many years, where she witnessed patients strapped into wheelchairs, "screaming because the restraints were too tight" (personal communication, 15 January 1999). "There was nothing other than a standard clump-down-the-hall walker and a wheelchair for the elderly in nursing homes. I'm a mom. When my kids were babies, they got around in little jump chairs on wheels. That's where I got the design—that concept. I came up with the Merry Walker®. Anybody who can ambulate with assistance can benefit from the Merry Walker."

The Merry Walker has four wheels on a rectangular metal frame, entered through a front gate, with a seat at the rear. With other rolling walkers, users push the device and its seat in front of them; it requires some physical dexterity to pivot and sit down. Merry Walker users can sit right down, without having to twist their bodies: "The minute they feel like they're going to fall or they get tired, they just sit. If people go backwards, boom! That seat is right there." The Merry Walker costs about $500, slightly more than other high-end rolling walkers, with a narrower model for home use.

Mary Harroun believes that her Merry Walker restores people's dignity. "The most haunting incident I ever had with the Merry Walker was a man who was a Holocaust survivor. I was called to a nursing home to show them how to use the Merry Walker. They had this man with Parkinson's and some dementia, nonverbal, who was standing up while strapped in his wheelchair and carrying the wheelchair on his back. He was probably 5 ft. 2 in. tall—a little, tiny guy. He had the tattoo on his arm from the concentration camp. I got him in the Merry Walker, and he smiled as he walked down the hall. I thought, I did it! I freed him a second time. If I did nothing else for the whole rest of the world, I've done that."

But Ms. Harroun had trouble convincing Medicare to cover the Merry Walker, to see it as better (and therefore worth paying more for) than the standard walker. "There is no Medicare billing code that adequately describes the Merry Walker. They've been trying to clean up Medicare. A lot

of durable medical equipment was sold through Medicare that was not necessary. So they really tried to tighten that down." Maybe the Merry
Walker was caught in the fallout. "The woman in charge of Medicare's cod-
ing system and I have become almost related, we've spent so many hours
on the phone. I met in Washington with two of her co-workers, arranged
through my congressman. That's the only way I could get the appointment. I brought a Merry Walker and another walker with the seat in front,
to show the difference." A year later, Medicare assigned the Merry Walker
its billing code, E0144.

Paying for Repairs or Replacement

Obtaining a mobility aid is only the first step. After equipment is delivered,
people frequently require mechanical adjustments to match their new
technology to their bodies and mobility needs (especially with sophisticated power wheelchairs). Insurers often do not support follow-up fine
tuning; pressure ulcers or other complications can result from ill-fitting
chairs (Scherer 1996, 163). When equipment fails, people typically encounter many difficulties getting and paying for repairs. Medicare and
Medicaid pay for replacement equipment only every five years.

The attorney Andrew Batavia, who has high quadriplegia and uses a sophisticated power wheelchair, typically replaces his equipment every five
to six years when it wears out and starts breaking down. Every time, he
girds for a "kabuki dance" with his insurer, a preferred provider organization (PPO) of Blue Cross–Blue Shield of Florida. In the most recent
switch, he felt caught in a catch-22. The insurer was willing to pay for re-
pairing his old wheelchair but not for purchasing a new one. Furthermore,
his physician's office manager argued, "How are we to know if you really
need a new chair or if the current chair can still be fixed? If we were to
write the prescription, and you do not really need a new chair, we could be
subject to claims of health care fraud" (1999, 176). Finally, the office manager admitted, "Do you know how much this new wheelchair will cost?
About $24,000. We all end up paying for that. The company has a right to
decide whether a new chair is needed or whether the current chair can be
repaired" (179). Batavia reminded her that his 20 percent copayment made
him well aware of the cost.

> My initial theory about why my PPO refused to purchase the new
> chair related to economics. Although the PPO is willing to pay for
> repairs, the amount it authorizes for them is quite limited. More-
> over, none of the DME . . . preferred providers on its network in my
> area has the expertise to repair my wheelchair. Therefore, I must pay
> the difference between the amount charged by my wheelchair repair

person and the amount authorized by the PPO. Because I pay the majority of the repair bill, it is obviously in the interest of the PPO not to pay for a new chair. Its liability for ongoing repairs is relatively small compared with the large cost of a new chair. . . .

Which takes longer—ordering a wheelchair or having a baby? After I fought with the PPO for two more months, it finally approved purchase of the chair. Unfortunately, the PPO approved payment of only $16,000, about two-thirds of the chair's actual cost. (180–81)

Tired of battle, Batavia chose not to contest this decision.

People with progressive chronic conditions face an additional problem, since insurers typically pay for only one piece of equipment per enrollee's lifetime (or time with the insurance) or—as Medicare and Medicaid do—for one piece every five years. Therefore, if debilities are increasing, people must think ahead to their needs a year or two hence and purchase equipment anticipating the worst. This situation is also very difficult financially and psychologically, as the occupational therapists noted during their focus group. "If insurance buys a wheelchair, then they won't pay for a walker," said Gina. Remember that a good rolling walker can cost $400.

"Right. If they pay for a walker, they won't pay for a cane," Joanne agreed.

"You send someone home with a wheelchair," Gina continued. "You tell them, 'All right. You can work toward getting out of the wheelchair to a walker, but you're going to have to buy the walker. You can then work toward using a cane, but you're going to have to buy the cane.' You can only get one piece of equipment."

"You can't argue," said Sherrie, "because that's the rule. Rules is rules."

"I had a MS patient who realized that she needed something—she wasn't safe with her walker anymore," Myra remembered. "She wanted a scooter. But because of the progression of her disease, a scooter is not the answer. Medicaid is only going to pay for one mobility aid for the next five years, and she's not going to be in a scooter for the next five years. She's going to need an electric four-wheeled wheelchair before that. It was really tough to get her to accept that wheelchair rather than a scooter because that's looking long-term down the road. That was a really hard decision. We convinced her that she needed the electric wheelchair to be safe."

Doing the Paperwork

Sally Ann Jones didn't have trouble getting Medicare to purchase her scooter. By the time she applied, her MS had progressed significantly; with her doctor's prescription, the scooter approval process went smoothly. Mrs.

Jones believes that her training as a social worker helped: "It's being educated in how things work. I always have worked with people who are cowed by the system before they'd even try it. They say that it can't be done, and they're afraid to ask." Another scooter user with arthritis was less sanguine: "The problem was getting it through Medicaid. I don't know how much paperwork they sat on! My partner called them time after time after time because I'd get so angry. It took months and months."

Andrew Batavia believes "that the process for approval of a wheelchair acquisition is at best haphazard and at worst arbitrary. In either case, only the educated, sophisticated consumer is likely to succeed. Others will probably be worn down by the process, and many will simply give up. The cynical among us would argue that this is the purpose of the process" (1999, 182). The medical director of a large western health insurer finds that only certain people appeal denials: "Educated people clearly have more technical knowledge and are more assertive than the nontechnical folks. Being educated is a benefit in getting what you want." Successful contestants "document everything that goes on. They usually have others state their case— not necessarily a lawyer, but that's often who it is."

Dr. Johnny Baker was Erna Dodd's primary care physician and dreads the time consumed by applying for equipment and appealing denials. "When this sort of thing comes along, I immediately get hold of a social worker and ask for help," said Dr. Baker, who works in an academic practice with social workers readily available. "Then she bombards me with all the papers that have to make their way to me, so I'm somewhat insulated." Most physicians do not have such support staff. Winnie Dowd, a physical therapist, finds that sometimes physicians provide inadequate help. She recalled a recent patient:

> This person had a stroke and really has no use of her right side. She has a manual wheelchair, but she's getting overuse injuries in her left arm now. She would definitely benefit from an electric wheelchair, but she has Medicare managed care. This person doesn't have $10,000 to shell out for an electric wheelchair. Odds are she won't get it unless her physician and myself and everyone go to bat as hard as we can. That's not the case. The physician isn't trying hard enough. The vendor isn't going to do anything unless they know they'll get paid. Medicare may say this woman's in a gray area where she doesn't need the electric wheelchair for just household distances. It's extremely frustrating.

Sometimes insurers seem motivated by good intentions, although their decisions run contrary to requests. One midwestern medical director said that he generally refuses scooters and authorizes only four-wheeled power wheelchairs. "Four-wheeled power chairs are a little more expensive but they are safer. If I have any influence, I push for the four-wheel over the scooter. I've seen too many three-wheeler types that tipped too easily."

Walter Masterson had three wheelchairs, two manual and one power. "What has been your experience with your insurance company paying for your wheelchairs?" I asked him.

"I have no experience. Quite frankly, I haven't gone to them for payment."

"Why?"

"When it's time to do something, I'm interested in the result, not in the process. So I've tended to rush into things. If you're going to deal through the insurance company, you don't do it that way." He itemized his three wheelchairs, including one he rented for so long that "the vendor couldn't, in good conscience, charge me rent on it anymore. They gave me title to it."

"So you've spent out-of-pocket for everything."

"Yeah, I have. But I'm going to buy another motorized chair—I've got an estimate from the vendor. For this one, I'm going to the insurance company and say I've got to have this. I have a prescription from my doctor. I'm going to play the game on this one. The vendor told me that, at the most, my insurance will only cover $1,200 a year for equipment." Mr. Masterson named a prominent local private health insurer.

"Would $1,200 cover what you've spent on equipment each year or what the new chair will cost?"

"No, not even close." Fortunately, Mr. Masterson had money.

HOME MODIFICATIONS

Dr. Jody Farr's health insurance bought her scooter, charging a 20 percent copayment. "But then I needed to spend $5,000 to allow the scooter to go into my garage and get up the four steps into my house." Insurance didn't pay for that. Dr. Farr could afford it, but others cannot. They would have the scooter but be unable to use it.

Health insurance rarely pays for home renovations and other environmental changes, large and small, meant to improve mobility and enhance safety. Medicare, for example, views many mobility-related aids as "personal comfort items" and therefore not reimbursable. It refuses payment for grab bars, seeing them as a "self-help device, not primarily medical in nature," and for raised toilet seats, labeled a "convenience item; hygienic equipment, not primarily medical in nature" (Pope and Tarlov 1991, 228). Depending on the state, Medicaid may cover some such items. The most common home adaptations are installing grab bars or special railings, ramps, extrawide doors, and raised toilet seats. According to a 1990 federal survey, people themselves pay for almost 78 percent of home accessibility improvements (LaPlante, Hendershot, and Moss 1992, 9).

To the occupational therapists, such policies seem short-sighted. Treating people who fall will cost insurers much more than grab bars, shower chairs, and raised toilet seats. "I just had two grab bars installed for someone," reported Joanne. "That's $108. Not covered, no, never."

"People just can't afford it," said Jennifer. "They're ill; they're not working. They say, 'I can't ask my family to pay for something else like that! My family's already taking time off work to help me with my shopping.' "

"Medicare covers anything that's a necessity," said Joanne. "That's the bottom line. That's what's covered—a necessity."

"Well, isn't bathing a necessity?" asked Myra, incredulous that insurers do not pay for shower chairs.

"You don't have to take a shower to be clean," Joanne retorted. "That's their argument. You can sponge-bathe. The same thing if you can't sit on a toilet normally. They won't pay for raised toilet seats, but they'll pay for a commode."

"That's a study they should do," Gina observed dryly. "How many accidents happen in bathrooms."

Coverage decisions could become even more restrictive in the future. Although health-care costs leveled off during the mid 1990s, recent signs suggest rapid rises ahead. Combined with pressures from expensive new medical discoveries, future costs may tighten coverage on items outside the acute medical paradigm. Stan Jones (personal communication, 6 February 1998) believes "we're seeing a retrenchment with regard to buying wheelchairs and a variety of assistive devices and other services" that aim toward improving daily functioning and quality of life.

> Competition among health plans based on their premiums is causing more and more conservative decisions and making it harder and harder for people to get these services. Sometimes there're no criteria anywhere defining what's covered under what circumstances. Sometimes plans just don't offer it or keep it in the background, not offering it unless the person asks. And if they ask, sometimes it's hard to get, or it takes a long time, so most people give up.

Mr. Jones believes that society must decide whether funding mobility aids is a priority, "because we're heading away from covering them." Dr. Patrick O'Reilley runs a neighborhood health center where all his patients are poor. His comment perhaps sums things up:

I'd hate to say this—it may sound really stupid—but rich people can have whatever they want. Like Christopher Reeve has a great wheelchair because he's a professional person; he has money. No insurance company is going to pay for a scooter for some of my patients. But if I think about it for a second, it's kind of crazy. Why wouldn't they pay for a scooter for someone who needs it? A relatively rich patient would decide on their own. They'd be reading the back of *Arthritis Today* and say, "Oh, I want that scooter!" They'd just go out and buy it.

15 Final Thoughts

A father called me recently to ask advice about his daughter Julie. The father is a physician, retired from practice but still well connected and vigorous. Julie, in her mid forties, had quit working several years ago because of MS. Her disease exhausts her, leaving her virtually bedridden on bad days. Without respite, it waxes and wanes, bringing disheartening new symptoms and giving her little peace. Julie's walking, however, had been reasonably good until now.

Julie's father didn't ask about cures for MS or techniques to improve her walking. Through his medical connections, she has seen the best neurologists and clinical specialists. After many years and countless but ultimately ineffective therapies, he and she are realistic. Instead, he wanted advice about improving her mobility for daily life, and he didn't know who to ask. Despite their extensive medical network and knowledge, they had not found practical advice sensitive to Julie's changing mobility needs and preferences. She is married with young children and lives in a house with bedrooms upstairs. Julie knows she needs help, but she has put it off, perhaps discouraged or embarrassed, unsure about how mobility aids would fit into her daily routine. How can Julie find mobility strategies that really work for her? Cost is fortunately not an issue.

I had only scattered suggestions for Julie's father. After many years exploring this topic and, more importantly, using mobility aids, my inept reply unnerved me. I knew what I wanted to recommend—one-stop shopping for all mobility-related services—but only scattered pieces of it exist. Here's what a one-stop Mobility Mart could offer:

- physical and occupational therapists working together on-site, to evaluate clients' mobility needs and preferences, with home assessments as necessary

- physiatrists, either on-site or on call, who are readily available for specialized assessments or planning mobility strategies

- networks of peer counselors or opportunities for support groups (on-site or online) for people and their families, addressing emotional concerns and sharing strategies for dealing with practical problems caused by mobility difficulties

- health insurance or resource specialists, skilled in navigating the insurance maze and knowledgeable about other potential funding opportunities (such as disease advocacy or faith-based organizations) for financing mobility aids, related equipment, home modifications, and assistance with daily activities

- diverse mobility aids—canes, crutches, walkers, manual and power wheelchairs, and scooters—which clients can try on-site and take home for weeklong trial runs and with technicians to customize aids for individual needs

- information about specialized mobility aids, such as wheelchairs for the beach or sports, through catalogs and on-site computers with Internet linkages to vendors' web pages

- information about other useful items, ranging from grab bars and shower seats to clapper devices for turning on lights to lifeline support systems (an emergency response when signaled using a small device) to ramps and stair lifts

- ongoing mobility aid training, with at least one home visit, workplace assessment (if necessary), and neighborhood tour to identify environmental barriers and devise strategies to improve daily movement

- information about community resources, ranging from instructions for getting handicapped parking placards and qualifying for local paratransit systems to information about accessible housing and transportation, legal advice around disability issues, shops with scooters, accessibility of local recreational and entertainment sites, and automobile dealers that adapt cars

- guides to local health-care providers and facilities, highlighting accessibility (such as automatically adjustable examination tables and X ray equipment, ease of navigating the office, parking), experience with persons with mobility problems, and satisfaction of prior patients

- a computerized record-keeping system, confidentially retaining not only contact information about clients but also their mobility needs and preferences, linked with e-mail or telephone systems for clients to submit questions and receive updates about new products or services as they wish
- information about community-based action and advocacy groups, enlisting diverse voices to improve physical access for everybody

This Mobility Mart would customize solutions to improve daily functioning and quality of life. Since the preponderance of clients have *progressive* chronic conditions, they would return to the Mobility Mart over time as their needs changed. When clients moved to new mobility equipment, they would return used items for credit, making recycled mobility aids available to others at lower costs. This Mobility Mart would serve clients regardless of their means, rich and poor. Located on accessible public transportation routes, it would have a spacious parking lot, with a free valet service so clients could be dropped off at the door. Although it would devise solutions for *individuals,* the Mobility Mart's universal design philosophy would advocate communitywide access for all.

This Mobility Mart is a daydream. Skeptics could reasonably ask, who would pay for it? Current public and private health insurance may reimburse selected items and services but not the entire package. It reaches outside health care, into housing, transportation, and other areas. But potentially millions of people, like Julie, would benefit greatly from a Mobility Mart. Today, for whatever reason, many persons whose walking fails live in needlessly difficult and constricted circumstances because of inadequate mobility-related services and equipment, as well as persisting environmental barriers.

WHAT IS BETTER

Despite this, some things have definitely improved. First, although few cures exist, significant strides have advanced therapies for certain chronic disorders, reducing their severity and effects on physical functioning and quality of life. Some may even save society money. For the millions with arthritis, for example, "total joint replacement emerges as a medical miracle of the late twentieth century," yielding substantial pain relief and improving function in over 90 percent of people with osteoarthritis and other hip problems. Despite costs per surgery of $25,000, representing $12 billion per year in the United States, joint replacement surgery saves money, considering the costs of assisting people disabled by arthritis with their daily activities (Katz 2001, 203).

People—at least those with health insurance—generally can choose whether to have expensive interventions like joint replacements. Public and private health insurers cover these costs, asking relatively few questions. Although rates of these procedures have grown, many people, like Mike Campbell, delay surgery as long as possible. Even among those with serious arthritis, less than 15 percent of people are willing to undergo joint replacement (Hawker et al. 2001, 212).[1] African American and Hispanic persons receive hip and knee replacements at half the rate as whites (Katz 2001, 205). Exactly why is unclear. Multiple factors probably contribute, including differences in access to care and personal preferences. In general, however, access to such major surgeries is certainly better in the United States than in some other countries.

Second, research in rehabilitation and physical and occupational therapy is progressing, yielding better understanding of how the brain and body interact to produce voluntary movement. Although more research is needed, especially on the benefits of conventional rehabilitation approaches, new discoveries could improve people's physical functional abilities even after severely debilitating conditions, like strokes. People themselves, like Jimmy Howard with his exercycle, have independently discovered the benefits of exercise. Across the general population, however, the fraction of people achieving recommended levels of physical activity remained unchanged from 1990 to 1998, at around 25 percent (Centers for Disease Control 2001a). Inadequate exercise combined with high rates of obesity (about 30 percent of people with mobility difficulties) are important public health targets for the next decade.

Third, diverse new mobility-related technologies offer creative options for satisfying daily demands and meeting specialized needs (e.g., for sports and recreation). Making lighter and more reliable batteries for power wheelchairs remains an important research goal, as does refining equipment's ability to surmount curbs, traverse uneven terrain, and avoid tipping. Computerized gyroscope techniques, like the revolutionary Ibot (chapter 14), offer tremendous potential for wheelchair users. For persons who can stand, the Segway Human Transporter, from Ibot's inventor, also employs gyroscope technology to carry users erect on tiny platforms, potentially transforming people's daily travels (Harmon 2001). From low- to high-tech, other gadgets and equipment can ease daily strains. As Cynthia Walker said, many useful devices are out there: the challenge is finding them.

Fourth, federal and state laws, like the ADA, have increased access and accommodation of people with impaired mobility in public spaces, transit systems, and workplaces. The universal design movement recognizes that many adaptations for people with disabilities help everybody, making sense from ergonomic to business perspectives. Although newly built public places are not always *welcoming* to wheelchair users, at least they are now generally reasonably accessible. As Eleanor Peters stated, "The money that's spent doesn't just help people with disabilities. Those curb cuts are not used only by wheelchairs. Everybody uses them—people with their baby carriages, bike riders, joggers, everybody."

Finally, the vast majority of people with mobility difficulties will not retreat into isolation. They shop, attend church, go to work or school, eat in restaurants, see movies, visit amusement parks, and make as few concessions to their mobility problems as possible. If treated by strangers with disrespect, they respond, generally by trying to educate. Although interviewees may not feel part of a larger "disability community," people recognize the victories and visibility of others with mobility difficulties. Everybody knows we have come a long way since Franklin Delano Roosevelt hid his wheelchair from public view.

WHAT IS UNCHANGED

In troubling ways, however, many things remain unchanged. People reporting mobility difficulties are more likely than others to be poor, uneducated, unemployed, and to live alone, despite their limitations in performing daily activities. Many have difficulties getting into their homes and navigating their neighborhoods. Walter Masterson, who had traveled extensively for business, observed,

> There are other countries that are far, far ahead of us in improving access. Maybe they don't do old streets real well, but they do houses a lot better—anyplace in Scandinavia, Germany, Netherlands. These people have thought it through. For example, I went into a toilet in either Frankfort or Amsterdam Airport. The toilet had a pulley system that could have lifted a car! There were five or six different ways you could use it depending on your condition when you encountered it. It was just there in a public restroom, and its only purpose was to get whoever needed it onto the toilet. Somebody had said, "Okay, we're going to build a toilet. Right. Here's all the people who have to use it." And so they built one that had a facility for all those people. They just did it. I've never seen a mechanism like that anywhere in the States for any purpose.

Mobility-related health-care policies also appear frozen in place, almost without change in nearly forty years. As with alms distribution in fourteenth-century Europe, these policies seemingly assume that people strive to bilk the system for private gain. Certainly, some "malingerers" use wheelchairs when they can really walk. Unscrupulous wheelchair vendors sometimes prey on people who cannot effectively use their items or services but can't say no. Nonetheless, the overwhelming majority of people see walking as more convenient than wheeled mobility. This practical reality, compounded by strong internal and societal pressures, suggests that relatively few people seek mobility aids unless they actually need them. The system is carefully structured to prevent abuses that people with mobility difficulties probably rarely commit, but it carries the unfortunate consequence of impeding or denying valid needs.[2]

Although insurers' "medical necessity" provisions try to draw bright lines between "medical" and other needs—paying only for services deemed medically necessary—boundaries often blur. Policies to ensure strict separations can save money, an important goal. But viewed systemwide, these policies don't make sense. Take someone like Jimmy Howard, in his late forties with a high school education. He was fired from his job because arthritis and foot problems prevented him from lifting heavy boxes, but he could do nonmanual work, especially with a power wheelchair to get around quickly and efficiently (arthritis in his hands and elbows makes manual wheelchairs infeasible). Jimmy has qualified for SSDI, but Social Security does not pay for assistive technologies, like a power wheelchair that could return him to "substantial gainful activity." Jimmy cannot afford a power wheelchair on his own.

Two years after receiving his first cash benefits, Jimmy will receive Medicare. He could then apply for a power wheelchair through Medicare but would almost certainly be denied: he does not need it at home, where he still navigates with his cane. So Jimmy draws dollars from Social Security and Medicare and neither contributes taxes nor builds his retirement pension. He is happy, home with his wife who also doesn't work: "Arthritis has put a hindrance on my life, but it hasn't stopped my life. I figure, as long as God can bless me to get up and see another day, hey, I'm ready to go." While Jimmy's strong faith assures him his basic needs will be met, sometimes he and his wife run short of money for private health insurance until Medicare kicks in. Jimmy presumably could live decades longer and, if employed, could perhaps improve both his financial standing and sense of contributing. He had worked ever since his hands were big enough to hold a snow shovel.

Jimmy Howard's story highlights several policy paradoxes. Although Social Security pays disability income, it does not cover assistive technology to permit work.[3] With Medicare coverage withheld until two years after SSDI cash flows, some people might delay needed medical services, worsening their functioning and possibly overall health (remember that, to qualify for SSDI, people must have medically documented disorders that will last at least twelve months). Finally, Medicare pays for power wheelchairs only if people must use them within their homes—not outside, where they might return to work and leave SSDI. Somebody like Jimmy Howard would not need highly sophisticated equipment. Perhaps a scooter with a basket would work well for him. Its cost, roughly $2,000 to $5,000, is relatively small.

Of course, $2,000 to $5,000 is not the total cost. Jimmy Howard would need to adapt his house, at a minimum installing a ramp or constructing a spot in his garage to recharge the batteries. He might need a new car with a large trunk and an automatic lift. Medicare would not reimburse either expense. A physician recently asked my advice about his patient Mrs. Abbott. Both her legs were amputated because of severe peripheral vascular disease, and she is too weak to propel herself in a manual wheelchair. Without question, her private health insurer paid for a power wheelchair, and she happily acquired her new wheels. Having anticipated being freed, however, Mrs. Abbott now felt stuck. Her elderly husband cannot put the wheelchair into their car, so she can't take it anywhere. Insurance refused to pay the $1,900 for an automatic car lift, which she and her husband can't afford. Without other options, Mrs. Abbott's family have pitched in and are buying the car lift on installment.

Even though these costs add up, they nevertheless fall far short of Jimmy Howard's income support or payment for people to run the errands Mrs. Abbott now does for herself. "Penny wise and pound foolish" aptly sums up some insurance policies, such as Medicare's refusal to pay for grab bars in bathrooms or shower seats—low-cost strategies for preventing expensive and life-threatening falls. Numerous contradictory policies include the following:

- reimbursement only for restorative physical therapy, not therapy to maintain function or prevent its decline

- limited coverage of mobility aids by private, employment-based health insurance (for which employers choose insurance benefits packages that should—in theory—restore mobility so that able employees could return to work and maximum productivity)

- payment for mobility aids but not for the training to show people how to use them daily in their homes and communities

- no allowance for trial runs with mobility aids to see if they are helpful (people generally abandon incompatible devices, rarely recycling them to someone who could really benefit)

- payment for only one assistive technology in a lifetime or over long periods, so people must get equipment anticipating future needs rather than devices appropriate to their current functioning

- no allowance for what are seen as expensive "extras," like special wheelchair cushions to prevent decubitus ulcers, but reimbursement for surgical treatment when ulcers occur

- withdrawal of coverage for home-health services when people get wheelchairs and leave home independently, without considerable and taxing effort

Policy analysts speak of "the woodwork effect"—once new benefits become available, untold numbers emerge from the woodwork, seeking the service. Predicting demand for services when policies change is therefore difficult. If, for example, insurers suddenly relax their policies and purchase power wheelchairs, how many requests would arise?

The answer is unclear. Currently, about 1.1 million adults use manual wheelchairs, about 109,400 use power wheelchairs, and 114,600 use scooters and expect to do so more than a year.[4] If one-fifth wanted to replace or upgrade their equipment—assuming an average wheelchair has a life span of five years—this translates into roughly 265,000 new equipment purchases per year. Among people reporting major mobility difficulties, almost 80 percent (an estimated 4.6 million adults) do not currently use wheeled mobility aids. Who knows how many of them would benefit from manual or power wheelchairs? If 10 percent, this translates into roughly 458,500 people; if 5 percent, approximately 229,200 people. With wheelchairs costing from about $1,500 to over $35,000 for the most technologically sophisticated models, potential costs are substantial, especially for the *one-time* expense of meeting unfilled needs.[5] Balanced against this outlay, however, are costs of daily personal care, lost work opportunities, mental health expenses, and treatment for injuries, not to mention improved quality of life and relief of family caregivers.

Additional costs are inevitable, especially for home modifications. Among people with major mobility problems, 11 percent say they need railings at home but do not have them, while just over 13 percent need bathroom modifications, 5 percent need kitchen modifications or automatic or easy-to-open doors, and around 4 percent need stair lifts or elevators, alerting devices, or accessible parking.[6] Counterbalancing the expense of these modifications are costs of building and moving people to new accessible housing and the medical and personal costs of injuries from falls. Quality of life should improve, but that's hard to quantify in dollars.

FINDING INFORMATION ON MEETING MOBILITY NEEDS

Julie's father and Mrs. Abbott's doctor didn't know who to ask for advice, so they turned to me. Appendix 2 suggests selected resources. I e-mailed Julie Internet addresses of prominent wheelchair manufacturers so she could study their offerings. Nowadays, hundreds of Internet sites relate to disability in general, with many specific to impaired mobility and pertinent diseases. If people do not have a Mobility Mart nearby, at least they can browse the Internet without leaving their homes. Gerald Bernadine found not only his bright red scooter on the Internet, but also the automatic scooter lift for his station wagon.

Wheelchair manufacturers offer Internet sites, as do vendors of various products, including adapted cars and vans, clothing for wheelchair users, travel agents for accessible vacations, and advocacy groups targeting specific conditions. Because mobility is an intensely physical experience, however, the virtual reality of the Internet only goes so far. Mr. Bernadine did not try his scooter before buying it; he had scoured the web and knew what he wanted. Most people need to examine potential purchases in person— sit in the chair, use the cane or walker, see how it feels and maneuvers.[7] The "information divide," separating the "haves" and "have nots" of Internet access, raises a new barrier. Entering the Internet and navigating it successfully may be especially hard for people who are poor and uneducated, as are many with mobility difficulties.[8]

Within communities, many new services, often catering to working people with busy lifestyles, make daily existence easier. Grocery stores, pharmacies, restaurants, and dry cleaners sometimes make home deliveries, albeit for a price. Catalog vendors and television shopping networks provide innumerable products, without people ever leaving their homes.

Perhaps the hardest need to fill is assistance with routine daily tasks. When family members can't help, who does? People are often unwilling to accept or request help for basic activities they have always performed for themselves. Almost 25 percent of people reporting major mobility difficulties say they need assistance with daily activities but have not tried hiring help, with up to 20 percent of these saying they don't want a stranger's aid (Table 18).[9] Among those not seeking help, 50 to 70 percent of those with

TABLE 18. People with Major Mobility Difficulties
Getting Help with Daily Activities

Need and Reason Not Met	(%)
Person needs help but hasn't tried to hire any	24
If person hasn't tried to get help, why not?	
Doesn't want a stranger for helper	16
Help is too expensive, can't afford it	47
Isn't sick enough to get help from agency	15
Income is too high to get help from agency	5
Type of help needed is probably not available	8
Doesn't know where to look for help	25
Is too sick to look for help	4

all levels of mobility difficulty say help is too expensive, and 25 percent report they do not know where to look.

As elsewhere in health care nowadays, people often must become their own advocates. Most doctors know little about mobility-related equipment and services, and even physical and occupational therapists may not appreciate the full menu of options. Sometimes social workers help, but Barbara Forrest wants a "daily living advocate—a worker that makes sure that you get all the services that you can, looks into things for you, like somebody to help with the shopping. There are a lot of programs out there, but they all have requirements. How do you know whether you'd get the service?" Advocate and ombuds programs have sprung up, especially to help elderly people with multiple health problems navigate the health insurance maze. For elderly persons, as well as for people with mobility problems, such advocates must reach beyond health care to other service sectors, including housing and transportation. Still, people like Barbara Forrest wonder why finding resources must be so complicated.

THE "BOOMERS" ARE COMING

With a wry smile, a colleague in his early fifties said that he was glad he'd had a bad back during much of his forties—it had prevented the vigorous exercise that puts so much wear and tear on knees. Now that his back is better, he is playing tennis and running while many contemporaries are having knee surgery, spending months in postoperative physical therapy. He anticipates that his knees too will give out—it's just a matter of time.

Predictions about how many people will have mobility difficulties in the decades ahead depend on several assumptions, most importantly whether patterns of diseases and treatments will change. If the prevalence of major chronic conditions remains unchanged, by the year 2049, the number of older Americans with functional limitations will rise by at least 311 percent (Boult et al. 1996, 1391).[10] Arthritis, which affects roughly 55 percent of elderly people, will cause more physical impairments than ischemic heart disease, cancer, and dementia, combined. By 2020, the number of people with arthritis will grow to sixty million, with twelve million having activity limitations (Centers for Disease Control 2001b, 334). Reducing fatal conditions like coronary heart disease and cancer could paradoxically increase the number of older persons with limited function—with many more people living into very old age, impairments will arrive after age ninety or even one hundred, following additional decades of vigorous life.

New generations of older persons will differ from their forbears. Sally Ann Jones feels that government officials have missed the obvious:

> It amazes me that nobody's gotten this notion yet: the "boomers" are coming. Despite MS and other diseases, they're going to live longer. We're not going to warehouse them in nursing homes. These "boomers" simply won't do that. They're not going to go quietly into the night.

Certainly, some may seek quiet solitude, at least for a time. An acquaintance in her early fifties recently underwent foot surgery for a bone spur, and beforehand she bought a cache of novels, relishing the notion of being laid up for a week or two, unable to get to work. When I teasingly suggested that she could rent a scooter to get into work, she was momentarily disconcerted but soon regained her composure. No, she would never think of that! Yes, she understood my point, but she looked forward to the socially acceptable postoperative respite. Afterward, she reported having enjoyed her novels and quiet time, although the scooter suggestion had made her think. One morning, on returning to work, she noticed that the elevators were broken at the South Station train stop. She could walk down the stairs to catch her subway, but what about someone using a wheelchair?

Although the 10 percent of adults reporting mobility difficulties remains a minority, it is a large minority—a group anyone can join at any time and which many will in the future. The good news is that ways to restore mobility exist, even in a mechanized form. The bad news is that the elevators at subway stations often don't work—the quintessential symbol of needless societal barriers. For many, health and other policies, public and private, still impede their way. In the future, I hope that members of my rolling focus group won't have to ask my advice—that they'll already know how to get what they need. Instead, they'll share stories about what they've seen and done.

"Why a red scooter?" I asked Gerald Bernadine when he finally paused, after zipping around his office suite. His boss had already jokingly suggested he affix a cowcatcher to the front of his scooter to scoop up wayward pedestrians. Exhaustion had enveloped Gerald at our first encounter: now he was a man transformed. He answered me with an impish grin.

"The exhilaration of speed. I feel the need for speed. That's why I got red. I've always wanted a red car with racing stripes. The scooter's like a Ferrari, you know," Gerald laughed. "To me it is. It has opened up a whole new vista for me." Yes, gravity does sometimes slow us down. But on wheels, we can also move fast and free.

Familiar Interviewees

All fifty-six interviewees with mobility difficulties said important and memorable things. I quote almost everybody at least once somewhere in this book. Yet I cite some people much more than others, and they become familiar voices, recurring across chapters. Here, I intersperse additional descriptions of several key interviewees with shorter sketches of others I frequently quote, listing them alphabetically but changing small details about their lives to protect their anonymity.

Arnis Balodis

Early sixties; white; never married; high-school education; retired from diverse jobs, including security guard; low income; amputations below the knees of both legs because of diabetes-related gangrene; walked with one or two canes. Several years after our interview, Arnis died suddenly from a heart problem, shortly after his mother's death.

Gerald Bernadine

Mr. Bernadine is in his late fifties and white, with a graduate degree in business. He had worked as the manager of a law practice before being fired from his job in the early 1990s after being diagnosed with MS. His wife works and their income is good; they live in a comfortable Boston suburb. Mr. Bernadine worries about the demands his debility has put on his wife. After losing his job, he taught part-time at a local university, where I went for both of our interviews. A slight man with curling wisps of white hair, Mr. Bernadine has a gentle demeanor and ironic sense of humor. He is deeply religious and feels that his MS has been, in many ways, a blessing.

I telephoned Mr. Bernadine recently to see how he is doing. His MS is progressing, and he now needs a brace for both legs (previously, he used only one brace). Learning to walk with the second brace has been slow and daunting. With the new brace, Mr. Bernadine can no longer operate his car with foot pedals, so he has installed hand controls—also something to learn. He still loves his bright red scooter, which had become encrusted with tree pollen from his springtime walks. "I don't know where I'd be without it," he said. "I go everywhere in my little scooter." Mr. Bernadine was planning to hire a neighborhood boy to give his scooter a wash and a shine.

Mike Campbell

Mid sixties; white; married to Betty, with several grown children and grandchildren; high-school education; retired from building maintenance; low income; arthritis from degenerative joint disease, had each knee replaced; used cane when in pain. Died about two years after the interview from pneumonia.

Lonnie Carter

Mrs. Carter was in her late forties and African American. Long-standing diabetes mellitus had made her almost blind and forced amputation of all five toes on one foot and three on the other; and she had had bilateral congenital hip displacements requiring surgical repair. Mrs. Carter died about six months after our interview.

Despite her significant illnesses, Mrs. Carter had a vital presence. We met in the clinic. When I went to find her, she was sitting in a chair in the lobby, her manual wheelchair by her side, its seat loaded with parcels. Mrs. Carter walked slowly pushing her wheelchair, refusing our offer to push her. During the interview, Lonnie didn't want to sit in her wheelchair—no surprise! It looked cheap and uncomfortable, befitting its bargain-basement price. One of Lonnie's eyes bore the opalescent blue of blindness behind thick glasses, but we maintained eye contact during the entire interview, she fixing me somewhat skeptically with her remaining eye. Most of her teeth were missing, and her hair had receded like a man's, the remainder a grizzled gray. She wore round-toed, clay-colored orthopedic shoes, her legs encased in gray support hose.

Mrs. Carter had a lot to say. She had completed two years of college and remained in school. She also worked part-time in various jobs, including as an advocate for minorities with disabilities. Despite that, she was poor, widowed, lived alone in a low-income housing complex, and received Medicaid health insurance. Mrs. Carter experienced the most blatant outright hostility reported by any interviewee, attributing this abuse to her disability. Teenage boys in her housing project taunted her, saying she shouldn't go out. Adult neighbors spoke discriminatory and hateful words. Lonnie dished it right back, for example, making a "citizen's arrest" of someone blocking a curb cut with their car and verbally contesting the teenage boys. Although Lonnie spoke at length, at the outset talking for twenty minutes without pause, I also sensed wariness.

Fred Daigle

Early sixties; white; married to Martha, with several grown children; seventh-grade education; retired from job as painter and handyman; low income; severe chronic lung disease related to asbestos exposure and smoking, heart disease; required supplemental oxygen; walked slowly short distances in home without assistance. Probably died soon after the interview.

Tina DiNatale

Mrs. DiNatale is in her mid forties, white, and of Italian descent—as she noted repeatedly. She had had MS for twenty years. We met on a hot, sunny afternoon at her modest one-story clapboard house in a middle-class town outside Boston. A small swimming pool shimmered in a fenced enclosure outside sliding doors along a kitchen wall. Tina was darkly tanned and dressed entirely in black (long-sleeved India cotton top, flowing pants), wearing black thong sandals with a slight heel. Her husband, Joe, a big, muscular man of the strong silent type, seemed anxious to slip out the door—he was working an early evening shift.

We talked in an open area with a circular table and rolling chairs adjacent to the kitchen. Mrs. DiNatale had designed the kitchen in a U-shape so that she wouldn't have far to walk to perform any task. She keeps a padded bar stool on the inner circumference of the U-shaped counter where she presides over meals; Joe calls her stool "control central." The kitchen was meticulously clean, with only a plate of fudge and another of cookies—offerings to her guests—on the shining countertop.

Tina got around her house by grabbing everything in sight and running her hands along the wall at shoulder height (chapter 11). Although Mrs. DiNatale has a college degree, she has not worked for almost twenty years, and she and Joe decided not to have children. She was frustrated with her experiences with Mass Rehab, exploring retraining to find a suitable job. She felt that they treated her very poorly: "Just because I had a college degree, I got nothing. Nothing. They were not helpful."

Mrs. DiNatale therefore spends much of her time alone at home, although she still drives short distances, occasionally seeing family and volunteering at her church. She searches the Internet and keeps abreast of current events but sometimes feels isolated. For our conversation, she had prepared a written list of talking points about her experiences and opinions on mobility problems. Mrs. DiNatale was searching for a doctor who suited her desires (someone who would listen to her concerns, respect her viewpoint, watch her walk, and not seem rushed) and for the perfect lightweight wheelchair. When I contacted her by e-mail about two years after our interview, she said she was doing about the same.

Erna Dodd

Mid fifties; black; several grown children, raising two grandchildren; fifth-grade education; retired from housekeeping jobs; low income; emphysema, diabetes requiring insulin, congestive heart failure, seizures, obesity, and arthritis from degenerative joint disease; used walker holding oxygen canister and sometimes used manual wheelchair. Died at home within a year of the interview, probably from lung failure.

Barney Fink

Early sixties; married to Rachel, with several grown children; graduate degree; retired from optometry practice; middle income; Parkinson's disease; no mobility aids but walks slowly. Several years after the interview, doing about the same.

Lester Goodall

Mr. Goodall is a black man in his mid fifties, with a long history of diabetes requiring insulin. Diagnosed with MS six years ago, he now uses a cane. He is married, has two teenage daughters, and works as a mid-level manager in a Fortune 500 company. He lives in suburban Boston but wants to move back into the city, to a nice urban neighborhood.

We met at Mr. Goodall's office in downtown Boston. Although I addressed him as Mr. Goodall, he immediately called me "Lisa," setting an affable, personal tone for the interview. He is an experienced focus group attendee, frequenting events at a marketing research firm down the street (recently evaluating a new sandwich—turkey with cranberry sauce). He is handsome, tall, and trim, with wavy dark hair graying slightly at the temples. He spoke confidently, with good humor. He became most impassioned in discussing today's low standards on television, which, in his view, should be family-friendly. Yet Mr. Goodall repeatedly mentioned his age (he is about fifteen years older than his wife) and his fears of burdening her. He frequently searches the Internet, looking for advances in treating MS. At the follow-up focus group, about eighteen months after our initial interview, his walking had worsened slightly.

Esther Halpern

Mid seventies; white; married to Harry, with one grown daughter; completed college; retired flute teacher; middle income; spinal stenosis (back problem); uses a four-wheeled rolling walker.

Mattie Harris

Ms. Harris is a black woman in her late forties with arthritis of her knees and hands and severe back pain. When we met at my office, she wore a plush purple pants suit, and her face was carefully made up, her hair arrayed in dozens of braids lengthened by hair extenders. Ms. Harris plunged into the interview with little introduction. She is in pain; she has issues; and she wanted to talk about them. She wasn't antagonistic—just emphatic and sure of the realities of her experiences.

Ms. Harris had earned her high-school equivalency diploma and had worked in a department store stockroom. But she left the job because of painful arthritis in her hands and is now unemployed and low income, receiving Medicaid. She lives in a first-floor apartment in a crowded working-class town near Boston. Ms. Harris works hard as a divorced single mother raising children: she had seven children living with her, two of them her biological children, and her older children come round to help care for the younger ones. Ms. Harris considers all these children as her own, treating this responsibility as central to her life. Even in this, racial issues surface. A Portuguese girl had recently left her care after three years. "Her family didn't like black people," said Ms. Harris, "but the girl loved me because I was the only one in her life that'd been a mother to her. She called me Ma. Her family told her, 'What you calling that black woman Ma for?' It was hard on her, and she left." Ms. Harris mourns her loss, knowing the girl now wanders the streets.

I recently asked Ms. Harris's doctor how she is doing, and he shook his head sadly. Her pain remains unrelieved (chapter 8).

Jimmy Howard

Mr. Howard is a black man in his late forties with arthritis. He has a high-school education and had done heavy lifting in ManuCo's warehouse for years before being fired (chapter 7). He and his wife never had children although he loves kids. His wife also doesn't work, and they therefore have little income, often worrying about whether they can afford essentials, like COBRA health insurance payments. The Howards live in a two-family home: they are downstairs, his mother-in-law upstairs. His mother-in-law spends much of her time lying on her sofa saying she cannot walk, asking her daughter, Mr. Howard's wife, to do all her chores. This aggravates Mr. Howard. "It's all in her mind," he claimed. "She can walk. She can walk great. Well, sir, she's got that old mentality, that if she don't want to do it, she doesn't do it!"

Nevertheless, Mr. Howard has an infectious laugh and a strong religious faith that carries him through dark moments. When we met at the clinic, he seemed completely at ease, unrushed, willing to answer any and all questions. He is a tall man, big all around, lumbering with a slow, knock-kneed gait in high-topped athletic shoes as he leaned on his "assistant," an aluminum cane. Mr. Howard wore heavy gold chains around his neck and several large rings on each hand; his hair, brushed out against its natural curl, hung several inches below his red baseball cap, and his round face was creased with smiles.

He repeatedly mentioned that his belief in God gets him through, but he hasn't always felt that way. Although he had been brought up in the church, as a young man, Mr. Howard "got rebellious. You sleep Sunday. You ain't got time to go to church. You ain't got time to give praise to the Lord." He and his wife started reading their Bible when their finances were especially bleak and everything seemed to be going awry: "We put God back in our lives. Everything just fell right back into place." Despite his arthritis pain and shaky finances, Mr. Howard feels that all will be well "as long as God can bless me to get up and see another day."

Mr. Howard's primary care doctor recently told me he now has severe wrist pain, perhaps from carpal tunnel syndrome, undoubtedly making it harder for him to lean on his "assistant." In addition, his diabetes is causing problems, especially with his feet. Mr. Howard frequently visits his podiatrist to treat the foot ulcers that could progress to gangrene and even amputation.

Myrtle Johnson

Early seventies; white; married with many children and grandchildren; several years of college; diverse jobs (e.g., in retail, housing rentals); low income; still attending school and volunteering at a local advocacy agency; arthritis from degenerative joint disease in both knees; using four-point cane, which she hopes to discard following knee replacement surgery. Doing about the same two years after the interview, although her husband's health was poor.

Sally Ann Jones

Mid fifties; white; widowed with two grown sons and grandchildren; master's degree in social work; retired social worker; middle income; MS for over three decades; uses scooter. Being unable to stand and pivot, Mrs. Jones is exploring technologies to lift her onto the toilet independently, since finding personal assistance is so difficult.

Walter Masterson

When I called Mr. Masterson a few years ago to schedule a meeting, he said it would have to wait: he and his wife, Nancy, were taking a cruise to a warm place. He thought the time was fast approaching when he would need a ventilator to help him breathe, and so he and Nancy tried to find opportunities to enjoy themselves. When Ron finally drove me to the Mastersons' house, the snow from the previous weekend had melted away in the early spring sunshine, and one had the exhilarating feeling that winter might actually end. They lived on a secluded hill west of Boston, with bare rock outcroppings bordering towering yet leafless trees. We entered the house through a lower level, steep narrow stairs leading up to the living quarters. I rode a chair lift to a sunny kitchen.

Mr. Masterson, a white man in his late fifties with silvering hair and a closely trimmed beard, had certainly been tall and attractive, in control of situations. When we met, he appeared ashen, thin and gaunt, seated in his wheelchair. Below baggy comfortable clothes, his body seemed emaciated from the progressive ALS. Nevertheless, he retained firm control of what he offered intellectually, his mind sharp and astute. He spoke well, periodically challenging me with reasoned arguments. But he was beginning to lose control of his voice—it had a gruffer edge than previously. Becoming unable to communicate was his greatest fear. Nancy left us alone for the interview. She was much younger and his second wife; they had no children. The house was filled with Nancy's artwork, crafted in a studio on an upper floor he had not visited in a long time.

Mr. Masterson spoke openly about the inevitability of death from ALS. He had told his primary care physician, Dr. Burton, that he would no longer want to live when he became ventilator-dependent. After the interview, I periodically asked Dr. Burton how Mr. Masterson was doing. He had soon moved to the ventilator and found it manageable, no longer wanting to die. He could communicate through various devices operated by his hands, then his eyes. Yet as his disease progressed—his mind still active but his body shutting down, as happens in ALS—Mr. Masterson thought more concretely about the moment of his death. Dr. Burton would, at his request, turn off his ventilator and, appropriately medicated for comfort, he would slip away. Almost three years after our interview, he decided it was time. With a hospice nurse in attendance, Dr. Burton went to the Mastersons' home to do as his patient wished. Nancy climbed into bed with her husband for the last time, the house hushed except for the soft sounds of Mozart. A few hours after Dr. Burton turned off the ventilator, Walter Masterson died.

Tom Norton

Early seventies; white; married to Nelda, with many grown children and grandchildren; some college; retired business executive; high income; motor neuron disease (neurologic condition causing weakness in foot and leg); uses cane.

Eleanor Peters*

Mid forties; black; several grandchildren; master's degree; works for state vocational rehabilitation agency; polio as child; uses power wheelchair. Several years after the interview, she's doing about the same.

Boris Petrov

Mid forties; white, divorced, has girlfriend; surgeon in former Soviet Union but can no longer operate; volunteers helping other Russian immigrants; low income; thromboangiitis obliterans causing multiple amputations; uses power wheelchair. Several years after the interview, Dr. Petrov's primary care physician says he is doing "great," exercising daily at a community center.

Stella Richards

Mid sixties; black; widowed, with one grown daughter; some college; retired accountant; middle income; spondylolisthesis (back problem); uses walker. Several years later, she's still in pain and using a walker.

Candy Stoops

Late thirties; married with one young son; some college; retired administrative assistant; upper-middle income; myasthenia gravis; does not use mobility aids but has "slow days."

Brianna Vicks

Mid forties; black; divorced, with several grown children; high-school education; retired as nurse's aid but taking vocational education classes in computer skills; recurring benign spinal tumors; uses power wheelchair. Several years later, she's attending school half-time and working as an administrative assistant half-time.

Cynthia Walker*

Mid thirties; white; married, with several young children; completed college; runs day care in home; arthritis (rheumatoid); periodically uses crutches.

Joe Warren

Early forties; white; divorced with two small children; high-school education; had worked in computers until accident; low income; had scoliosis, curvature of the spine, as a young adult; now is disabled by partial spinal cord injury from a car accident; has been unemployed since then and suffering from pain and pressure ulcers; uses manual wheelchair.

*These persons participated only in focus groups, while all others had individual interviews (from which I collected more biographical information than during focus groups).

Selected Resources

This appendix suggests sources people can contact to obtain information about function-related services, assistive technologies, laws and public policies concerning disability in general, and other selected topics. The list is not exhaustive, and the contact information is current as of July 2002. I grouped resources into four broad categories: health care professionals and providers; federal agencies and national organizations; links to information on the Internet; and state assistive technology projects. Other useful information emerges continually, especially through disease-specific organizations and the Internet. Appearance on this list does not imply an endorsement of specific organizations. Each person seeking information will have his or her own specific needs, and some sources will be more useful to individuals than other sources.

HEALTH CARE PROFESSIONALS AND PROVIDERS

American Academy of Physical Medicine and Rehabilitation
One IBM Plaza, Suite 2500
Chicago, IL 60611–3604
Phone: (312) 464–9700
Fax: (312) 464–0227
http://www.aapmr.org

American Occupational Therapy Association
4720 Montgomery Lane
P.O. Box 31220
Bethesda, MD 20824–1220
Phone: (301) 652–2682
TDD: (800) 377–8555
Fax: (301) 652–7711
http://www.aota.org

American Physical Therapy Association
1111 North Fairfax Street
Alexandria, VA 22314–1488
Phone: (703) 684-APTA (2782) or (800) 999-APTA (2782)
TDD: (703) 683–6748
Fax: (703) 684–7343
http://www.apta.org

Medicare
Centers for Medicare & Medicaid Services
7500 Security Boulevard
Baltimore, MD 21244–1850
Phone: (800) MEDICARE
http://www.cms.gov

Rehabilitation Engineering and Assistive Technology Society
   of North America (RESNA)
RESNA Technical Assistance Project
1700 North Moore Street, Suite 1540
Arlington, VA 22209–1903
Phone: (703) 524–6686
TTY: (703) 524–6639
Fax: (703) 524–6630
http://www.resna.org

FEDERAL AGENCIES AND NATIONAL ORGANIZATIONS

Social Security Administration
6401 Security Boulevard
Baltimore, MD 21235–0001
Phone: (800) 772–1213
http://www.ssa.gov

U.S. Department of Justice
ADA Information
950 Pennsylvania Avenue, NW
Civil Rights Division
Disability Rights Section—NYAVE
Washington, D.C. 20530
Phone: (800) 514–0301
TTY: (800) 514–0383
http://www.usdoj.gov/crt/ada/adahom1.htm

U.S. Equal Employment Opportunity Commission
1801 L Street, NW
Washington, D.C. 20507

Phone: (800) 669–4000
TTY: (800) 669–6820
http://www.eeoc.gov

U.S. Department of Transportation
400 7th Street, SW
Washington, D.C. 20590
Phone: (202) 366–4000
http://www.dot.gov

Architectural and Transportation Barrier Compliance Board
The Access Board
1331 F Street NW, Suite 1000
Washington, DC 20004–1111
Phone: (800) 872–2253
TTY: (800) 993–2822
Fax: (202) 272–5447
http://www.access-board.gov

Office on Disability and Health
National Center of Birth Defects and Developmental Disabilities
Centers for Disease Control and Prevention
U.S. Department of Health and Human Services
4770 Bufford Highway
Atlanta, GA 30341
Phone: (770) 488–7150
Fax: (770) 488–7156
http://www.cdc.gov/ncbddd/dh/default.htm

National Women's Health Information Center
The Office on Women's Health
U.S. Department of Health and Human Services
8550 Arlington Boulevard, Suite 300
Fairfax, VA 22031
Phone: (800) 994-WOMAN
http://www.4women.gov

National Institute on Disability and Rehabilitation Research
U.S. Department of Education
400 Maryland Avenue, S.W.
Washington, DC 20202–2572
Phone: (202) 205–8134
TTY: (202) 205–4475
http://www.ed.gov/offices/OSERS/NIDRR/index.html

President's Committee on Employment of People with Disabilities
Job Accommodations Network
West Virginia University
P.O. Box 6080
Morgantown, WV 26506–6080
Phone/TTY: (304) 293–7186
Phone/TTY: (800) 526–7234
Phone/TTY: (800) ADA-WORK
Fax: (304) 293–5407
http://www.jan.wvu.edu

National Council on Disability
1331 F Street NW, Suite 850
Washington, DC 20004
Phone: (202) 272–2004
TTY: (202) 272–2074
Fax: (202) 272–2022
http://www.ncd.gov

Alliance for Technology Access
2175 E. Francisco Boulevard, Suite L
San Rafael, CA 94901
Phone: (415) 455–4575
TTY: (415) 455–0491
http://www.ataccess.org

LINKS TO INFORMATION ON THE INTERNET

ABLEDATA
8630 Fenton Street, Suite 930
Silver Spring, MD 20910
Phone: (800) 227–0216
TTY: (301) 608–8912
Fax: (301) 608–8958
http://www.abledata.com

Links to information on assistive technology

Untangling the Web
International Center for Disability Information
West Virginia University
http://www.icdi.wvu.edu/others.htm

Links to wide-ranging information about disability, from legal issues to recreation and travel to assistive technology to employment

National Center for the Dissemination of Disability Research
Southwest Educational Development Laboratory (SEDL)
211 East Seventh Street, Room 400
Austin, TX 78701–3281
Phone/TTY: (512) 476–6861
Phone/TTY: (800) 266–1832
Fax: (512) 476–2286
http://www.ncddr.org/index.html

Links to disability-related research on various topics, including employment, health care, and assistive technology

STATE ASSISTIVE TECHNOLOGY PROJECTS

These offices are funded under the federal Technology-Related Assistance for Individuals with Disabilities Act of 1998 (P.L. 105–394). Each state develops its own program, which may be more or less applicable to adults with mobility limitations. These "Tech Act Projects" do not typically provide AT but instead offer information, support networks, demonstration centers, links to other state services, and other educational materials. Programs appear here alphabetically by state (current contact information on these programs is maintained at http://www.trace.wisc.edu or http://www.resna.org/taproject/at/statecontacts .html).

Alabama STAR System for Alabamians with Disabilities
2125 East South Boulevard
P.O. Box 20752
Montgomery, AL 36120–0752
Phone: (334) 613–3480
Phone: (800) STAR656 (in state)
Fax: (334) 613–3485
http://www.rehab.state.al.us/star/default.htm

Assistive Technologies of Alaska
1016 W. 6th, Suite 200
Anchorage, AK 99501
Phone: (907) 269–3570
Phone: (800) 478–4378 (in state)
Fax: (907) 269–3632
http://www.labor.state.ak.us/at/index.htm

Arizona Technology Access Program (AzTAP)
N. Arizona University
P.O. Box 5630

Flagstaff, AZ 86011
Phone: (520) 523–7035
TDD: (520) 523–1695
Fax: (520) 523–9127
http://www.nau.edu/ihd/aztap

Arkansas Increasing Capabilities Access Network (ICAN)
2201 Brookwood, Suite 117
Little Rock, AR 72202
Phone: (501) 666–8868
Phone: (800) 828–2799 (in state)
Fax: (501) 666–5319
http://www.arkansas-ican.org

California Assistive Technology System (CATS)
California Department of Rehabilitation
2000 Evergreen Street
Sacramento, CA 95815
Phone: (916) 263–8687
Fax: (916) 263–8683
http://interwork.sdsu.edu/catsca

Assistive Technology Partners (Colorado)
University of Colorado Health Sciences Center
1245 E. Colfax Avenue, Suite 200
Denver, CO 80218
Phone: (303) 315–1280
Fax: (303) 837–8964
http://www.uchsc.edu/atp

Connecticut Assistive Technology Project
Department of Social Services, BRS
25 Sigourney Street, 11th Floor
Hartford, CT 06106
Phone: (860) 424–4881
Fax: (860) 424–4850
http://www.techact.uconn.edu

Delaware Assistive Technology Initiative
Center for Applied Science & Engineering
University of Delaware/duPont Hospital for Children
1600 Rockland Road, Room 117E
P.O. Box 269
Wilmington, DE 19899
Phone: (302) 651–6790

Fax: (302) 651–6793
http://www.asel.udel.edu/dati

University Legal Services (ULS) Assistive Technology Program for the
  District of Columbia
300 I Street, NE
Suite 202
Washington, DC 20002
Phone: (202) 547–0198
TDD: (202) 547–2657
http://www.atpdc.org

Florida Alliance for Assistive Services and Technology
1020 E. Lafayette Street, Suite 110
Tallahassee, FL 32301–4546
Phone/TDD: (850) 487–3278
Fax: (850) 487–2805
http://faast.org

Georgia Tools for Life
Division of Rehabilitation Services
1700 Century Circle, Suite 300
Atlanta, GA 30345
Phone: (800) 497–8665
http://www.gatfl.org

Assistive Technology Resource Centers of Hawaii
414 Kuwili Street, Suite 104
Honolulu, HI 96817
Phone/TDD: (808) 532–7110
Fax: (808) 532–7120
http://www.atrc.org

Idaho Assistive Technology Project
129 W. Third Street
Moscow, ID 83843
Phone: (208) 885–3559
Fax: (208) 885–3628
http://www.icdri.org/idaho.htm

Illinois Assistive Technology Project
1 W. Old State Capitol Plaza, Suite 100
Springfield, IL 62701
Phone/TDD: (217) 522–7985

Fax: (217) 522–8067
http://www.iltech.org

ATTAIN, Inc. (Indiana)
Assistive Technology Through Action in Indiana
2346 South Lynhurst Drive, Suite 507
Indianapolis, IN 46241
Phone: (317) 486–8808
Phone: (800) 486–8246
Fax: (317) 486–8809
http://www.attaininc.org

Iowa Program for Assistive Technology (IPAT)
Center for Disabilities and Development
100 Hawkins Drive, Room 5295
Iowa City, IA 52242–1011
Phone: (319) 356–0550
Phone: (800) 331–3027
http://www.uiowa.edu/infotech

Assistive Technology for Kansas Project
2601 Gabriel
Parsons, KS 67357
Phone/TDD: (620) 421–8367
Phone: (800) 526–3648
Fax: (620) 421–0954
http://www.atk.lsi.ukans.edu

Kentucky Assistive Technology Services (KATS) Network
Charles McDowell Rehabilitation Center
8412 Westport Road
Louisville, KY 40242
Phone: (502) 327–0022
Phone: (800) 327–5287 (in state)
TDD: (502) 327–9855
Fax: (502) 327–9974
http://www.katsnet.org

Louisiana Assistive Technology Project
3042 Old Forge Drive
Baton Rouge, LA 70898
Phone/TDD: (225) 925–9500
Phone/TDD: (800) 270–6185
Fax: (225) 925–9560
http://www.latan.org

Maine CITE Coordinating Center
University of Maine System University College
46 University Drive
Augusta, ME 04330
Phone: (207) 621–3195
TDD: (207) 621–3482
Fax: (207) 621–3193
http://www.mainecite.org

Maryland Technology Assistance Project (TAP)
Governor's Office for Individuals with Disabilities
2301 Argonne Drive, Room T-17
Baltimore, MD 21218
Phone/TDD: (800) 832–4827
http://www.mdtap.org

Massachusetts Assistive Technology Partnership (MATP) Center
MATP Center, Children's Hospital
1295 Boylston Street, Suite 310
Boston, MA 02215
Phone: (617) 355–7820
Phone/TDD: (800) 848–8867 (in state)
Fax: (617) 355–6345
http://www.matp.org

Michigan TECH 2000
Michigan Assistive Technology Project
241 East Saginaw Highway, Suite 450
East Lansing, MI 48823
Phone: (517) 333–2477
Phone: (800) 760–4600 (in state)
Fax: (517) 333–2677
http://www.copower.org

Minnesota STAR Program
658 Cedar Street, Room 360
St. Paul, MN 55155
Phone: (612) 296–2771
Phone: (800) 657–3862
TDD: (612) 296–9478
http://www.state.mn.us/ebranch/admin/assistivetechnology/index.html

Mississippi Project START
P.O. Box 1698
Jackson, MS 39215–1000

Phone/TDD: (601) 987–4872
Fax: (601) 364–2349
E-mail: spower@mdrs.state.ms.com

Missouri Assistive Technology Project
4731 South Cochise, Suite 114
Independence, MO 64055–6975
Phone: (816) 373–5193
Phone: (800) 647–8557 (in state)
Fax: (816) 373–9314
http://www.dolir.state.mo.us/matp

MonTech (Montana)
Rural Institute on Disabilities
University of Montana
634 Eddie Avenue
Missoula, MT 59812
Phone: (406) 243–5676
Phone: (800) 732–0323
Fax: (406) 243–4730
http://ruralinstitute.umt.edu/HDC/montech.htm

Nebraska Assistive Technology Project
5143 South 48th Street, Suite C
Lincoln, NE 68516–2204
Phone: (402) 471–0734
Phone: (888) 806–6287 (in state)
Fax: (402) 471–0117
http://www.nde.state.ne.us/ATP

Nevada Assistive Technology Collaborative
Rehabilitation Division, Community-Based Services Development
711 South Stewart Street
Carson City, NV 89710
Phone: (775) 687–4452
TDD: (775) 687–3388
Fax: (775) 687–3292
E-mail: nvreach@powernet.net

New Hampshire Technology Partnership Project
Institute on Disability
#14 Ten Ferry Street
The Concord Center
Concord, NH 00301
Phone/TDD: (603) 224–0630

Phone: (800) 427–3338 (in state)
Fax: (603) 226–0389
http://iod.unh.edu

New Jersey Technology Assistive Resource Program
New Jersey Protection and Advocacy, Inc.
210 South Broad Street, 3rd Floor
Trenton, NJ 08608
Phone: (609) 633–7106
Phone: (800) 342–5832 (in state)
Fax: (609) 341–3327
http://www.njpanda.org

New Mexico Technology Assistance Program (NMTAP)
435 St. Michael's Drive, Building D
Sante Fe, NM 87505
Phone/TDD: (505) 954–8539
Phone/TDD: (800) 866–2253
Fax: (505) 954–8562
http://www.nmtap.com

New York State TRAID Project
Office of Advocate for Persons with Disabilities
One Empire State Plaza, Suite 1001
Albany, NY 12223–1150
Phone: (518) 474–2825
TDD: (518) 473–4231
Phone/TDD: (800) 522–4369 (in state)
Fax: (518) 473–6005
http://www.advoc4disabled.state.ny.us/TRAID_Project/technlog.htm

North Carolina Assistive Technology Project
Division of Vocational Rehabilitation Services
1110 Navaho Drive, Suite 101
Raleigh, NC 27609
Phone/TDD: (919) 850–2787
Fax: (919) 850–2792
http://www.mindspring.com/~ncatp

North Dakota Interagency Program for Assistive Technology
P.O. Box 743
Cavalier, ND 58220
Phone/TDD: (701) 265–4807
Fax: (701) 265–3150
http://www.ndipat.org

Ohio T.R.A.I.N.
Ohio Super Computer Center
1224 Kinnear Road
Columbus, OH 43212
Phone/TDD: (614) 292–2426
Phone: (800) 784–3425 (in state)
Fax: (614) 292–5866
http://www.atohio.org

Oklahoma ABLE Tech
Oklahoma State University Wellness Center
1514 W. Hall of Fame Road
Stillwater, OK 74078–2026
Phone: (405) 744–9748
Phone/TDD: (800) 257–1705
Fax: (405) 744–2487
http://okabletech.okstate.edu

Oregon TALN Project
Access Technologies, Inc
3070 Lancaster Drive NE
Salem, OR 97305
Phone/TDD: (503) 361–1201
Phone: (800) 677–7512 (in state)
Fax: (503) 370–4530
http://www.taln.org

Pennsylvania's Initiative on Assistive Technology Project (PIAT)
Institute on Disabilities/UAP
Ritter Annex 423
Temple University
Philadelphia, PA 19122
Phone: (215) 204–1356
Phone: (800) 204–7428
TDD: (800) 750–7428
Fax: (215) 204–9371
http://www.temple.edu/inst_disabilities/piat

Rhode Island Assistive Technology Access Project
Rhode Island Department of Human Services
Office of Rehabilitation Services
40 Fountain Street
Providence, RI 02903–1898
Phone: (401) 421–7005
TTY: (401) 421–7016

Fax: (401) 222–3574
http://www.atap.state.ri.us

South Carolina Assistive Technology Project
USC School of Medicine
Center for Developmental Disabilities
Columbia, SC 29208
Phone/TDD: (803) 935–5263
Fax: (803) 935–5342
http://www.sc.edu/scatp

DakotaLink (South Dakota)
1925 Plaza Boulevard
Rapid City, SD 57702
Phone: (605) 394–1876
Phone: (800) 645–0673 (in state)
Fax: (605) 394–5315
http://dakotalink.tie.net

Tennessee Technology Access Project (TTAP)
Citizens Plaza Office Building
400 Deadrick Street
Nashville, TN 37248
Phone: (615) 532–3122
Phone: (800) 732–5059 (in state)
TDD: (615) 741–4566
Fax: (615) 532–6719
http://www.state.tn.us/mental/ttap.html

Texas Assistive Technology Partnership
University of Texas at Austin
SZB 252 D5100
Austin, TX 78712–1290
Phone: (800) 828–7839
TDD: (512) 471–1844
http://tatp.edb.utexas.edu

Utah Assistive Technology Program
Center for Persons with Disabilities
6588 Old Main Hill
Logan, UT 84322–6588
Phone/TDD: (435) 797–3824
Fax: (435) 797–2355
http://www.uatpat.org

Vermont Assistive Technology Program
103 South Main Street
Weeks Building, First Floor
Waterbury, VT 05671–2305
Phone: (802) 241–2620
TTY: (802) 241–1464
Fax: (802) 241–2174
http://www.dad.state.vt.us/atp

Virginia Assistive Technology System (VATS)
8004 Franklin Farms Drive
P.O. Box K-300
Richmond, VA 23288–0300
Phone/TDD: (804) 662–9990
Phone: (800) 435–8490
Fax: (804) 662–9478
http://www.vats.org

Washington Assistive Technology Alliance
Center for Technology and Disability Studies
University of Washington
Box 357920
Seattle, WA 98195–7920
Phone: (206) 685–4181
TDD: (206) 616–1396
Fax: (206) 543–4779
http://wata.org

West Virginia University Center for Excellence in Disabilities
    (WVUCED)
Research & Office Park
955 Hartman Run Road
Morgantown, WV 26505
Phone: (800) 841–8436
TDD: (304) 293–4692
Fax: (304) 293–7294
http://www.ced.wvu.edu/Programs/Community/WVATS/Frontpage.htm

Wisconsin Assistive Technology Program (WisTech)
Office for People with Physical Disabilities
1 W. Wilson Street, Room 450
Madison, WI 53707
Phone: (608) 266–1794
TTY: (608) 267–9880
Fax: (608) 267–3203
http://www.wistech.org

Wyoming's New Options in Technology (WYNOT)
University of Wyoming
1465 North 4th Street, Suite 111
Laramie, WY 82072
Phone/TDD: (307) 766–2084
Phone/TYY: (800) 861–4312
Fax: (307) 721–2084
http://wind.uwyo.edu/wynot

Notes

1. MOBILITY LIMITS

1. Looking beyond individuals to populations, public-health experts since the mid 1800s have focused on eliminating specific threats to population health, including infectious, environmental, occupational, nutritional, and other causes of disease or injury. But "public health messages have often depicted people with disabilities as the negative result of 'unhealthy' actions" and many people with disabilities therefore "rejected public health as inimical to their very existence" (Lollar 2001, 754). Public health today explores the linkage between disability and socioeconomic disadvantage, trying to erase health disparities between people with and without disabilities, prevent secondary conditions, and carry out wellness programs.

2. To minimize the risk of presenting "the response to chronic illness and disability . . . [as] less social and collective and more and more rooted in the psychological, cognitive, and existential world of the individual" (Williams 2001, 132), I focus on experiences shared by at least several interviewees (i.e., specific settings and subjects may vary, but the general point is the same). Yet because these experiences are described by a convenience sample, we cannot generalize from them to all people in similar circumstances.

2. WHO HAS MOBILITY DIFFICULTIES

1. Most people with walking difficulties live in the community—rather than in nursing homes or long-term care settings, where most residents also have mobility problems. Among roughly 2.1 million Medicare beneficiaries in institutions in 1997, over 87 percent had mobility limitations. Rates ranged from 48 percent for persons under age 65 (i.e., who qualify for Medicare explicitly because of disability) to just over 95 percent for persons age 85 and older (Sharma et al. 2001, 62).

2. Only about 2 percent report that their problems began at birth or very early childhood, caused by congenital or genetic conditions such as cerebral

palsy, spina bifida, or muscular dystrophy. Of those who say their mobility difficulties began at age 75+, the percentages are 12 for minor; 13 for moderate; and 23 percent for major (these numbers come from the 1994–95 National Health Interview Survey—Disability [NHIS-D Phase I]).

3. These numbers on gender and race come from the 1994–95 NHIS-D Phase I and are adjusted for age differences (gender figures) and age and sex differences (race figures).

4. Manton and Gu (2001) take their figures from the National Long-Term Care Survey, which draws its sample from Medicare beneficiaries age 65+. They supplemented these figures with results from the National Nursing Home Survey. They define functional impairments by limitations in activities of daily living or ADLs (feeding, bathing, dressing, toileting, moving around home); limitations in instrumental ADLs (e.g., cleaning house, shopping, preparing meals); or being institutionalized in a long-term care facility. These types of limitations generally indicate fairly severe impairments.

5. "Arthritis" encompasses diverse conditions, such as osteoarthritis (degenerative joint disease associated with aging, by far the most common kind of arthritis), rheumatoid arthritis, and arthritis associated with such illnesses as sickle cell disease and systemic lupus erythematosus (an autoimmune disorder affecting many organ systems, as well as joints). Similarly, numerous conditions can cause back pain, including herniation of a disc, spinal stenosis (narrowing of the spinal canal, impinging on nerve roots), compression fractures of vertebra, tumors inside and outside the spinal canal, and spondylolisthesis (forward slippage of one vertebra on another, straining the ligaments and intervertebral joints). Each specific clinical entity has its own natural history and implications for treatment, yet mobility problems are common consequences of all. Throughout this book, I discuss broad categories of conditions, rather than specific entities.

6. The falls and accident categories do not include spinal cord injuries resulting in paralysis of the lower body (paraplegia) or upper and lower body (quadriplegia). The NHIS-D counted paraplegia and quadriplegia separately and, respectively, they account for 0.3 and 0.2 percent of people with mobility difficulties.

7. The NHIS-D asked only people with major mobility problems whether their difficulties would persist twelve or more months, and about 88 percent replied that they would. Among people reporting major *long-term* mobility problems, the percentages identifying specific causes by age are very similar to those in Table 2, generally differing by only a few tenths of a percent.

8. The NHIS-D does not list obesity separately as a specific reason for mobility problems.

9. Exact percentages of obese persons by level of mobility difficulty are 15 for no mobility difficulty; 31 for minor; 33 for moderate; and 29 percent for major difficulty. Some people with major mobility problems are much more likely to be underweight—almost 12 percent, compared to around 5 percent for other people—perhaps relating to serious illnesses such as cancer or certain severe lung diseases, which cause weakness and wasting away, thus compromis-

ing people's mobility (these figures come from the NHIS-D 1994–95 Phase I). We judged weight using the body mass index (BMI): (body weight in kilograms)/(height in meters)^2. Obesity is defined as BMI $\geq$ 30 kg/m^2, while underweight is BMI $<$ 18.5 kg/m^2.

3. SENSATIONS OF WALKING

1. Another condition that cuts across the four causal categories is pressure ulcers (decubitus ulcers), which occur where bony structures press into surrounding tissues of people who are immobilized, seated, or bedridden for long periods. Pressure ulcers can become profoundly debilitating and life-threatening, particularly among institutionalized persons with severely impaired mobility. But among people living in the community, less than 4 percent of those with major mobility problems report pressure ulcers, as do 0.4 and 1 percent of those with minor and moderate difficulties, respectively (1994–95 NHIS-D Phase II).

2. For people with amputations above the knee, the prosthesis must include not only a foot-ankle complex but also a knee joint, allowing persons to sit, climb stairs, walk up and down inclines. Complicated biomechanics make this prosthesis more difficult and expensive to devise, and it requires more training to use than below-the-knee prostheses. Sophisticated prostheses can substantially restore mobility, even permitting performance in rigorous competitive sports among athletes with high amputations.

3. The NHIS-D asked about sensory and other physical functions (Table 3) but did not indicate whether mobility difficulty caused or resulted from problems.

4. These data on use of cigarettes, snuff, and chewing tobacco come from the 1994 Healthy People 2000 supplemental questionnaire administered along with the 1994 NHIS-D. Exact percentages are 28 for minor, 30 for moderate, and 29 for persons with major mobility difficulties.

5. Among people age 65+, 86.2 persons/1,000 population were injured by falls in 1997: 47.2/1,000 men and 114.5/1,000 women (Warner, Barnes, and Fingerhut 2000, 18).

6. For some people, difficulties with voiding become life-threatening. Before broad-spectrum antibiotics became available, urinary tract infections killed many people with spinal cord injuries, who generally must use catheters or other instrumentation to evacuate their bladders. Today, these infections remain the leading reason for medical services, with more than half of people with spinal cord injuries developing urinary tract infections each year (Berkowitz et al. 1998, 44).

4. SOCIETY'S VIEWS OF WALKING

1. I write this revision just over a year after the 11 September 2001 terrorist attacks on the United States. What future airport security will entail is still evolving, as it becomes a federal responsibility. I resumed traveling by air about a month after the attacks and found that little had actually changed for

me when passing through airport security, although the request to remove my shoes is physically difficult and seems perhaps excessive. I had always been "patted down" manually by security personnel. Anecdotal reports suggest that airlines' performance was mixed when it came to accommodating passengers using wheelchairs even before 11 September. "For an industry trying to adjust to the new demands, the terrorist attacks only compounded the problem" (Canedy 2002, A12).

2. Recent Supreme Court decisions limit the reach of the ADA. In *Toyota Motor Manufacturing Inc. v. Williams,* decided 8 January 2002, a unanimous court ruled against Ella Williams, who had argued that her carpal tunnel syndrome prevented her from performing her job at a Toyota manufacturing plant. The justices argued that Ms. Williams was not "disabled" because she could still perform routine tasks at home, such as brushing her teeth and gardening—in other words, that her condition did not limit "major life activities" (thus implicitly viewing employment as outside "major life activities," the standard used by the ADA to describe disabling conditions). Another important case was *Board of Trustees of the University of Alabama et al. v. Garrett et al.* decided by a split court (5-to-4) on 21 February 2001. In this case, two employees of Alabama sued the state for money damages under Title I of the ADA. Patricia Garrett, a registered nurse, had been employed as a director of nursing at the University of Alabama in Birmingham Hospital when she developed breast cancer. During treatment for her cancer, she took extensive leave from work, and when she returned, her supervisor told Garrett that she had been transferred to a lower-paying job as a nurse manager. In a separate suit, Milton Ash had worked as a security officer for the Alabama Department of Youth Services. Because of asthma and at his physician's recommendation, Ash requested that his employer limit his exposure to cigarette smoke and carbon monoxide; Ash later developed sleep apnea and requested reassignment to daytime shifts. His employer denied Ash's requests. The Supreme Court ruled that individuals cannot bring lawsuits for money damages against states under the ADA. Writing for the majority, Chief Justice William H. Rehnquist asserted that, in passing the ADA, Congress had failed to show a convincing pattern of discrimination by states against people with disabilities, as would be required for these persons to meet the "equal protection" assurances of the Fourteenth Amendment. Rehnquist continued, "Thus, the Fourteenth Amendment does not require States to make special accommodations for the disabled, so long as their actions toward such individuals are rational. They could quite hardheadedly—and perhaps hardheartedly—hold to job-qualification requirements which do not make allowance for the disabled." Writing for the four dissenting justices, Justice Stephen G. Breyer rejected Rehnquist's assertion: "The powerful evidence of discriminatory treatment throughout society in general, including discrimination by private persons and local governments, implicates state governments as well, for state agencies form part of that larger society."

3. The Professional Golfers Association appealed a lower court's decision to the Supreme Court, which ruled 7-to-2 for Martin on 29 May 2001. The Supreme Court majority held that walking 5 miles or so around a golf course

is not fundamental to the game and therefore Martin (given his serious physical impairment) merits that accommodation. In his dissent, Justice Antonine Scalia described the majority's opinion as a misguided intrusion of compassion into the rule of law (and the rules of golf) rather than as a matter of justice.

4. Section 3 of the ADA defines disability as "(A) a physical or mental impairment that substantially limits one or more of the major life activities . . . ; (B) a record of such impairment; or (C) being regarded as having such an impairment." This definition thus explicitly encompasses both personal circumstances and external perceptions—society's views. The courts are struggling to define "major life activities."

5. In *Sutton et al. v. United Air Lines, Inc.,* twin sisters with uncorrected vision of 20/200 who see normally with glasses sued the airline for refusing to hire them as commercial pilots. In *Murphy v. United Parcel Service, Inc.,* a mechanic with hypertension controlled by medication sued after being fired from his job. The sisters and the mechanic alike lost by votes of 7 to 2.

5. HOW PEOPLE FEEL ABOUT THEIR DIFFICULTY WALKING

1. The NHIS-D did not ask what people feared when they reported being fearful and anxious.

2. These results come from a multivariable logistic regression using 1994–95 NHIS-D Phase I data with being frequently depressed or anxious as the dichotomous outcome (dependent) variable and the following as predictor (independent) variables: mobility level (none, minor, moderate, major); age group; sex; race (white, black, other nonwhite); ethnicity (Hispanic); education (high school or less, college, more than college); marital status (married, divorced, widowed, never married); cannot work because of health condition; currently unemployed; household income (less than $15,000, $15,000–$30,000, $30,000–$50,000, $50,000+); and self-perceived health status (excellent, very good, good, fair, poor). Because employment is an important factor, this analysis considered only people age 18–64. The adjusted odds ratios of reporting being depressed or anxious are significantly higher for those who live alone (50 percent higher than for others); are divorced (70 percent), widowed (40 percent), or never married (30 percent); cannot work because of health (140 percent); are currently unemployed (40 percent); have an annual income less than $15,000 (70 percent); or perceive health status to be fair (670 percent) or poor (1,120 percent). Factors that statistically significantly reduce the adjusted odds ratio of reporting being depressed or anxious include older age (for example, persons 60–64 have a 50 percent lower adjusted odds ratio than persons 18–25); black race (40 percent lower); other nonwhite race (30 percent); high school education or less (20 percent); and college education (compared to graduate school, 20 percent).

3. Table 6 shows responses among people who answered the NHIS-D themselves as opposed to having a proxy answer the questions. The NHIS-D does not indicate whether proxy-respondents accurately represent the views of the person for whom they are responding.

4. Women, racial minorities, and Hispanic respondents are much less likely to say they are disabled than men and white and non-Hispanic respondents; low-income persons are much more likely to perceive disability than those with high incomes (Iezzoni et al. 2000b). Complex cultural factors could explain these differences. If people expect to develop mobility problems, impairments may seem "normal" or "part of life," not something "deviant" or "disabled." If people feel disenfranchised because of membership in a racial or linguistic minority group, they may be unwilling to identify with yet another group perceived as excluded—persons with disabilities; their perceptions may reflect a desire for respect they do not associate with the disability identity. Poor persons may be more likely to perceive themselves as disabled because they need to qualify for financial support and governmental programs (e.g., health insurance, vocational training) tied to disability.

6. AT HOME—WITH FAMILY AND FRIENDS

1. These figures (adjusted for age group and sex) come from the 1994–95 NHIS-D Phase I, which asked about six activities of daily living (ADLs: bathing or showering; dressing; eating; getting in and out of bed or chairs; using the toilet, including getting to the toilet; and getting around inside the home) and four mobility-related instrumental ADLs (IADLs: preparing their own meals; shopping for personal items like toiletries or medicine; doing heavy work around the house like scrubbing floors, washing windows, and doing heavy yardwork; and doing light work around the house like doing dishes, light cleaning, or taking out the trash). Among persons without mobility difficulties, 0.2 percent or fewer report any ADL problems; among those with mild or moderate mobility difficulties, many fewer than 10 percent report problems with all ADLs except bathing or showering, which is difficult for 11 percent of persons with moderate mobility problems. Among persons with major mobility difficulties, the ADL presenting the least problem is eating (13 percent have problems), while the most troubling ADLs are bathing, dressing, getting in and out of chairs and around inside the home (31 to 34 percent reporting difficulties). Heavy housework is the most problematic IADL, causing difficulties for 28 and 52 percent of people with mild and moderate mobility problems, respectively.

2. Most existing private properties predate federal and state accessibility laws. The Fair Housing Amendments Act of 1988 added people with disabilities as a group protected from discrimination in private housing, representing the first time antidiscrimination provisions for people with disabilities extended to the private sector (West 1991a, 18–19). The 1988 amendments prohibit homeowners from refusing to rent or sell housing to someone because of disability, or to charge them higher rents, sales prices, or security deposits (Pelka 1997, 119–20). In addition, the law mandates physical accessibility of new construction of multifamily dwellings with four or more units and ensures that disabled people can adapt their residences to meet their needs.

3. These rates come from the 1994 Healthy People 2000 supplemental survey and are adjusted for age group and sex. Almost 25 percent of people with

major mobility problems live in apartments or condominiums (vs. houses or townhouses), as do 24 percent of people without any mobility difficulties and about 31 percent of those reporting minor and moderate impairments. Just over 4 percent of persons reporting major mobility difficulties say they were denied housing within the last year because of their physical impairment (these age-and-sex adjusted rates come from the 1994–95 NHIS-D Phase II).

4. Centers for Independent Living (CILs) are located in communities nationwide. Originating during the 1970s, many CILs help people with disabilities find community-based assistance with wide-ranging needs, including ADLs, IADLs, housing, vocational training, and employment. The 1994–95 NHIS-D Phase II asked specific questions about use of CIL services. Only 29 (0.3 percent) of 8,926 respondents with mobility difficulties indicated that they received CIL services, with 23 of these having major mobility problems. This number of respondents is too small for meaningful analysis or derivation of population estimates.

5. These rates come from the 1994–95 NHIS-D Phase I and look at people reporting assistance with ADLs. For IADLs, the percentages with paid help are 22 for minor, 23 for moderate, and 27 percent for major mobility difficulties.

6. These rates come from the 1994–95 NHIS-D Phase I and look at people reporting assistance with ADLs. Around 20 percent did not get any help with ADLs. For IADLs, just over one third got help only from a spouse, parent, or child across the three groups with mobility difficulties, with roughly 20 percent not receiving any assistance with IADLs.

7. These rates come from the 1994–95 NHIS-D Phase I and are adjusted for age group and sex.

8. Differences in marital status occur especially at younger ages. Among persons age 18–44, 74 percent of those without mobility difficulties are married, compared to only 57 percent of those with major mobility problems. In the same age range, 13 percent of persons without mobility difficulties are divorced, compared to 20 percent of those with major mobility difficulties (these figures come from the NHIS-D Phase I and are adjusted for age group and sex).

9. Neither Phase I nor II of the NHIS-D directly asked how many children respondents had. Phase II did ask if respondents had at least one *living* child. The percentages responding that they had at least one living child were 31, 37, and 30 for people age 45–64 with mild, moderate, and major mobility problems, respectively. Of people age 65+ with mild, moderate, and major mobility problems, 51, 47, and 61 percent, respectively, have at least one living child.

10. Among people age 18–44, 91 percent with minor mobility difficulties have at least one living parent, as do 82 and 87 percent of those with moderate and major mobility problems, respectively (these rates are taken from the 1994–95 NHIS-D Phase II and adjusted for age group and sex).

7. OUTSIDE HOME—AT WORK AND IN COMMUNITIES

1. These rates come from the 1994–95 NHIS-D Phase II and are adjusted for age group and sex.

2. Of working-age persons who had worked or still work, 12 to 13 percent are self-employed, regardless of mobility status (1994–95 NHIS-D and 1994–95 Family Resources supplement). Of persons still working, 6 to 8 percent have more than one job, regardless of mobility. For persons now age 65+, the percentage who had been self-employed is much higher than for younger persons: 33 for people with no difficulties; and 29 for mild, 32 for moderate, and 40 percent for major mobility difficulties.

3. Among people who work as employees (i.e., are not self-employed), the percentage working 40 or more hours per week is 75 percent with no mobility difficulty; and 70, 65, and 62 percent with mild, moderate, and major difficulties, respectively (1994–95 NHIS-D Phase I and 1994–95 Family Resources supplement, figures adjusted for age group and sex).

4. Additional information drawn from the 1994–95 NHIS-D Phase I reinforces perceptions that poverty increases with worsening mobility impairments. About 3 percent of working-age people without impaired mobility report they receive welfare payments (primarily Aid to Families with Dependent Children; this survey was performed before "welfare reform" produced Temporary Aid to Needy Families), compared to 8 to 11 percent of persons with mobility difficulties. Only 11 percent of working-age people without mobility problems receive food stamps, compared to over 30 percent for those with impaired mobility.

5. The percentage of working-age people reporting disability pensions other than Social Security or railroad retirement is 1 for people with no difficulties; and 4 for mild, 7 for moderate, and 6 percent for major mobility difficulties. The percentage of persons age 65+ reporting disability pensions is 2, 3, 4, and 5 for people with no mobility problems and minor, moderate, and major difficulties, respectively.

6. Social Security amendments of 1956 introduced cash benefits for disabled workers between age 50–65; the 1958 amendments granted cash benefits to children and dependent spouses of disability recipients; the 1960 amendments extended benefits to workers under age 50; and the 1965 amendments changed the definition of "permanent disability" to one "expected to continue for at least 12 months" (Stone 1984, 78). Supplemental Security Income passed in 1972 and extended coverage to persons disabled before age 22 who had never worked (Pelka 1997, 285).

7. People with short-term limitations can obtain cash benefits through state-sponsored temporary disability programs or through sickness or accident insurance purchased privately by individuals or their employers. Persons with work-related injuries receiving payments from employer-financed workers' compensation programs run by states generally have their Social Security benefits cut by that amount. Cash from private long-term disability insurance or pensions purchased through employers or by workers themselves can supplement Social Security payments.

8. As of December 2000, just over 5 million people (2.8 million men and 2.2 million women) received SSDI (Martin, Chin, and Harrison 2001). In 2000, the SSA awarded 610,700 disabled workers benefits. The most common single rea-

son was musculoskeletal problems such as arthritis (25 percent), followed by mental disorders (24 percent), circulatory conditions such as heart disease (12 percent), cancer (10 percent), and disorders involving the nervous system or sensory organs (8 percent).

9. Among people with major mobility difficulties who have applied to the SSA for disability, 60 percent have applied once, 22 percent twice, 15 percent three to four times, and 5 percent five or more times (percentage exceeds 100 because of rounding error; these figures come from the 1994–95 NHIS-D Phase I and 1994–95 Family Resources supplement and are adjusted for age and sex).

10. People could qualify for SSA disability because of disabling conditions other than impaired mobility, such as serious mental illness. Because SSDI cash benefits reflect contributions to the Social Security trust fund, disabled workers receive varying payments. Nationwide, the average monthly SSDI benefit in 2000 was about $834, with $948 for men and $701 for women (Martin, Chin, and Harrison 2001). In 2000, average monthly payments for those receiving SSI were about $373, although most states supplement these amounts.

11. The Ticket to Work and Work Incentives Improvement Act of 1999 gives SSDI and SSI recipients a "ticket" to purchase vocational rehabilitation at public or private agencies, rewarding agencies with a portion of the benefits saved when people work. It also prolongs Medicare coverage for SSDI recipients and extends state Medicaid programs for SSI recipients.

12. Under the Consolidated Omnibus Budget Reconciliation Act (COBRA) of 1985, most companies must offer former employees (and certain dependents) the opportunity to continue purchasing group health insurance for some period after terminating employment.

13. Persons with progressive chronic conditions are often in late middle age or nearing retirement, and other clinical aspects of their medical conditions frequently preclude employment. They are therefore less likely candidates for vocational rehabilitation referrals than young disabled people, especially those with sudden impairments (e.g., spinal cord injury). Of working-age people, just under 18 percent of those with major mobility difficulties report ever having received vocational rehabilitation, compared to 8 with moderate, 6 with minor, and 1 percent with no mobility impairments. Relatively few people report job-related training, although among those who do, roughly 50 percent involves state rehabilitation agencies. These rates are taken from the 1994–95 NHIS-D Phase I for persons age 18–64 and adjusted for age group and sex.

14. Section 504 of the 1973 Rehabilitation Act pioneered the notion that, with "reasonable accommodations," otherwise qualified individuals with disabilities can perform essential functions of a job (Feldblum 1991). Unlike the ADA, Section 504 applied only to entities receiving federal funds, and it precipitated Supreme Court challenges (*Southeastern Community College v. Davis* in 1979, *Alexander v. Choate* in 1985) to delineate what were *reasonable* accommodations and determine when discrimination had actually occurred.

The bottom line was that the diversity of disabilities, jobs, and potential accommodations precludes a single standard approach: solutions must be customized individually. The ADA adopted this practical framework.

15. JAN's Internet web site address (http://www.jan.wvu.edu) is based at West Virginia University.

16. Estimates on how often people with impaired mobility experience employment discrimination are difficult to obtain. Lawsuits and formal complaints to governmental agencies certainly underestimate the numbers of incidents. The NHIS-D occurred in 1994–95, only a few years after passage of the ADA. According to Phase II responses among persons age 18–64 who currently work, 10 percent of those with major mobility problems report having been fired or forced to resign in the past five years because of an ongoing health problem, as have 9 percent with moderate and 5 percent with minor difficulties. Among those reporting major and moderate mobility difficulties, 5 percent had been refused a promotion in the past five years because of ongoing health problems, as had 2 percent with minor difficulties. These figures are adjusted for age group and sex.

17. Special programs have experimented with assistive technology purchases. SSI's PASS work incentive allows recipients to accumulate cash to purchase such equipment, but the allowable amount falls far below the costs of power wheelchairs. Both SSDI and SSI deduct impairment-related work expenses from income figures when people return to work, so that cash benefits are not reduced by these amounts. But if people do not have the equipment to start working, this helpful provision of the work incentive program becomes moot.

18. Among those who had received special aids or technologies for vocational rehabilitation, the percentage obtaining equipment from state rehabilitation agencies is 26 for minor, 44 for moderate, and 28 percent for major mobility difficulties (these rates come from the 1994–95 NHIS-D Phase II and are adjusted for age group and sex).

19. These rates come from the 1994–95 NHIS-D Phase II and are adjusted for age group and sex.

20. Among people with major mobility problems, 26 percent have hand controls, as do 8 percent with moderate mobility difficulties. For people with major mobility problems, other common car adaptations include hand rails, straps, ramps, lifts, or special handles (30 percent). These rates come from the 1994–95 NHIS-D Phase II and are adjusted for age group and sex.

21. Several prior laws aimed to improve access to public transportation for people with disabilities, including the Urban Mass Transportation Act of 1970, Section 504 of the Rehabilitation Act of 1973, and the Air Carrier Access Act of 1986. Court challenges by the transit industry, which successfully argued excessive costs, slowed movement toward fully accessible systems.

22. These rates come from the 1994–95 NHIS-D Phase II and are adjusted for age group and sex.

23. The percentages of people reporting difficulties using public transportation are 13, 33, and 38 for those with minor, moderate, and major mobil-

ity problems, respectively. By far, the most common reason for trouble using public transportation is difficulty walking (53, 74, and 81 percent of those with minor, moderate, and major mobility problems, respectively). Of people with major mobility limitations 27 percent cite access problems with their wheelchair or scooter. Cost is rarely a problem (less than 2 percent). These rates come from the 1994–95 NHIS-D Phase II and are adjusted for age group and sex.

8. PEOPLE TALKING TO THEIR PHYSICIANS

1. Nobody really knows how well the health-care system does this job. Although federal and local governments collect detailed statistics about deaths and specific diseases (National Center for Health Statistics 2000), no source routinely gathers data about how people function physically in their daily lives, except for periodic surveys like the NHIS-D.

2. Percentages for people age 65+ reporting they have a usual source of health care are 92 for no mobility problems; and 95 for mild, 96 for moderate, and 95 percent for major mobility difficulties. Percentages for people age 18–64 reporting they have a usual source of health care are 81 for no mobility problems; and 87 for mild, 88 for moderate, and 93 percent for major mobility difficulties (these rates come from the 1994–95 NHIS-D Phase I and Family Resources supplements).

3. The percentages of people age 18–64 who had two or more physician visits in the last year are 47, 78, 84, and 83 percent for persons with no, minor, moderate, and major mobility difficulties, respectively. Among persons age 65+, the percentages are 66, 82, 86, and 87 percent for those with no, minor, moderate, and major mobility difficulties, respectively (these figures come from the 1994–95 NHIS-D Phase I and are adjusted for age group and sex).

4. The NHIS-D did not indicate the reason for hospitalizations. Impaired mobility alone is not typically an acute condition demanding round-the-clock nursing care and medical oversight (requirements for general hospital admissions) unless it is caused by some cataclysmic event (e.g., injury, spinal cord compression by a tumor). From being sedentary, people can develop life-threatening conditions such as pressure ulcers or pulmonary emboli (clots generally formed in leg veins that lodge in the lungs, blocking blood flow). Falls with major fractures certainly require hospitalization. The most likely reasons for admissions are surgery (e.g., joint replacement for arthritis, corrective operations for back problems) or exacerbations of cardiorespiratory or cerebrovascular diseases and diabetes—leading chronic causes of impaired mobility.

5. "General medical doctors" include family physicians, general practitioners, internists, and pediatricians.

6. The percentages of people age 18–64 who use specialists as their usual source of care are 4, 12, 16, and 22 percent for persons with no, minor, moderate, and major mobility difficulties, respectively. Among persons age 65+, the percentages are 7, 9, 12, and 12 percent for those with no, minor, moderate, and major mobility difficulties, respectively (these figures come from the 1994–95

NHIS-D Phase I and 1994–95 Family Resources supplement and are adjusted for age group and sex).

7. For persons age 65+, the most common explanation for not having a usual source of care is that they don't need a doctor, cited by 58 percent of those without mobility difficulties and by 39, 15, and 23 percent with minor, moderate, and major difficulties, respectively. Persons 18–64 without a usual source of care also often said they didn't need one: 52, 19, 9, and 13 percent for those with no, minor, moderate, and major mobility difficulties, respectively (these figures come from the 1994–95 NHIS-D Phase I and 1994–95 Family Resources supplement and are adjusted for age group and sex).

8. In 1999, the pharmaceutical industry released its latest pain medication, COX-2 (type 2 cyclooxygenase) inhibitors. With a blitz of advertisements, the manufacturer appealed directly to consumers to request this drug from their physicians. COX-2 inhibitors are expensive, have side effects (as do all pain medications), and their marginal benefits for pain control remain controversial.

9. PHYSICIANS TALKING TO THEIR PATIENTS

1. An exception involves training at osteopathic medical schools in musculoskeletal conditions and associated mobility problems.

2. The American Association of Medical Colleges (AAMC) maintains an on-line database (CurrMIT) listing curricular offerings (accessed on 13 October 2000 at www.aamc.org). CurrMIT represents curricula at 128 U.S. medical schools (including the University of Puerto Rico) and 16 Canadian medical schools. Annually, to populate the CurrMIT database, medical schools voluntarily submit information to AAMC about course names and educational methods (the AAMC does not independently confirm their accuracy or completeness). We searched using key words "rehabilitation" and "physical medicine" and found that few institutions require students to complete clerkships in physical medicine and rehabilitation (PM&R). Only nine require PM&R clerkships, some combined with sports medicine, chronic care, neurologic diseases, cardiac or orthopedic rehabilitation, or geriatrics; less than a dozen others offer elective rehabilitation rotations.

3. Some primary care residencies, including family medicine and general practitioner programs, may offer more training in functional concerns than others.

4. State medical licensure laws require physicians to document "continuing medical education" (CME), furnishing periodic proof of certified CME credits. CME typically concentrates on updating or refreshing knowledge of topics taught in medical school and residencies, such as management of acute clinical problems or new treatments for diseases. Only rarely do physicians seek entirely new knowledge through CME. Few general medical CME courses offer training on assessing mobility or functional abilities.

5. To qualify as disabled, the Social Security Administration specifically requires evidence of "medically determinable" impairments, defined as "An im-

pairment that results from anatomical, physiological, or psychological abnormalities which can be shown by medically acceptable clinical and laboratory diagnostic techniques. A physical or mental impairment must be established by medical evidence consisting of signs, symptoms, and laboratory findings—not only by the individual's statement of symptoms" (SSA 1998, 3). The SSA and workers' compensation programs use different processes for evaluating disability: the SSA's "blue book," *Disability Evaluation Under Social Security* (1998) for SSDI and SSI; and the American Medical Association's *Guides to the Evaluation of Permanent Impairment* (1993; Cocchiarella and Andersson 2001), used for workers' compensation disability determinations in most states.

6. *Up-to-Date* is an online medical text, continuously updated and also available on CD ROMs, accessed online 17 December 2001 (http://www.upto dateonline.com).

7. These questions were asked only of people who reported having had a routine physical examination within the previous three years. The percentage reporting having been asked by their physicians about trouble with ADLs is 10 percent of those without mobility problems and 13, 19, and 27 percent with minor, moderate, and major difficulties, respectively. Questioning about IADL problems is similar: 10, 15, 24, and 26 percent for those with no, minor, moderate, and major mobility difficulties, respectively (these figures come from the 1994 NHIS-D Phase I and 1994 Healthy People 2000 supplement and are adjusted for age group and sex).

8. We performed multivariable logistic regressions separately for men and women, controlling for age group, race, Hispanic ethnicity, education, and household income. The reference group was persons without mobility problems. The adjusted odds ratio (95 percent confidence interval) for being asked about contraception for persons with major mobility problems expected to last at least 12 months are 0.3 (0.1, 0.8) for women; and 1.4 (0.5, 4.2) for men. Although not statistically significant, the slightly higher odds ratio for men was provocative and could relate to physicians' concerns about male patients' physical abilities to be sexually active (e.g., erectile function).

9. These figures represent adjusted odds ratios and come from the 1994 NHIS-D and Healthy People 2000 supplement, which queried people who had had a routine health-care visit in the last three years (Iezzoni et al. 2000a). Women over age 49 were asked if they had had mammograms in the prior two years. Women age 18–75 who had not had a hysterectomy were asked if they had had a Pap smear in the last three years. Persons of all ages were asked about smoking. Adjusted odds ratios control for age group, sex (smoking analyses only), race, Hispanic ethnicity, education, income, health insurance, and having a usual source of care. The reference group was persons without mobility difficulties. Adjusted odds ratios (95 percent confidence intervals) for persons with major mobility problems were 0.7 (0.5, 0.9) for mammography; 0.6 (0.4, 0.9) for Pap smears; and 0.8 (0.6, 1.0) for smoking, smokers only analyzed (P = 0.05).

10. These rates come from the 1994–95 NHIS-D and are adjusted for age group and sex.

11. Specialized geriatric assessment programs began in England in the 1930s, their success leading to establishment of geriatric assessment units as entry points for elderly into the British National Health Service (Urdangarin 2000, 384). In the United States since the early 1980s, geriatric researchers have explored better ways to care for frail elderly people who have multiple health problems, typically including impaired mobility. At issue is whether comprehensive evaluations (of diagnoses, medications, rehabilitation potential, living arrangements) improve outcomes, such as by lowering death rates and enhancing functional abilities and quality of life. Early efforts showed positive results, although later studies proved mixed. Many studies, however, were small and poorly designed, contrasting geriatric evaluation programs with ill defined usual care. Comprehensive geriatric assessment, "the multidisciplinary evaluation and care planning of older adults by more than one health professional, has become a cornerstone of geriatric care systems" (Urdangarin 2000, 383), although it remains unclear how widely these services are used in routine practice. Medicare has paid relatively poorly for these services (Boult et al. 1998).

12. Harvard Medical School, the academic origin of about half of the physician interviewees, did not have a PM&R program until the mid 1990s. A physician familiar with Harvard's deliberations feels that questions about the scientific basis of PM&R caused the delays. Another physician said that "turf battles" with other clinical specialties within major Harvard teaching hospitals also contributed.

13. The American Occupational Therapy and American Physical Therapy Associations were established in 1917 and 1921, respectively, while the American Congress of Rehabilitation Medicine was founded only in 1933 and the PM&R Academy in 1938 (Brandt and Pope 1997, 31).

14. Roosevelt personally lobbied AOA members and recruited the New York orthopedist LeRoy Hubbard to oversee the progress of Warm Springs patients. Dr. Hubbard's positive report convinced the AOA to endorse the Warm Springs hydrotherapeutic center in 1927.

10. PHYSICAL AND OCCUPATIONAL THERAPY

1. Some people get physical or occupational therapy specifically for vocational rehabilitation. Of people with major mobility limitations, just over 20 percent report having received physical therapy specifically for vocational rehabilitation, as do 13 percent of those with moderate and 11 percent of persons with mild impairments. Among those who received physical therapy for vocational rehabilitation, the percentage obtaining these services from state rehabilitation agencies is 16 for minor, 24 for moderate, and 23 percent for major mobility difficulties. Of people reporting major mobility problems, just over 7 percent received occupational therapy for vocational purposes, as did 3 percent of those with mild and moderate impairments. Among those who received occupational therapy for vocational rehabilitation, the percentage obtaining these services from state rehabilitation agencies is 27 for minor, 32 for moder-

ate, and 26 percent for major mobility difficulties (these figures come from the 1994–95 NHIS-D Phase II and are adjusted for age group and sex).

2. The mean (standard deviation) number of PT visits in the last year is 19 (17), 20 (18), and 21 (21) for persons with minor, moderate, and major mobility difficulties, respectively. The mean (standard deviation) number of OT visits in the last year is 24 (15), 19 (16), and 18 (15) for persons with minor, moderate, and major mobility difficulties, respectively (these figures come from the 1994–95 NHIS-D Phase II and are adjusted for age group and sex).

3. These ranges reflect percentages for persons with minor to major mobility difficulties (the findings come from the 1994–95 NHIS-D Phase II and are adjusted for age group and sex).

4. As of 1990, only 79 percent of U.S. hospitals (regardless of type) report offering physical therapy, with just 53 percent providing occupational therapy (Punwar 1994, 109).

5. This study surveyed working-age persons with physical disabilities at an outpatient vocational rehabilitation facility in New York City. The five most common causes of disability among respondents were paraplegia and quadriplegia, low back pain, hemiplegia, MS, and cerebral palsy.

11. AMBULATION AIDS

1. As expected, use of mobility aids is especially high among people reporting being unable to walk 3 city blocks, climb 10 stairs without resting, or stand 20 minutes: among these persons, 33 percent use canes, 4 percent crutches, 22 percent walkers, and 26 percent wheelchairs (these figures come from the 1994–95 NHIS-D Phase I).

2. According to the 1994–95 NHIS-D Phase I, the following percentages (estimated millions of people) anticipate using mobility aids for twelve months or longer: 2 (estimated 3.91 million) use canes; 0.1 (0.14 million) use crutches; 0.7 (1.33 million) use walkers; 0.66 (1.23 million) use wheelchairs or scooters; and 0.6 percent (1.18 million) use more than one mobility aid.

3. People with strokes or MS are most likely to use wheelchairs, while cane use is highest among people with amputations, and walker use is highest for people with diabetes. People with back problems are least likely to use wheelchairs. However, within specific chronic condition groups, responses about mobility aid use are often missing. Therefore, it is unclear whether the remaining people (i.e., 100 percent minus the percentage reporting mobility aid use) do not use any mobility aids or did not respond to the question.

4. For persons reporting major mobility difficulties, patterns of mobility aid use also vary by selected demographic characteristics. Older people use canes significantly more often than younger people but are much less likely to use crutches or wheelchairs. Women are significantly less likely than men to use canes, crutches, or wheelchairs, and much more likely to use walkers. Black people use canes more frequently than whites or people of other races. These findings come from four multivariable logistic regression analyses of 1994–95 NHIS-D Phase I data using each of the four mobility aids as the outcome (de-

pendent) variable and the following predictor (independent) variables: age group; sex; race (white, black, other nonwhite); ethnicity (Hispanic); education (high school or less, college, graduate school); living alone; living in a rural area; household income (less than $15,000, $15,000–$30,000, $30,000–$50,000, and $50,000+); and having health insurance.

5. Some believe (based largely on conventional wisdom) that "quad" or four-point canes offer superior stability to single-point canes. One study involving only 14 stroke patients found no advantage for the four-point cane (Milczarek et al. 1993). Some people like the four-point cane because it can stand on its own (e.g., next to someone's chair), while others find it unwieldy and cumbersome.

12. WHEELED MOBILITY

1. The federal Justice Department brought an antitrust lawsuit against E&J in the late 1970s, charging it with monopoly practices and setting artificially high prices. After the lawsuit was settled, E&J was slow to tap into the new market of independent wheelchair users who pushed consumer empowerment (Shapiro 1994, 216). It finally retooled its operations and tried new lightweight plastic composites.

2. Even the name "Quickie" is a lighthearted double entendre, mocking the assumption that sex life ends when legs stop working.

3. The population estimate of wheelchairs currently in use is 1.35 million manual wheelchairs, 128,700 power wheelchairs, and 129,400 scooters (1994–95 NHIS-D Phase I). Estimates for people expected to use their wheelchairs for 12 months or more are slightly lower (chapter 15).

4. The average age of power wheelchair users (54 years) is younger than that of manual wheelchairs (66 years) and scooters (62 years), according to the 1994–95 NHIS-D Phase I. For power wheelchair users, more time had elapsed since the onset of their mobility difficulties (16 years) than for manual wheelchair or scooter users (both 10 years). These figures suggest that power wheelchair users, on average, have significantly debilitating conditions that occur in early middle age, such as MS and ALS, or have had disabling injuries in their youth.

5. Airlines pack wet-cell batteries in protective boxes; some airlines refuse to allow wet-cell batteries on board certain airplanes because if batteries spill, they can erode through the fuselage. Because scooters routinely use gel-cell batteries, they are easier to take on airplanes than wheelchairs using wet-cell batteries. Most airlines leave the gel-cell batteries attached to my scooter's platform.

6. Advanced prosthetic technologies, with sophisticated bioengineering aided by new lightweight materials, have dramatically improved since Cleland's rehabilitation in the 1960s. Today he might make the same decision to use the wheelchair, but he would have more choices. High costs prevent many people with amputations, like Arnis Balodis, from taking full advantage of these new technologies.

13. WHO WILL PAY?

1. Most Medicare recipients purchase private supplemental insurance to reimburse some uncovered services, including deductibles and coinsurance. Perhaps for this reason, only 6 to 7 percent of people age 65+ with major and moderate mobility difficulties report having delayed needed care, as did 3 percent of those with no or mild impairments. In this age range, percentages of recipients who report needing prescription drugs they could not afford are 1 percent among people without mobility difficulties; and 2, 3, and 4 percent among people with minor, moderate, and major difficulties, respectively. In contrast, just over 13 percent of younger persons reporting major mobility problems could not afford prescription medications, compared to roughly 2 percent of those without mobility limitations (these rates come from the 1994–95 NHIS-D Phase I and 1994–95 Family Resources supplement).

2. This finding comes from a multivariable logistic regression analysis using 1994–95 NHIS-D Phase I data with wheelchair use as the outcome (dependent) variable and the following predictor (independent) variables: age group; sex; race (white, black, other nonwhite); ethnicity (Hispanic); education (high school or less, college, graduate school); living alone; living in a rural area; household income (less than $15,000, $15,000–$30,000, $30,000–$50,000, and $50,000+); and having health insurance. An identical multivariable logistic regression was performed with walker use as the dependent variable.

3. Legislative reports and statements made during congressional deliberations give guidance for interpreting the ADA. Several examples include the following (Feldblum 1991, 101): first, employers may not refuse to hire persons because they will have higher insurance or health-care costs. Second, employers and health insurers may keep "preexisting condition clauses" in their health plans, even if such provisions deny benefits for specified times to people with disabilities. For instance, an employer's health plan could exclude diabetes care for some time for workers with preexisting diabetes. Third, employers and health insurers may limit coverage for specified procedures or treatments. Finally, employers may not, however, allow health plans to completely deny coverage to people because of their diagnoses. Even if plans exclude payments for preexisting conditions or specified therapies, they must cover other health problems, procedures, or treatments.

4. By definition, to qualify as disabled under Social Security and be eligible for SSDI (and Medicare) or SSI (and Medicaid), people must demonstrate they cannot be employed (i.e., cannot perform a "substantial gainful activity," chapter 7). So probably being unemployed and having Medicare or Medicaid are tightly linked among working-age persons.

5. The percentages of people denied health insurance when they applied for coverage is 1 percent for people without mobility difficulties and 4, 5, and 5 percent among those with minor, moderate, and major problems, respectively. Among these people, the most common reason for being denied coverage is preexisting health conditions (46, 60, 62, and 77 percent of persons with none, minor, moderate, and major mobility difficulties, respectively). The second most common reason is poor health risks, such as smoking or being overweight

(8, 11, 4, and 11 percent across the four groups). These figures come from the 1994–95 NHIS-D Phase I and 1994–95 Family Resources supplement and are adjusted for age group and sex.

6. An important exception was enactment of Medicare's End Stage Renal Disease (ESRD) program in 1972. However, the political rationale and structure of the ESRD program proved unique: "The ESRD program did not foreshadow universal coverage or even reveal a new sensitivity to the tough policy issues raised by chronic disease" (Fox 1993, 77).

7. All C.F.R. references are dated 1 October 1999.

8. Recent changes grant Medicare coverage of palliative hospice care for persons in the last six months of life with terminal illnesses, and selected preventive services, such as certain immunizations and screening mammograms.

9. As of 1982, Medicare added health maintenance organizations (HMOs) to traditional indemnity coverage. Many of these plans provided prescription drugs and other benefits not covered by traditional Medicare, but they also tended to recruit healthier Medicare beneficiaries than average. The Balanced Budget Act of 1997 and the Balanced Budget Refinement Act of 1999 introduced new types of health plans, managed care organizations (MCOs), and reimbursement policies (risk adjustment and new ways of setting local payment rates). Many MCOs are revising their benefits packages, with some eliminating the additional services, while others are dropping Medicare enrollees. As of 1 January 2001, Medicare MCOs dropped over 933,000 elderly and disabled beneficiaries, leaving beneficiaries scrambling to find new health plans (Thomas 2000). Among people dropped from Medicare MCOs, 43 percent now worry about paying their health-care bills (Laschober et al. 1999, 155).

10. Eligibility for SSI (enacted in 1972 and implemented in 1974) immediately confers Medicaid coverage, although details of benefits vary state-to-state. States may follow the so-called 209(b) option, which allows tightening of Medicaid eligibility requirements beyond the standard SSI disability or means tests (Tanenbaum 1989). States may also liberalize Medicaid eligibility under Section 1619 of the 1980 Social Security Act Amendments, which aims to encourage work among SSI recipients.

11. Evidence clearly suggests that Medicare MCOs have systematically sought "healthier" members, avoiding persons with chronic disease and disability. Advertising campaigns featuring vigorous elders, swimming at health clubs, square dancing, or playing golf, convey a subtle message that the physically fit should apply. Whether health club memberships provided through health plans include personal trainers or customized exercise programs for people with mobility difficulties is not widely known.

12. Medicare originally explicitly did not cover orthopedic shoes. However, Mrs. Johnson's knowledge of Medicare is up to date, although her comment about arthritis is probably correct only in limited situations. According to a specialist at 1–800-MEDICARE (contacted 5 January 2001), as of March 1998 an amendment to the Medicare Medical Policy Manual allows coverage of orthopedic shoes for persons with diabetes or when the shoe is attached to a leg

brace. In either case, physicians must submit a prescription for the shoes, indicating correctly the relevant diagnosis.

13. In California: "Medically Necessary means reasonable and necessary services to protect life, to prevent significant illness or significant disability, or to alleviate severe pain through the diagnosis or treatment of disease, illness, or injury" (Rosenbaum et al. 1998, 2:694).

In Pennsylvania: "the service or benefit will, or is reasonably expected to, prevent the onset of an illness, condition, or disability . . . reduce or ameliorate the physical, mental, or developmental effects of an illness, condition, injury, or disability . . . assist the individual to achieve or maintain maximum functional capacity in performing daily activities" (Rosenbaum et al. 1998, 2:711–12).

In South Carolina: "those medical services which . . . are essential to prevent, diagnose, prevent the worsening of, alleviate, correct or cure medical conditions that endanger life, cause suffering or pain, cause physical deformity or malfunction, threaten to cause or aggravate a handicap, or result in illness or infirmity" (Rosenbaum et al. 1998, 2:715).

14. In clarifying the "homebound definition," Section 507 of the Beneficiary Improvement and Protection Act (P.L. 106–554, enacted 21 December 2000) eliminated the phrase that "absences from home are infrequent or of relatively short duration or are attributable to receiving medical treatment." The following text was inserted: "Any absences of an individual from the home attributable to the need to receive health care . . . shall not disqualify an individual from being considered to be 'confined to his home.' Any other absence of an individual from the home shall not so disqualify an individual if the absence is of infrequent or of relatively short duration. . . . Any absence for the purpose of attending a religious service shall be deemed to be an absence of infrequent or short duration."

15. Every interviewee had some health insurance: Medicare, either because of age or SSDI; Medicaid, qualifying by poverty with or without disability (SSI); or private, employment-based insurance, by themselves, through their spouse, through disability or retirement pensions, or through COBRA provisions following job loss.

14. WHAT WILL BE PAID FOR?

1. Two bills submitted to Congress (HR 1490 and S 2085) would have created the Homebound Clarification Act of 2001. Supporters hoped these bills would be added to a Medicare reform bill at the end of the 2002 congressional session. HR 1490 would have eliminated the language of the homebound definition added in 2000 (see chapter 13 note 14) and replaced it with the following: "Any other absence of an individual from the home, including any absence for the purpose of attending a religious service, shall not so disqualify the individual." These bills and President George W. Bush's declaration on 26 July 2002 were motivated by a grassroots campaign largely spurred by David Jayne, a Georgia resident who had developed ALS in 1988 at age twenty-seven. Over the years Mr. Jayne had become totally incapacitated, and in 1997 Medicare

started paying for skilled nursing care in his home. However, in 2000, Mr. Jayne traveled out of town with a college friend to watch a Georgia Bulldog football game. The trip and Mr. Jayne's story appeared in an Atlanta newspaper, and shortly thereafter his home health agency discharged him for violating the homebound definition. His local congressman, Mac Collins, arranged for Mr. Jayne's services to be reinstated, but Mr. Jayne began campaigning to reform the homebound definition. He founded the National Coalition to Amend the Medicare Homebound Restriction and proved an exceptional lobbyist, although now he speaks only with the aid of a computer.

2. The president's statement comes from the White House web site (http://www.whitehouse.gov/news/releases/2002/07/20020726-8.html) accessed on 27 July 2002.

3. Medicare also explicitly limits treatment in rehabilitation hospitals, reimbursing care only for patients viewed as likely to benefit from intensive physical, occupational, and/or speech-language therapy and to return home soon afterward. Patients must be sufficiently ill to require hospital-level services, defined as needing round-the-clock skilled nursing care overseen by physicians. In 1982 HCFA stipulated that all persons admitted to rehabilitation hospitals must receive physical therapy and occupational therapy at least 3 hours a day, 5 days a week, with slightly reduced hours on weekends (Gillick 1995, 203). These policies effectively exclude persons who are too debilitated for 3-hour daily therapy sessions.

4. Medicare Part A covers home-based physical and occupational therapies, while outpatient therapies (services provided at a clinic or office) "when they are medically necessary" fall under Part B. Medicare beneficiaries pay nothing out-of-pocket for home health services and 20 percent copayments for outpatient services. Although administrative details differ for home health and outpatient services, the basic intent is identical (these provisions also address speech-language therapy, as someone might need after a stroke). First, Medicare's home-care regulations state that "physical and occupational therapy and speech-language pathology services must relate directly and specifically to a treatment regimen (established by the physician, after any needed consultation with the qualified therapist) that is designed to treat the beneficiary's illness or injury" (42 C.F.R. Sec. 409.44[c][1]). Physicians must review and sign the plan of care at least every 62 days for home-health services (42 C.F.R. Sec. 409.43[e]) and at least every 30 days for outpatient services (42 C.F.R. Sec. 410.61[e]). The therapy must be "reasonable and necessary" (42 C.F.R. Sec. 409.44[c][2]).

5. For outpatient therapy, the 1997 Balanced Budget Act (BBA) imposed two annual $1,500 caps: one for physical therapy and speech-language pathology and another for occupational therapy, excluding services provided by hospital outpatient departments. The 1999 Balanced Budget Refinement Act (BBRA) delayed implementation of some BBA provisions, including a two-year moratorium on the $1,500 cap on outpatient therapy, which was extended through 2002.

6. Legislation has been submitted to allow people to pay the difference between Medicare's allowed cost and the actual price for medical equipment.

7. Although some people receive DME and home modifications through state-sponsored vocational rehabilitation programs, vocational rehabilitation generally targets only those deemed "employable" and often excludes middle-aged people with progressive chronic conditions. In addition, many states have significantly reduced funding for DME and related services (Karp 1998, 28).

8. Even the phrase "power operated vehicle" suggests a car or other mode of voluntary transportation, rather than a wheelchair a person requires for mobility.

9. Medicare covers power wheelchairs only when necessary based on the beneficiary's "medical and physical condition." The equipment must meet safety specifications promulgated by CMS (42 C.F.R. Sec. 410.38[c]). Medicare accepts prescriptions for these wheelchairs only from specialists in physical medicine, orthopedic surgery, neurology, or rheumatology (or from the beneficiary's regular physician if specialists are distant or the person's medical condition prevents travel to a specialist). Vendors must have physicians' prescriptions in hand before they supply the equipment.

10. The other three questions on Form HCFA 850(4/96) and OMB no. 0938–0679 are "Is the physician signing this form a specialist in physical medicine, orthopedic surgery, neurology, or rheumatology?"; "Is the patient more than one day's round trip from a specialist in physical medicine, orthopedic surgery, neurology, or rheumatology?"; and "Does the patient's physical condition prevent a visit to a specialist in physical medicine, orthopedic surgery, neurology, or rheumatology?"

11. Medicare makes coverage decisions at the national level for important new technologies with widespread implications (for other new interventions, the dozens of contractors that process Part A and B claims around the country make decisions). Major national coverage decisions involve analyzing medical evidence and posting proposed rules in the *Federal Register*, soliciting public comment. Medicare's decision to cover liver transplants, for example, took four to five years. Local Medicare billing contractors make decisions more idiosyncratically, often relying on regional medical opinions rather than explicit evidence.

12. Although Medicare's policies are still evolving, proposed rules for making coverage decisions echo medical necessity standards, following four sequential steps (HCFA 2000b, 31127).

Step 1—medical benefit: Does sufficient evidence demonstrate that the item or service medically benefits a defined population?

Step 2—added value: For this defined patient population, do medically beneficial alternatives exist that are currently covered by Medicare and within the same clinical modality?

Step 3—added value: How does the benefit of the item or service compare to the Medicare-covered alternative?

Step 4—added value: Will costs of the item or service be equivalent or lower for the Medicare population than the Medicare-covered alternative?

15. FINAL THOUGHTS

1. This study comes from Ontario. Canada's health-care system differs significantly from that in the United States: all Canadians have health insurance.

2. Dishonest or disingenuous equipment vendors and therapists undoubtedly do bilk the system, urging people to purchase unnecessary items or services. Policies should aim to prevent these abuses, not to withhold needed devices or therapies.

3. Along with many other middle-aged people with progressive chronic conditions, Jimmy Howard has not been referred to state vocational rehabilitation. Purchases of assistive technology and required training through state vocational rehabilitation programs appear idiosyncratic.

4. Numbers represent population estimates from the 1994–95 NHIS-D Phase I for people reporting they will use the equipment for at least 12 months.

5. The NHIS-D gives cross-sectional prevalence estimates—the number of people who experience mobility difficulties—not incidence estimates (the number of people who develop mobility difficulties each year). If a new program purchased wheelchairs this year for all people with major mobility problems who need them, next year the program would have to buy equipment only for those newly developing difficulties, a much smaller number.

6. These findings come from the 1994–95 NHIS-D Phase II and are adjusted for age group and sex.

7. As elsewhere on the Internet, charlatans may misstate or exaggerate claims. The federal National Institute on Disability and Rehabilitation Research in the U.S. Department of Education has a web site that covers a variety of mobility-related topics, including equipment, with the content examined for accuracy (www.ed.gov/offices/OSERS/NIDRR/index.html).

8. Many conditions that impair mobility, such as arthritis, MS, and Parkinson's disease, also limit fine-motor movements involving the hands, such as using a keyboard or moving a mouse to position the cursor on the computer screen. Although new technologies allow "hands-free" use of computers, these devices are not widely available, are expensive, and may be affected by speech or language disorders.

9. Percentages for persons with mild and moderate mobility problems are similar to those for people with major difficulties.

10. These projections derive from the Longitudinal Study of Aging and consider six common chronic conditions: arthritis, stroke, diabetes, coronary artery disease, cancer, and confusion.

References

Albrecht, G. L., K. D. Seelman, and M. Bury, eds. 2001. *Handbook of Disability Studies.* Thousand Oaks, Calif.: Sage Publications.

Alexander, N. B. 1996. Gait Disorders in Older Adults. *Journal of the American Geriatrics Society* 44, no. 4:434–51.

Altman, B. M. 2001. Disability Definitions, Models, Classification Schemes, and Applications. In *Handbook of Disability Studies,* ed. G. L. Albrecht, K. D. Seelman, and M. Bury, 97–122. Thousand Oaks, Calif.: Sage Publications.

American Academy of Physical Medicine and Rehabilitation. 2000. http://www.aapmr.org, accessed 27 March.

American Medical Association, Department of Geriatric Health. 1996. *Guidelines for the Use of Assertive Technology: Evaluation, Referral, Prescription.* 2d ed. Chicago.

American Occupational Therapy Association. 2001. http://www.aota.org, accessed 14 February.

American Physical Therapy Association. 2001. http://www.apta.org, accessed 14 February.

Andriacchi, R. 1997. Primary Care for Persons with Disabilities: The Internal Medicine Perspective. *American Journal of Physical Medicine and Rehabilitation* 76, no. 3 (Supplement):S17–S20.

Atkinson, R. L. 2000. A 33-year-old Woman with Morbid Obesity. *Journal of the American Medical Association* 283, no. 24:3236–43.

Barker, L. R., J. R. Burton, and P. D. Zieve, eds. 1999. *Principles of Ambulatory Medicine.* 5th ed. Baltimore: Williams and Wilkins.

Barnard, D. 1995. Chronic Illness and the Dynamics of Hoping. In *Chronic Illness: From Experience to Policy,* ed. S. K. Toombs, D. Barnard, and R. D. Carson, 38–57. Bloomington: Indiana University Press.

Barnes, C., G. Mercer, and T. Shakespeare. 1999. In *Exploring Disability: A Sociological Introduction.* Cambridge: Polity Press.

Batavia, A. I. 1999. Of Wheelchairs and Managed Care. *Health Affairs* 18, no. 6:177–82.

———. 2000. Ten Years Later: The ADA and the Future of Disability Policy. In *Americans with Disabilities: Exploring Implications of the Law for Individuals and Institutions,* ed. L. P. Francis and A. Silvers, 283–92. New York: Routledge.

Baynton, D. C. 2001. Disability and the Justification of Inequality in American History. In *The New Disability History: American Perspectives,* ed. P. K. Longmore and L. Umansky, 33–57. New York: New York University.

Benjamin, A. E. 2001. Consumer-Directed Services at Home: A New Model for Persons with Disabilities. *Health Affairs* 20, no. 6:80–95.

Berger, J. T., F. Rosner, P. Kark, and A. J. Bennett, for the Committee on Bioethical Issues of the Medical Society of the State of New York. 2000. Reporting by Physicians of Impaired Drivers and Potentially Impaired Drivers. *Journal of General Internal Medicine* 15, no. 9:667–72.

Berkowitz, E., and D. M. Fox. 1989. The Politics of Social Security Expansion: Social Security Disability Insurance, 1935–1986. *Journal of Policy History* 1, no. 3:233–60.

Berkowitz, M., P. K. O'Leary, D. L. Kruse, and C. Harvey. 1998. *Spinal Cord Injury: An Analysis of Medical and Social Costs.* New York: Demos Medical Publishing.

Bickenbach, J. E. 2001. Disability Human Rights, Law, and Policy. In *Handbook of Disability Studies,* ed. G. L. Albrecht, K. D. Seelman, and M. Bury, 565–84. Thousand Oaks, Calif.: Sage Publications.

Blanck, P. D. 2000. Studying Disability, Employment Policy and the ADA. In *Americans with Disabilities: Exploring Implications of the Law for Individuals and Institutions,* ed. L. P. Francis and A. Silvers, 209–20. New York: Routledge.

Bockenek, W. L., N. Mann, I. S. Lanig, G. DeJong, and L. A. Beatty. 1998. Primary Care for Persons with Disabilities. In *Rehabilitation Medicine: Principles and Practice,* ed. J. A. DeLisa and B. M. Gans, 905–28. Philadelphia: Lippincott-Raven Publishers.

Boult, C., M. Altmann, D. Gilbertson, C. Yu, and R. L. Kane. 1996. Decreasing Disability in the 21st Century: The Future Effect of Controlling Six Fatal and Nonfatal Conditions. *American Journal of the Public Health* 86, no. 10:1388–93.

Boult, C., L. Boult, L. Morishita, S. L. Smith, and R. L. Kane. 1998. Outpatient Geriatric Evaluation and Management. *Journal of the American Geriatrics Society* 46, no. 3:296–302.

Branch, W. T., Jr., ed. 1994. *Office Practice of Medicine.* 3d ed. Philadelphia: W. B. Saunders.

Brandt, E. N., Jr., and A. M. Pope, eds. 1997. In *Enabling America: Assessing the Role of Rehabilitation Sciences and Engineering.* Washington, D.C.: Institute of Medicine.

Burns, T. J., A. I. Batavia, Q. W. Smith, and G. DeJong. 1990. Primary Health Care Needs of Persons with Physical Disabilities: What Are the Research and Service Priorities? *Archives of Physical Medicine and Rehabilitation* 71, no. 2:138–43.

Byrom, B. 2001. A Pupil and a Patient: Hospital-Schools in Progressive America. In *The New Disability History: American Perspectives,* ed. P. K. Longmore and L. Umansky, 133–56. New York: New York University.

Calkins, D. R., L. V. Rubenstein, P. D. Cleary, A. R. Davies, A. M. Jette, A. Fink, J. Kosecoff, R. T. Young, R. H. Brook, and T. L. Delbanco. 1991. Failure of Physicians to Recognize Functional Disability in Ambulatory Patients. *Annals of Internal Medicine* 114, no. 6:451–54.

———. 1994. Functional Disability Screening of Ambulatory Patients: A Randomized Controlled Trial in a Hospital-Based Group Practice. *Journal of General Internal Medicine* 9, no. 10:590–92.

Canedy, D. 2002. Wheelchair Users Fly More, and Airlines Try to Adapt. *New York Times,* 2 January:YNE A12.

Cassell, E. J. 1997. *Doctoring. The Nature of Primary Care Medicine.* New York: Oxford University Press.

Centers for Disease Control and Prevention. 1994. Arthritis Prevalence and Activity Limitations—United States, 1990. *Journal of the American Medical Association* 272, no. 5:346–47.

———. 2001a. Physical Activity Trends—United States, 1990–1998. *Morbidity and Mortality Weekly Report* 50, no. 9:166–69.

———. 2001b. Prevalence of Arthritis—United States, 1997. *Morbidity and Mortality Weekly Report* 50, no. 17:334–36.

Chan, L., J. N. Doctor, R. F. MacLehose, H. Lawson, R. A. Rosenblatt, L. M. Baldwin, and A. Jha. 1999. Do Medicare Patients with Disabilities Receive Preventive Services? A Population-Based Study. *Archives of Physical Medicine and Rehabilitation* 80, no. 6:642–46.

Charlton, J. I. 1998. *Nothing About Us Without Us: Disability Oppression and Empowerment.* Berkeley: University of California Press.

Chirikos, T. N. 1991. The Economics of Employment. In *The Americans with Disabilities Act: From Policy to Practice,* ed. J. West, 150–79. New York: Milbank Memorial Fund.

Cleland, M. 1989. *Strong at the Broken Places.* Atlanta: Cherokee Publishing.

Cocchiarella, L., and G. B. J. Andersson, eds. 2001. *Guides to the Evaluation of Permanent Impairment.* 5th ed. Chicago: American Medical Association.

Cooper, B., P. Rigby, and L. Letts. 1995. Evaluation of Access to Home, Community, and Workplace. In *Occupational Therapy for Physical Dysfunction,* ed. C. A. Trombly, 55–72. 4th ed. Baltimore: Williams and Wilkins.

Covinsky, K. E., L. Goldman, E. F. Cook, R. Oye, N. Desbiens, D. Reding, W. Fulkerson, A. F. Connors, Jr., J. Lynn, and R. S. Phillips for the SUPPORT Investigators. 1994. The Impact of Serious Illness on Patients' Families. *Journal of the American Medical Association* 272, no. 23:1839–44.

Currie, D. M., K. Hardwick, and R. A. Marburger. 1998. Wheelchair Prescription and Adaptive Seating. In *Rehabilitation Medicine: Principles and Practice,* ed. J. A. DeLisa, and B. M. Gans, 763–88. 3d ed. Philadelphia: Lippincott-Raven Publishers.

Curry, R. L. 1995. The Exceptional Family: Walking the Edge of Tragedy and Transformation. In *Chronic Illness: From Experience to Policy*, ed. S. K. Toombs, D. Barnard, and R. D. Carson, 24–37. Bloomington: Indiana University Press.

Cutler, D. M. 2001. Declining Disability among the Elderly. *Health Affairs* 20, no. 6:11–27.

Cwynar, D. A., and T. McNerney. 1999. A Primer on Physical Therapy. *Primary Care Practice* 3, no. 4:451–59.

DeJong, G. 1997. Primary Care for Persons with Disabilities: An Overview of the Problem. *American Journal of Physical Medicine and Rehabilitation* 76, no. 3 (Supplement):S2-S8.

DeLisa, J. A., D. M. Currie, and G. M. Martin. 1998. Rehabilitation Medicine: Past, Present, and Future. In *Rehabilitation Medicine: Principles and Practice*, ed. J. A. DeLisa and B. M. Gans, 3–32. 3d ed. Philadelphia: Lippincott-Raven Publishers.

Dickens, C. 1981. *Christmas Books.* Oxford: Oxford University Press.

Dolan, P. 1996. The Effect of Experience of Illness on Health State Valuations. *Journal of Clinical Epidemiology* 49, no. 5:551–64.

Douard, J. W. 1995. Disability and the Persistence of the "Normal." In *Chronic Illness: From Experience to Policy*, ed. S. K. Toombs, D. Barnard, and R. D. Carson, 154–75. Bloomington: Indiana University Press.

Edgman-Levitan, S. 1993. Providing Effective Emotional Support. In *Through the Patient's Eyes*, ed. M. Gerteis, S. Edgman-Levitan, J. Daley, and T. L. Delbanco, 154–77. San Francisco: Jossey-Bass Publishers.

Eisenberg, D. M., R. C. Kessler, C. Foster, F. E. Norlock, D. R. Calkins, and T. L. Delbanco. 1993. Unconventional Medicine in the United States: Prevalence, Costs, and Patterns of Use. *New England Journal of Medicine* 328, no. 4:246–52.

Eisenberg, D. M., R. B. Davis, S. L. Ettner, S. Appel, S. Wilkey, M. Van Rompay, and R. C. Kessler. 1998. Trends in Alternative Medicine Use in the United States, 1990–1997: Results of a Follow-up National Survey. *Journal of the American Medical Association* 280, no. 18:1569–75.

Eklund, V. A., and M. L. MacDonald. 1991. Descriptions of Persons with Multiple Sclerosis, with an Emphasis on What is Needed from Psychologists. *Professional Psychology: Research and Practice* 22:277–84.

Ellenberg, D. B. 1996. Outcomes Research: The History, Debate, and Implications for the Field of Occupational Therapy. *American Journal of Occupational Therapy* 50, no. 6:435–41.

Ellers, B. 1993. Innovations in Patient-Centered Education. In *Through the Patient's Eyes*, ed. M. Gerteis, S. Edgman-Levitan, J. Daley, and T. L. Delbanco. 96–118. San Francisco: Jossey-Bass Publishers.

Feinglass, J., J. L. Brown, A. LoSasso, M. W. Sohn, L. M. Manheim, S. J. Shah, and W. H. Pearce. 1999. Rates of Lower-Extremity Amputation and Arterial Reconstruction in the United States, 1979 to 1996. *American Journal of Public Health* 89, no. 8:1222–27.

Feldblum, C. R. 1991. Employment Protections. In *The Americans with Disabilities Act: From Policy to Practice,* ed. J. West, 81–110. New York: Milbank Memorial Fund.

Feldman, P. H. 1997. Labor Market Issues in Home Care. In *Home-Based Care for a New Century,* ed. D. M. Fox and C. Raphael, 155–83. New York: Milbank Memorial Fund.

Figg, L., and J. Farrell-Beck. 1993. Amputation in the Civil War: Physical and Social Dimensions. *Journal of the History of Medicine and Allied Sciences* 48, no. 4:454–75.

Fine, M., and A. Asch, eds. 1988. *Women with Disabilities. Essays in Psychology, Culture, and Politics.* Philadelphia: Temple University Press.

Fisher, B., and R. Galler. 1988. In Friendship and Fairness: How Disability Affects Friendship Between Women. In *Women with Disabilities. Essays in Psychology, Culture, and Politics,* ed. M. Fine and A. Asch, 172–94. Philadelphia: Temple University Press.

Foley, M. P., B. Prax, R. Crowell, and T. Boone. 1996. Effects of Assistive Devices on Cardiorespiratory Demands in Older Adults. *Physical Therapy* 76, no. 12:1313–19.

Foote, S. M., and C. Hogan. 2001. Disability Profile and Health Care Costs of Medicare Beneficiaries Under Age Sixty-Five. *Health Affairs* 20, no. 6:242–53.

Fox, D. M. 1989. Policy and Epidemiology: Financing Health Services for the Chronically Ill and Disabled, 1930–1990. *Milbank Quarterly* 67, suppl. 2, pt. 2:257–87.

———. 1993. *Power and Illness: The Failure and Future of American Health Policy.* Berkeley: University of California Press.

Francis, L. P., and A. Silvers, eds. 2000. *Americans with Disabilities: Exploring Implications of the Law for Individuals and Institutions.* New York: Routledge.

Freedman, V. A., and L. G. Martin. 1998. Understanding Trends in Functional Limitations Among Older Americans. *American Journal of Public Health* 88, no. 10:1457–62.

Freudenheim, M. 1999. Employers Focus on Weight as Workplace Health Issue. *New York Times,* 6 September, YNE A11.

Friedson, E. 1970. *Professional Dominance: The Social Structure of Medical Care.* Chicago: Aldine Publishing.

Gaal, R. P., N. Rebholtz, R. D. Hotchkiss, and P. F. Pfaelzer. 1997. Wheelchair Rider Injuries: Causes and Consequences for Wheelchair Design and Selection. *Journal of Rehabilitation Research and Development* 34, no. 1:58–71.

Gallagher, H. G. 1994. *FDR's Splendid Deception.* Arlington, Va.: Vandamere Press.

———. 1998. *Black Bird Fly Away: Disabled in an Able-Bodied World.* Arlington, Va.: Vandamere Press.

Gans, B. M., N. R. Mann, and B. E. Becker. 1993. Delivery of Primary Care to the Physically Challenged. *Archives of Physical Medicine and Rehabilitation* 74, no. 12:S15-S19.

Geiringer, S. R. 1998. Interactions with the Medico Legal System. In *Rehabilitation Medicine: Principles and Practice,* ed. J. A. DeLisa and B. M. Gans, 231–38. 3d ed. Philadelphia: Lippincott-Raven Publishers.

Gerteis, M., S. Edgman-Levitan, J. Daley, and T. L. Delbanco, eds. 1993. *Through the Patient's Eyes.* San Francisco: Jossey-Bass Publishers.

Gilbert, M. 1991. *Churchill: A Life.* New York: Henry Holt.

Gillick, M. R. 1995. The Role of the Rules: The Impact of the Bureaucratization of Long-Term Care. In *Chronic Illness: From Experience to Policy,* ed. S. K. Toombs, D. Barnard, and R. D. Carson, 189–211. Bloomington: Indiana University Press.

Goffman, E. 1963. *Stigma: Notes on the Management of Spoiled Identity.* New York: Simon and Schuster.

Goodwin, D. K. 1994. *No Ordinary Time: Franklin and Eleanor Roosevelt: The Home Front in World War II.* New York: Simon and Schuster.

Goroll, A. H., L. A. May, and A. G. Mulley, Jr., eds. 1995. *Primary Care Medicine: Office Evaluation and Management of the Adult Patient.* 3d ed. Philadelphia: J. B. Lippincott.

Guide to Physical Therapist Practice. 2001. *Physical Therapy.* 2d ed. Vol. 8:9–744.

Hall, J. A., M. A. Milburn, D. L. Roter, and L. H. Daltroy. 1998. Why Are Sicker Patients Less Satisfied with Their Medical Care? Tests of Two Explanatory Models. *Health Psychology* 17, no. 1:70–75.

Hall, J. A., D. L. Roter, M. A. Milburn, and L. H. Daltroy. 1996. Patients' Health as a Predictor of Physician and Patient Behavior in Medical Visits: A Synthesis of Four Studies. *Medical Care* 34, no. 12:1205–18.

Harmon, A. 2001. An Inventor Unveils His Mysterious Personal Transportation Device. *New York Times,* 13 December:C1.

Harris Interactive. 2000. *2000 National Organization on Disability/Harris Survey of Americans with Disabilities.* Conducted for the National Organization on Disability. New York: Harris Interactive.

Hawker, G. A., J. G. Wright, P. C. Coyte, J. I. Williams, B. Harvey, R. Glazier, A. Wilkins, and E. M. Badley. 2001. Determining the Need for Hip and Knee Arthroplasty: The Role of Clinical Severity and Patients' Preferences. *Medical Care* 39, no. 3:206–16.

Health Care Financing Administration, United States Department of Health and Human Services. 2000a. *Medicare and You 2001.* Publication no. HCFA-10050. Baltimore, September.

———. 2000b. Medicare Program: Criteria for Making Coverage Decisions. *Federal Register* 65, no. 95 (16 May):31124–29.

Hockenberry, J. 1995. *Moving Violations: War Zones, Wheelchairs, and Declarations of Independence.* New York: Hyperion.

Hoenig, H. 1993. Educating Primary Care Physicians in Geriatric Rehabilitation. *Clinics in Geriatric Medicine* 9, no. 4:883–93.

Hoenig, H., C. Pieper, M. Zolkewitz, M. Schenkman, and L. G. Branch. 2002. Wheelchair Users Are Not Necessarily Wheelchair Bound. *Journal of the American Geriatrics Society* 50, no. 4:645–54.

Holm, M. B., J. C. Rogers, and A. B. James. 1998a. Treatment of Activities of Daily Living. In *Willard and Spackman's Occupational Therapy*, ed. M. E. Neistadt and E. B. Crepeau, 323–64. 9th ed. Philadelphia: Lippincott Williams and Wilkins.

Holm, M. B., J. C. Rogers, and R. G. Stone. 1998b. Person-Task-Environment Interventions: A Decision-Making Guide. In *Willard and Spackman's Occupational Therapy*, ed. M. E. Neistadt and E. B. Crepeau, 471–98. 9th ed. Philadelphia: Lippincott Williams and Wilkins.

Holman, H. 1996. What Would Ideal Care Look Like? In *Changing Health Care Systems and Rheumatic Disease*, ed. F. J. Manning, and J. A. Barondess, 35–49. Washington, D.C.: National Academy Press.

Iezzoni, L. I. 1999. Boundaries. *Health Affairs* 18, no. 6:171–76.

Iezzoni, L. I., E. P. McCarthy, R. B. Davis, and H. Siebens. 2000a. Mobility Impairments and Use of Screening and Preventive Services. *American Journal of Public Health* 90, no. 6:955–61.

Iezzoni, L. I., E. P. McCarthy, R. B. Davis, and H. Siebens. 2000b. Mobility Problems and Perceptions of Disability by Self-Respondents and Proxy-Respondents. *Medical Care* 38, no. 10:1051–57.

Iezzoni L. I., E. P. McCarthy, R. B. Davis, and H. Siebens. 2001. Mobility Difficulties Are Not Only a Problem of Old Age. *Journal of General Internal Medicine* 16, no. 4:235–43.

Illingworth, P., and W. E. Parmet. 2000. Positively Disabled. The Relationship Between the Definition of Disability and Rights Under the American Disability Act. In *Americans with Disabilities: Exploring Implications of the Law for Individuals and Institutions*, ed. L. P. Francis and A. Silvers, 3–17. New York: Routledge.

Inman, V. T., H. J. Ralston, and F. Todd. 1981. *Human Walking*. Baltimore: Williams and Wilkins.

Institute of Medicine, Committee on Quality of Health Care in America. 1999. *To Err Is Human: Building a Safer Health System*. Washington, D.C.: National Academy Press.

———. 2001a. *Crossing the Quality Chasm: A New Health System for the 21st Century*. Washington, D.C.: National Academy Press.

———. Committee on the Consequences of Uninsurance. 2001b. *Coverage Matters: Insurance and Health Care*. Washington, D.C.: National Academy Press.

Jefferson, T. 1984. Notes on the State of Virginia. In *Thomas Jefferson: Writings*, 123–325. New York: The Library of America.

Jeka, J. J. 1997. Light Touch Contact as a Balance Aid. *Physical Therapy* 77, no. 5:476–87.

Jones, J. G., J. McCann, and M. N. Lassere. 1991. Driving and Arthritis. *British Journal of Rheumatology* 30, no. 5:361–64.

Jones, N. L. 1991. Essential Requirements of the Act: A Short History and Overview. In *The Americans with Disabilities Act: From Policy to Practice*, ed. J. West. 25–54. New York: Milbank Memorial Fund.

Joyce, B. M., and R. L. Kirby. 1991. Canes, Crutches and Walkers. *American Family Physician* 43, no. 2:535–42.

Kamenetz, H. L. 1969. *The Wheelchair Book: Mobility for the Disabled.* Springfield, Ill.: Charles C. Thomas.

Kane, R. A., R. L. Kane, and R. C. Ladd. 1998. *The Heart of Long-Term Care.* New York: Oxford University Press.

Kaplan, S. H., and L. M. Sullivan. 1996. Maximizing the Quality of the Physician-Patient Encounter. *Journal of General Internal Medicine* 11, no. 3:187–88.

Karp, G. 1998. *Choosing a Wheelchair: A Guide for Optimal Independence.* Sebastopol, Calif.: O'Reilley and Associates.

———. 1999. *Life on Wheels: For the Active Wheelchair User.* Sebastopol, Calif.: O'Reilley and Associates.

Katz, J. N. 2001. Preferences, Quality, and the (Under)utilization of Total Joint Arthroplasty. *Medical Care* 39, no. 3:203–5.

Katzmann, R. A. 1991. Transportation Policy. In *The Americans with Disabilities Act: From Policy to Practice,* ed. J. West, 214–37. New York: Milbank Memorial Fund.

Kerrigan, D. C., M. Schaufele, and M. N. Wen. 1998. Gait Analysis. In *Rehabilitation Medicine: Principles and Practice,* ed. J. A. DeLisa and B. M. Gans, 67–187. 3d ed. Philadelphia: Lippincott-Raven Publishers.

Kleinman, A. 1988. *The Illness Narratives.* New York: Basic Books.

Krauss, H. H., C. Godfrey, J. Kirk, and D. M. Eisenberg. 1998. Alternative Health Care: Its Use by Individuals with Physical Disabilities. *Archives of Physical Medicine and Rehabilitation* 79, no. 11:1440–47.

Kuan, T. S., J. Y. Tsou, and F. C. Su. 1999. Hemiplegic Gait of Stroke Patients: The Effect of Using a Cane. *Archives of Physical Medicine and Rehabilitation* 80, no. 7:777–84.

Kumar, R., M. C. Roe, and O. U. Scremin. 1995. Methods for Estimating the Proper Length of a Cane. *Archives of Physical Medicine and Rehabilitation* 76, no. 12:1173–75.

Kutner, N. G., M. G. Ory, D. I. Baker, K. B. Schechtman, M. C. Hornbrook, and C. D. Mulrow. 1992. Measuring the Quality of Life of the Elderly in Health Promotion Intervention Clinical Trials. *Public Health Reports* 107, no. 5:530–39.

Lang, A. E., and A. M. Lozano. 1998a. Parkinson's Disease: First of Two Parts. *New England Journal of Medicine* 339, no. 15:1044–53.

———. 1998b. Parkinson's Disease: Second of Two Parts. *New England Journal of Medicine* 339, no. 16:1130–43.

LaPlante, M. P., G. E. Hendershot, and A. J. Moss. 1992. Assistive Technology Devices and Home Accessibility Features: Prevalence, Payment, Need, and Trends. *Advanced Data: Vital and Health Statistics* 217:1–11.

Laschober, M. A., P. Neuman, M. S. Kitchman, L. Meyer, and K. M. Langwell. 1999. Medicare HMO Withdrawals: What Happens to Beneficiaries. *Health Affairs* 18, no. 6:150–57.

Law, S. A. 1974. *Blue Cross: What Went Wrong?* New Haven: Yale University Press.

Leonard, J. A., Jr., and R. H. Meier, III. 1998. Upper and Lower Extremity Prostheses. In *Rehabilitation Medicine: Principles and Practice,* ed. J. A. DeLisa and B. M. Gans, 669–96. 3d ed. Philadelphia: Lippincott-Raven Publishers.

Levine, C., ed. 2000. *Always on Call: When Illness Turns Families Into Caregivers.* New York: United Hospital Fund.

Lewis, V. L., Jr. 1996. Pressure Sores. In *Medical Management of Long-Term Disability,* ed. D. Green, D. A. Olson, and H. B. Betts, 263–73. 2d ed. Boston: Butterworth-Heinemann.

Linton, S. 1998. *Claiming Disability: Knowledge and Identity.* New York: New York University Press.

Lollar, D. J. 2001. Public Health Trends in Disability: Past, Present, and Future. In *Handbook of Disability Studies,* ed. G. L. Albrecht, K. D. Seelman, and M. Bury, 754–71. Thousand Oaks, Calif.: Sage Publications.

Longmore, P. K., and L. Umansky. 2001. *The New Disability History: American Perspectives.* New York: New York University Press.

Maeda, A., K. Naskamura, A. Otomo, S. Higuchi, and Y. Motohashi. 1998. Body Support Effect on Standing Balance in the Visually Impaired Elderly. *Archives of Physical Medicine and Rehabilitation 79,* no. 8:994–97.

Mairs, N. 1987. On Being a Cripple. In *With Wings,* ed. M. S. Saxton and F. Howe, 118–27. New York: The Feminist Press at the City University of New York.

———. 1996. *Waist-High in the World.* Boston: Beacon Press.

Malanga, G., and J. A. DeLisa. 1998. Clinical Observation. In *Gait Analysis in the Science of Rehabilitation,* ed. J. A. DeLisa, 1–10. Washington, D.C.: Department of Veterans Affairs, Veterans Health Administration, Rehabilitation Research and Development Service, Scientific and Technical Publications Section, Monograph 002.

Manning, F. J., and J. A. Barondess, eds. 1996. *Changing Health Care Systems and Rheumatic Disease.* Washington, D.C.: National Academy Press.

Manton, K. G., L. Corder, and E. Stallard. 1997. Chronic Disability Trends in Elderly United States Populations: 1982–1994. *Proceedings of the National Academy of Sciences 94,* no. 6:2593–98.

Manton, K. G., and X. Gu. 2001. Changes in the Prevalence of Chronic Disability in the United States Black and Nonblack Population Above Age 65 from 1982 to 1999. *Proceedings of the National Academy of Sciences 98,* no. 11:6354–59.

Marmor, T. R. 2000. *The Politics of Medicare.* 2d ed. New York: Aldine de Gruyter.

Marottoli, R. A., C. F. Mendes de Leon, T. A. Glass, C. S. Williams, L. M. Cooney, Jr., L. F. Berkman, and M. E. Tinetti. 1997. Driving Cessation and Increased Depressive Symptoms: Prospective Evidence from the New Haven EPESE. *Journal of the American Geriatrics Society 45,* no. 2:202–6.

Marottoli, R. A., E. D. Richardson, M. H. Stowe, E. G. Miller, L. M. Brass, L. M. Cooney, Jr., and M. E. Tinetti. 1998. Development of a Test Battery to Identify Older Drivers at Risk for Self-Reported Adverse Driving Events. *Journal of the American Geriatrics Society 46,* no. 5:562–68.

Martin, L., C. Chin, and C. A. Harrison. 2001. *Annual Statistical Report on the Social Security Disability Insurance Program, 2000.* http://www.ssa.gov/statistical/di_asr/2000/index.html. Accessed 28 December 2001.

Mathias, S., U. S. Nayak, and B. Isaacs. 1986. Balance in Elderly Patients: The "Get Up & Go" Test. *Archives of Physical Medicine and Rehabilitation 67,* no. 6:387–89.

McCarthy, H. 1988. Attitudes that Affect Employment Opportunities for Persons with Disabilities. In *Attitudes Toward Persons with Disabilities,* ed. H. E. Yuker, 246–61. New York: Springer Publishing.

McClellan, M., and S. Kalba. 1999. Benefit Diversity in Medicare: Choice, Competition, and Selection. In *Medicare HMOs: Making Them Work for the Chronically Ill,* ed. R. Kronick and J. de Beyer, 133 60. Chicago: Health Administration Press.

Medicare Payment Advisory Commission. 1999. *Report to the Congress: Selected Medicare Issues.* Washington, D.C., June.

Meyer, J. A., and P. J. Zeller. 1999. *Profiles of Disability: Employment and Health Coverage.* Washington, D.C.: Henry J. Kaiser Family Foundation.

Milczarek, J. J., R. L. Kirby, E. R. Harrison, and D. A. MacLeod. 1993. Standard and Four-Footed Canes: Their Effect on Standing Balance of Patients with Hemiparesis. *Archives of Physical Medicine and Rehabilitation 74,* no. 3:281–85.

Minow, M. 1990. *Making All the Difference: Inclusion, Exclusion, and American Law.* Ithaca, New York: Cornell University Press.

Morris, J. 1996a. *Pride Against Prejudice: Transforming Attitudes to Disability.* London: The Women's Press.

———. 1996b. The Fall. In *What Happened to You? Writing by Disabled Women,* ed. L. Keith, 167–71. New York: The New Press.

Murphy, R. F. 1990. *The Body Silent.* New York: W. W. Norton.

National Center for Health Statistics. 2000. *Health United States, 2000: With Adolescent Health Chartbook.* Hyattsville, Md.: United States Department of Health and Human Services, Centers for Disease Control and Prevention, National Center for Health Statistics. DHHS Publication no. (PHS) 00–232.

Neistadt, M. E., and E. B. Crepeau, eds. 1998. *Willard and Spackman's Occupational Therapy.* 9th ed. Philadelphia: Lippincott Williams and Wilkins.

Nelson, E., B. Conger, R. Douglass, D. Gephart, J. Kirk, R. Page, A. Clark, K. Johnson, K. Stone, J. Wasson, and M. Zubkoff. 1983. Functional Health Status Levels of Primary Care Patients. *Journal of the American Medical Association* 249, no. 24:3331–38.

Noble, J., ed. 2001. *Textbook of General Medicine and Primary Care.* 3d ed. St. Louis: Mosby.

Nordin, M., and M. Campello. 1999. Physical Therapy. Exercises and the Modalities: When, What and Why? *Neurologic Clinics of North America* 17, no. 1:75–89.

Oliver, M. 1996. *Understanding Disability: From Theory to Practice.* New York: St. Martin's Press.

Olkin, R. 1993. Crips, Gimps and Epileptics Explain it All to You. *Readings* 8:13–17.

———. 1999. *What Psychotherapists Should Know About Disability*. New York: The Guildford Press.

Pearson, V. I. 2000. Assessment of Function in Older Adults. In *Assessing Older Persons: Measures, Meaning, and Practical Applications,* ed. R. L. Kane and R. A. Kane, 17–48. New York: Oxford University Press.

Pelka, F. 1997. *The ABC-CLIO Companion to the Disability Rights Movement.* Santa Barbara, Calif.: ABC-CLIO.

Perry, M., and N. Robertson. 1999. *Individuals with Disabilities and Their Experiences with Medicaid Managed Care: Results from Focus Group Research.* Washington, D.C.: Henry J. Kaiser Family Foundation.

Pipher, M. 1999. *Another Country: Navigating the Emotional Terrain of Our Elders.* New York: Riverhead Books.

Pope, A. M., and A. R. Tarlov. 1991. *Disability in America: Toward a National Agenda for Prevention.* Washington, D.C.: National Academy Press, Institute of Medicine.

President's Advisory Commission on Consumer Protection and Quality in the Health Care Industry. 1997. *Consumer Bill of Rights and Responsibilities.* Washington, D.C., November.

———. 1998. *Quality First: Better Health Care for All Americans.* Washington, D.C.: U.S. Government Printing Office.

Price, R. 1995. *A Whole New Life: An Illness and a Healing.* New York: Plume.

Punwar, A. J. 1994. *Occupational Therapy: Principles and Practice.* 2d ed. Baltimore: Williams and Wilkins.

Radcliffe, C. W. 1994. Prosthetics. In *Human Walking,* ed. J. Rose and J. G. Gamble, 165–99. Baltimore: Williams and Wilkins.

Ragnarsson, K. T. 1998. Lower Extremity Orthotics, Shoes, and Gait Aids. In *Rehabilitation Medicine: Principles and Practice,* ed. J. A. DeLisa and B. M. Gans, 651–67. 3d ed. Philadelphia: Lippincott-Raven Publishers.

Reeve, C. 1998. *Still Me.* New York: Random House.

Regenstein, M., and C. Schroer. 1998. *Medicaid Managed Care for Persons with Disabilities: State Profiles.* Washington, D.C.: Henry J. Kaiser Family Foundation.

Reinhardt, U. E. 1999. Employer-Based Health Insurance: A Balance Sheet. *Health Affairs* 18, no. 6:124–32.

Resnick, N. M. 1996. An 89-Year-Old Woman with Urinary Incontinence. *Journal of the American Medical Association* 276, no. 22:1832–40.

Rice, T. 1999. Should Medicare Managed Care Plans and Medigap Policies Have a Coordinated Open Enrollment Period? In *Medicare HMOs: Making Them Work for the Chronically Ill,* ed. R. Kronick and J. de Beyer, 109–31. Chicago: Health Administration Press.

Rimmer, J. H. 1999. Health Promotion for People with Disabilities: The Emerging Paradigm Shift from Disability Prevention to Prevention of Secondary Conditions. *Physical Therapy* 79, no. 5:495–502.

Robinson, J. C. 1999. *The Corporate Practice of Medicine: Competition and Innovation in Health Care.* Berkeley: University of California Press.

Rogers, J. C., and M. B. Holm. 1998. Evaluation of Activities of Daily Living (ADL) and Home Management. In *Willard and Spackman's Occupational Therapy,* ed. M. E. Neistadt and E. B. Crepeau, 185–208. 9th ed. Philadelphia: Lippincott Williams and Wilkins.

Rondinelli, R. D., J. P. Robinson, S. J. Scheer, and S. M. Weinstein. 1998. Occupational Rehabilitation and Disability Determination. In *Rehabilitation Medicine: Principles and Practice,* ed. J. A. DeLisa and B. M. Gans, 213–30. 3d ed. Philadelphia: Lippincott-Raven Publishers.

Rose, J., H. J. Ralston, and J. G. Gamble. 1994. Energetics of Walking. In *Human Walking,* ed. J. Rose and J. G. Gamble, 45–72. Baltimore: Williams and Wilkins.

Rosenbaum, S., B. M. Smith, P. Shin, M. H. Zakheim, K. Shaw, C. A. Sonosky, and L. Repasch. 1998. *Negotiating the New Health System: A Nationwide Study of Medicaid Managed Care Contracts.* Vol. 2, part 1. Ed. K. A. Johnson. Washington, D.C.: Center for Health Policy Research, George Washington University.

Rosenbaum, S., D. M. Frankford, B. Moore, and P. Borzi. 1999. Who Should Determine When Health Care Is Medically Necessary? *New England Journal of Medicine* 340, no. 3:229–32.

Roszak, T. 1998. *America the Wise.* Boston: Houghton Mifflin.

Sacks, O. 1993. *A Leg to Stand On.* New York: Harper Perennial.

Samuels, R. 2001. Ibot Update: The Future Beckons. *New Mobility* 12, no. 97:22.

Scherer, M. J. 1996. Outcomes of Assistive Technology Use on Quality of Life. *Disability Rehabilitation* 18, no. 9:439–48.

———. 2000. *Living in the State of Stuck: How Technology Impacts the Lives of People with Disabilities.* 3d ed. Cambridge, Mass.: Brookline Books.

Scotch, R. K. 2001. American Disability Policy in the Twentieth Century. In *The New Disability History: American Perspectives,* ed. P. K. Longmore and L. Umansky, 375–95. New York: New York University Press.

Scully, R. M., and M. R. Barnes, eds. 1989. *Physical Therapy.* Philadelphia: J. B. Lippincott.

Shapiro, J. P. 1994. *No Pity: People with Disabilities Forging a New Civil Rights Movement.* New York: Times Books.

Sharma, R., S. Chan, H. Liu, and C. Ginsberg. 2001. *Health and Health Care of the Medicare Population: Data from the 1997 Medicare Current Beneficiary Survey.* Rockville, Md.: Westat.

Silvers, A. 2000. The Unprotected: Constructing Disability in the Context of Anti-Discrimination Law. In *Americans with Disabilities: Exploring Implications of the Law for Individuals and Institutions,* ed. L. P. Francis and A. Silvers, 126–45. New York: Routledge.

Singer, S. J., and L. A. Bergthold. 2001. Prospects for Improved Decision Making About Medical Necessity. *Health Affairs* 20, no. 1:200–206.

Social Security Administration, Office of Disability. 1998. *Disability Evaluation Under Social Security.* SSA Publication no. 64–039. Washington, D.C.

Sontag, S. 1990. *Illness as Metaphor; and AIDS and Its Metaphors.* New York: Anchor Books.

Stein, M. A. 2000. Market Failure and ADA Title I. In *Americans with Disabilities: Exploring Implications of the Law for Individuals and Institutions,* ed. L. P. Francis and A. Silvers, 193–208. New York: Routledge.

Stewart, M. A., and C. W. Buck. 1977. Physicians' Knowledge of and Response to Patients' Problems. *Medical Care* 15, no. 7:578–85.

Stone, D. A. 1984. *The Disabled State.* Philadelphia: Temple University Press.

Stone, R. I. 2000. *Long-term Care for the Elderly with Disabilities: Current Policy, Emerging Trends, and Implications for the Twenty-First Century.* New York: Milbank Memorial Fund.

Sudarsky, L. 1994. Parkinsonism, Tremors, and Gait Disorders. In *Office Practice of Medicine,* ed. W. T. Branch, Jr., 761–69. 3d ed. Philadelphia: W. B. Saunders.

Tanenbaum, S. 1989. Medicaid and Disability: The Unlikely Entitlement. *Milbank Quarterly* 67, suppl. 2, pt. 2:288–310.

Thomas, J. 2000. H.M.O.'s to Drop Many Elderly and Disabled People. *New York Times,* 31 December:A14.

Tinetti, M. E. 1986. Performance-Oriented Assessment of Mobility Problems in Elderly Patients. *Journal of the American Geriatrics Society* 34, no. 2:119–26.

Tinetti, M. E., D. I. Baker, P. A. Garrett, M. Gottschalk, M. L. Koch, and R. I. Horwitz. 1993. Yale FICSIT: Risk Factor Abatement Strategy for Fall Prevention. *Journal of the American Geriatrics Society* 41, no. 3:315–20.

Tinetti, M. E., D. I. Baker, G. McAvay, E. B. Claus, P. Garrett, M. Gottschalk, M. L. Koch, K. Trainor, and R. I. Horwitz. 1994. A Multifactorial Intervention to Reduce the Risk of Falling Among Elderly People Living in the Community. *New England Journal of Medicine* 331, no. 13:821–27.

Tinetti, M. E., and S. F. Ginter. 1988. Identifying Mobility Dysfunctions in Elderly Patients. *Journal of the American Medical Association* 259, no. 8:1190–93.

Tinetti, M. E., W. L. Liu, and E. B. Claus. 1993. Predictors and Prognosis of Inability to Get Up After Falls Among Elderly Persons. *Journal of the American Medical Association* 269, no. 1:65–70.

Tinetti, M. E., and M. Speechley. 1989. Prevention of Falls Among the Elderly. *New England Journal of Medicine* 320, no. 16:1055–59.

Tinetti, M. E., and C. S. Williams. 1997. Falls, Injuries Due to Falls, and the Risk of Admission to a Nursing Home. *New England Journal of Medicine* 337, no. 18:1279–84.

Toombs, S. K. 1995. Sufficient Unto the Day: A Life with Multiple Sclerosis. In *Chronic Illness: From Experience to Policy,* ed. S. K. Toombs, D. Barnard, and R. D. Carson, 3–23. Bloomington: Indiana University Press.

Trombly, C. A. 1995a. *Occupational Therapy for Physical Dysfunction.* 4th ed. Baltimore: Williams and Wilkins.

———. 1995b. Theoretical Foundations for Practice. In *Occupational Therapy for Physical Dysfunction,* ed. C. A. Trombly, 15–27. 4th ed. Baltimore: Williams and Wilkins.

U.S. Census Bureau. 1999a. http://www.census.gov/hhes/www/housing/poms/multifam/mfunit/mftab18.html. Accessed 7 September 2000.

———. 1999b. http://www.census.gov/hhes/www/housing/poms/singlefam/sfunit/sftab18.html. Accessed 7 September 2000.

U.S. Department of Health and Human Services, Public Health Service, Centers for Disease Control and Prevention, National Center for Health Statistics. 1995. *Healthy People 2000, Review 1994*. DHHS Publication no. (PHS) 95–1256–1. Hyattsville, Md., July.

U.S. Department of Health and Human Services. 2000. *Healthy People 2010: With Understanding and Improving Health and Objectives for Improving Health*. 2 vols. 2d ed. Washington, D.C.: U.S. Government Printing Office.

U.S. General Accounting Office. 1996a. *SSA Disability: Program Redesign Necessary to Encourage Return to Work*. GAO/HEHS-96–62. Washington, D.C.

———. 1996b. *Social Security: Disability Programs Lag in Promoting Return to Work*. GAO/HEHS-96–147. Washington, D.C.

———. 1997a. *Social Security Disability: Improving Return-to-Work Outcomes Important, but Trade-offs and Challenges Remain*. GAO/HEHS-97–186. Washington, D.C.

———. 1997b. *Medicare Post-Acute Care: Cost Growth and Proposals to Manage It Through Prospective Payment and Other Controls*. GAO/T-HEHS-97–106. Washington, D.C.

———. 2000. *Medicare Home Health Care: Prospective Payment System Could Reverse Recent Declines in Spending*. GAO/HEHS-00–176. Washington, D.C.

U.S. Preventive Services Task Force. 1996. *Guide to Clinical Preventive Services*. 2d ed. Baltimore: Williams and Wilkins.

Urdangarin, C. F. 2000. Comprehensive Geriatric Assessment and Management. In *Assessing Older Persons: Measures, Meaning, and Practical Applications*, ed. R. L. Kane and R. A. Kane, 383–405. New York: Oxford University Press.

Verbrugge, L. M., C. Rennert, J. H. Madans. 1997. The Great Efficacy of Personal and Equipment Assistance in Reducing Disability. *American Journal of Public Health* 87, no. 3:384–92.

Vladeck, B. C., E. O'Brien, T. Hoyer, and S. Clauser. 1997. Confronting the Ambivalence of Disability Policy: Has Push Come to Shove? In *Disability: Challenges for Social Insurance, Health Care Financing, and Labor Market Policy*, ed. V. P. Reno, J. L. Mashaw, and B. Gradison, 83–1000. Washington, D.C.: National Academy of Social Insurance.

Walker, J. D. 1993. Enhancing Physical Comfort. In *Through the Patient's Eyes*, ed. M. Gerteis, S. Edgman-Levitan, J. Daley, and T. L. Delbanco, 119–53. San Francisco: Jossey-Bass Publishers.

Warner, M., P. M. Barnes, and L. A. Fingerhut. 2000. Injury and Poisoning Episodes and Conditions: National Health Interview Survey, 1997. *Vital and Health Statistics* 10, no. 202.

Warren, C. G. 1990. Powered Mobility and Its Implications. *Journal of Rehabilitation Research and Development* 2, clinic. suppl.:74–85.

Wartman, S. A., L. L. Morlock, F. E. Malitz, and E. Palm. 1983. Impact of Divergent Evaluations by Physicians and Patients of Patients' Complaints. *Public Health Reports* 98, no. 2:141–45.

Welner, S. L. 1998. Caring for Women with Disabilities. In *Textbook of Women's Health*, ed. L. A. Wallis, 87–92. Philadelphia: Lippincott-Raven Publishers.

———. 1999. *A Provider's Guide for the Care of Women with Physical Disabilities and Chronic Medical Conditions*. Raleigh: North Carolina Office on Disability and Health.

Welner, S. L., C. C. Foley, M. A. Nosek, and A. Holmes. 1999. Practical Considerations in the Performance of Physical Examinations on Women with Disabilities. *Obstetrics and Gynecology Survey* 54, no. 7:457–62.

West, J. 1991a. The Social and Policy Context of the Act. In *The Americans with Disabilities Act: From Policy to Practice*, ed. J. West, 3–24. New York: Milbank Memorial Fund.

———, ed. 1991b. *The Americans with Disabilities Act: From Policy to Practice*. New York: Milbank Memorial Fund.

Wickizer, T. M. 1995. Controlling Outpatient Medical Equipment Costs Through Utilization Management. *Medical Care* 33, no. 4:383–91.

Williams, G. 2001. Theorizing Disability. In *Handbook of Disability Studies*, ed. G. L. Albrecht, K. D. Seelman, and M. Bury, 123–44. Thousand Oaks, Calif.: Sage Publications.

World Health Organization. 1980. *International Classification of Impairments, Disabilities, and Handicaps*. Geneva.

———. 2001. *International Classification of Functioning, Disability and Health*. Geneva.

Wright, D. L., and T. L. Kemp. 1992. The Dual-Task Methodology and Assessing the Attentional Demands of Ambulation with Walking Devices. *Physical Therapy* 72, no. 4:306–12.

Yelin, E. H. 1991. The Recent History and Immediate Future of Employment Among Persons with Disabilities. In *The Americans with Disabilities Act: From Policy to Practice*, ed. J. West, 129–49. New York: Milbank Memorial Fund.

Young, J. M. 1997. *Equality of Opportunity: The Making of the Americans with Disabilities Act*. Washington, D.C.: National Council on Disability.

Young, I. M. 2000. Disability and the Definition of Work. In *Americans with Disabilities: Exploring Implications of the Law for Individuals and Institutions*, ed. L. P. Francis and A. Silver, 169–73. New York: Routledge.

Zola, I. K. 1982. *Missing Pieces: A Chronicle of Living with a Disability*. Philadelphia: Temple University Press.

———. 1989. Toward the Necessary Universalizing of a Disability Policy. *Milbank Quarterly* 67, suppl. 2, pt. 2:401–28.

Index

abandonment: of mobility aids, 215, 218–19; of prostheses, 210

accessibility, 264; architecture of, 53–55, 69, 87–90, 116, 125–26, 264, *Plate 2*; economics of, 88, 116, 117, 123, 224, 258, 266, 267–68; of health-care facilities, 125–26, 156, 261; home, 87–90, 173, 174, 175, 257–59, 302n2; job, 115–17; laws, 53–55, 123–24, 125, 264, 302n2, 306n21; Mobility Mart information about, 261, 262; parking spots, 55, 122, 123, 268; public spaces, 125–26, 214–15, 264, *Plates 2, 4, 5, 7, 8*; transportation, 8, 123–24, 306–7nn21,23; wheelchair, 53–55, 69, 88, 89, 116, 125–26, 214–15, 219, 264. *See also* mobility aids; modifications, for accessibility

accidents, 120, 298n6. *See also* falls; injuries; safety; traumatic conditions

activities of daily living (ADLs), 84–87, 264, 302–3, 307n1; comparative difficulty of various, 302n1; help with, 81–82, 90–93, 96, 101–3, 128, 136, 268–69, 269 *table*, 303n6; housework, 28, 84, 302n1; instrumental (IADLs), 84, 153, 302n1, 303n6; marriage and, 81–82, 91–92, 96; meal preparation, 84, 86, 101; Mobility Mart and, 262; parents/adult children and, 101–3, 276;

physicians and, 128, 136–37, 143–46, 147, 153, 157–60, 163, 309n7; PTs/OTs and, 163–73, 243–44; time for, 18, 86–87. *See also* home; mobility aids; physical functioning; transportation; walking

activity: defined by *ICF*, 8. *See also* activities of daily living (ADLs)

acupuncture, 177–79

ADA. *See* Americans with Disabilities Act

addiction, drug, 139, 140

adjustment, to mobility difficulties, 52–53, 68–69, 78–79. *See also* positive attitudes

ADLs. *See* activities of daily living

advertisements: drug, 308n8; health insurance, 314n11; wheelchair, 212

advocacy: daily living, 269; self-advocacy, 79, 211, 236, 269. *See also* rights

African Americans. *See* blacks

age/aged: chronic diseases associated with, 19, 20; drivers with accidents, 120; falls and, 18, 41, 299n5; geriatric assessment programs, 310n11; housing with elderly/younger disabled people, 89; incontinence, 45; without insurance, 226–27; marital status, 303n8; mobility-aid choices, 311n4, 312n4; mobility difficulties, 4, 12, 13 *fig*, 18, 19–20, 226–27,

335

Compositor:	Impressions Book and Journal Services, Inc.
Indexer:	Barbara Roos
Text:	10/13 Aldus
Display:	Aldus
Printer and binder:	Sheridan Books, Inc.